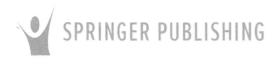 SPRINGER PUBLISHING

T0093219

GET THE MOST FROM YOUR BOOK

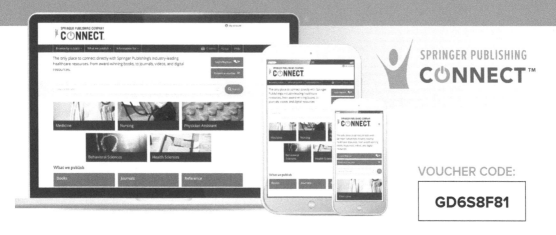

SPRINGER PUBLISHING
CONNECT™

VOUCHER CODE:

GD6S8F81

Online Access

Your print purchase of *Infectious Disease Epidemiology: An Introduction*, includes **online access via Springer Publishing Connect**™ to increase accessibility, portability, and searchability.

Insert the code at http://connect.springerpub.com/content/book/978-0-8261-5674-7 today!

Having trouble? Contact our customer service department at cs@springerpub.com

Instructor Resource Access for Adopters

Let us do some of the heavy lifting to create an engaging classroom experience with a variety of instructor resources included in most textbooks SUCH AS:

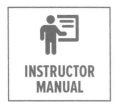
INSTRUCTOR MANUAL

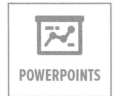
POWERPOINTS

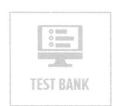
TEST BANK

Visit **https://connect.springerpub.com/** and look for the **"Show Supplementary"** button on your **book homepage** to see what is available to instructors! First time using Springer Publishing Connect?

Email **textbook@springerpub.com** to create an account and start unlocking valuable resources.

INFECTIOUS DISEASE EPIDEMIOLOGY

Eyal Oren, PhD, MS, holds an undergraduate degree in neurobiology and behavior from Cornell University and PhD and MS degrees in epidemiology from the University of Washington. He is the director of the School of Public Health at San Diego State University. He is a tenured professor of epidemiology and a core-investigator at the Institute for Behavioral and Community Health, and for many years was a lead infectious disease epidemiologist in one of the largest metropolitan health departments in the United States. He is trained as an infectious disease and social epidemiologist, with expertise in respiratory infections, and has worked at the interface of infectious etiologies and chronic disease outcomes. He has taught infectious disease epidemiology at the undergraduate level and introduction to epidemiology and social epidemiology to graduate students.

Heidi E. Brown, PhD, MPH, received her undergraduate degree in psychology from Virginia Tech, followed by an MPH in international health promotion from George Washington University and her PhD in the epidemiology of microbial diseases from Yale University. She conducted post-doctoral studies in zoology at Oxford University and the Bacterial Diseases Branch at the Centers for Disease Control and Prevention's Division of Vector-Borne Diseases. She is a tenured associate professor of public health in the Mel and Enid Zuckerman College of Public Health at the University of Arizona. Her research focuses on environmental influences on vector-borne diseases and on infectious causes of cancer. In addition to a graduate level spatial epidemiology course and a data analysis and communication course, she has been teaching undergraduate epidemiology since 2013. She engages in evidence-based learning to improve student learning.

INFECTIOUS DISEASE EPIDEMIOLOGY

An Introduction

Eyal Oren, PhD, MS

Heidi E. Brown, PhD, MPH

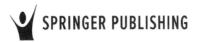 SPRINGER PUBLISHING

Springer Publishing Company, LLC
11 West 42nd Street, New York, NY 10036
www.springerpub.com
connect.springerpub.com/

Senior Acquisitions Editor: David D'Addona
Director, Content Development: Taylor Ball
Production Editor: Joseph Stubenrauch
Compositor: Amnet

ISBN: 978-0-8261-5673-0
ebook ISBN: 978-0-8261-5674-7
DOI: 10.1891/9780826156747

SUPPLEMENTS:

A robust set of instructor resources designed to supplement this text is located at http://connect.springerpub.com/content/book/978-0-8261-5674-7. Qualifying instructors may request access by emailing textbook@springerpub.com.

Qualified instructors may request supplements by emailing textbook@springerpub.com
Instructor Manual ISBN: 978-0-8261-5677-8
Instructor PowerPoints ISBN: 978-0-8261-5675-4
Instructor Test Bank ISBN: 978-0-8261-5676-1

22 23 24 25 / 5 4 3 2 1

Library of Congress Cataloging-in-Publication Data

Names: Oren, Eyal, 1976- author. | Brown, Heidi E., author.
Title: Infectious disease epidemiology : an introduction / Eyal Oren, Heidi E. Brown.
Description: New York, NY : Springer Publishing Company, [2023] | Includes bibliographical references and index.
Identifiers: LCCN 2022040880 (print) | LCCN 2022040881 (ebook) | ISBN 9780826156730 (paperback) | ISBN 9780826156747 (ebook)
Subjects: MESH: Communicable Diseases—epidemiology | Epidemiologic Methods | Disease Transmission, Infectious | Disease Outbreaks | Communicable Disease Control
Classification: LCC RA643 (print) | LCC RA643 (ebook) | NLM WC 100 | DDC 362.1969—dc23/eng/20221104
LC record available at https://lccn.loc.gov/2022040880
LC ebook record available at https://lccn.loc.gov/2022040881

Contact sales@springerpub.com to receive discount rates on bulk purchases.

Printed in the United States of America by Gasch Printing.

We dedicate this book to our family, colleagues, and students, who provided inspiration through writing this first, and we hope not last, edition of the text. EO thanks Jenny, Jacob, and Ari for their support and Heidi for the wonderful collaboration. HEB thanks Jono, Demsey, and Til for their patience and Eyal and the Springer team for making writing fun.

CONTENTS

FOREWORD

Readers of this comprehensive and well-written new textbook about infectious disease epidemiology were almost certainly born no earlier than the 1990s. As a result, they can be forgiven if they are unaware that many experts writing in the 1950s and 1960s were confidently predicting the end of infectious diseases as a significant threat, leaving us free to focus our energies and research on "chronic diseases," such as cardiovascular disease, cancer, and diabetes mellitus. This view developed simultaneous to the increasing availability of diverse antimicrobial agents for treating infectious diseases, particularly bacterial infections, and the development of new vaccines, such as the vaccines against polio and measles. The elimination of infectious diseases as a threat to human populations seemed tantalizingly close.

It was in the 1970s and 1980s that the emergence or re-emergence of various infectious diseases—such as HIV/AIDS and multidrug-resistant tuberculosis—brought the realization that infectious diseases had not, in fact, been conquered as a result of advances in diagnosis, treatment, and prevention of such diseases. And anyone who has lived through the recent COVID-19 pandemic and outbreak of monkeypox will clearly understand that infectious diseases are most decidedly *not* in our rearview mirror. Furthermore, we now understand that the distinction between "infectious diseases" and "chronic diseases" was always predicated on a lack of understanding of the critical role of chronic infection in diseases such as cancer of the stomach, liver, cervix, and other parts of the body, along with the tantalizing hypothesis concerning the possible role of infection or chronic infection in the pathogenesis of neurologic and psychiatric illnesses, cardiovascular disease, and other "chronic diseases." Thus, there remains a need to train a new generation of public health professionals and academic researchers in the concepts and methods required to understand, investigate, and inform prevention and mitigation efforts targeting a wide variety of infectious diseases.

Infectious Disease Epidemiology: An Introduction by Eyal Oren, PhD, MS, and Heidi E. Brown, PhD, MPH, is a valuable offering for instructors and students in a variety of settings. Key concepts and principles underlying infectious disease epidemiology are presented in an organized manner, and important activities such as disease surveillance and outbreak investigation are well-described. Those beginning their study of infectious disease epidemiology, as well as those working to train the next generation of prevention and control experts, will find this volume valuable and instructive.

Arthur Reingold, MD
Professor of Epidemiology
Chair, Epidemiology Division
School of Public Health
University of California, Berkeley
Berkeley, California

PREFACE

The field of infectious disease epidemiology has been front-and-center for the past few years. With the COVID-19 pandemic, an opportunity arose to provide "armchair epidemiologists" with a deeper understanding of the population-level impacts of infectious diseases, and the tools available to control them. This field has its own unique culture and set of tools and rules. We will utilize a whole new vocabulary in this book, from how to consider transmission—with the idea of a disease reproductive rate—to how disease is dispersed or clustered, and to how to design a study. As the reader will see, infectious disease epidemiologists seek to learn who is sick, why they are sick, and when and where they became sick.

This text aims to provide a unique introduction and perspective to the field of infectious disease epidemiology. We geared the text for students in public health programs or students in other majors with an interest in the field both in the United States and globally, with the goal of introducing both interesting and timely content as well as key methodology used in the field. We designed this book as an introduction to infectious disease epidemiology with the student learners and the instructors supporting their learning in mind. This book provides an approachable introduction to the field, utilizing a combination of intuitive case studies, popular media examples, and didactic exercises. In each chapter, learners are introduced to major conceptual approaches in the field, as well as key factors that enable us to mitigate disease spread. We are both instructors of large and small undergraduate classes. As we incorporated active learning techniques into our classrooms, we looked around for a book that would match the learning we observed in the classroom. Each chapter is structured to include key terms, a helpful narrative, "Heads Up" sections that help to allay conceptual confusion, highlights on a key figure in history, and a section with lessons learned from the classroom and questions to foster further investigation. The "Teaching Corner" and the "Heads Up" boxes come directly from our experiences in the classroom, observing and trying to address student misconceptions. Chapters include an introduction to key methods used in infectious disease epidemiology. Instructors will find key supplementary resources online as well as linkages to materials and websites that help model transmission, analyze data, and allow more advanced students to read primary source material. We structured the book into four parts that walk learners through the world of infectious disease epidemiology, first covering *disease emergence and basics*, moving on to *modes of transmission and types of diseases*, then proceeding to *infectious diseases in context*, and finally *disease control, eradication and emergence*. We hope that both the integrated approach and content of the book provide an exciting entrée into a field that is rich in its complexity, dynamicism, and multidisciplinary leanings.

We would like to thank a number of individuals for their support and time. Without them, this book would not have been possible. Thank you to the students and instructors who tested preliminary chapters in their classroom in the Fall of 2021. Your feedback was invaluable to improving the utility and interest level of the book. We also thank our colleagues who generously volunteered their time to review the chapters for content, advice, and accuracy. Among these colleagues we include Jijun Zhao (Qingdao University), Jonathan Mayer (University of Washington), Erika

Austhof (University of Arizona), Judith Harbertson (San Diego State University and Naval Health Research Center), and Hannah Gould (NY Department of Health).

We are additionally indebted to many other luminaries and authors in public health, epidemiology, and infectious diseases whose scholarship and ceaseless leadership forms the basis for this textbook. Finally, we give a special thank you to the publishing team at Springer Publishing, specifically David D'Addona and Taylor Ball, who have believed in this work from the first moment and have contributed continuing encouragement and energy to make this book a reality.

Eyal Oren, PhD, MS
Heidi E. Brown, PhD, MPH

INSTRUCTOR RESOURCES

 A robust set of instructor resources designed to supplement this text is located at http://connect.springerpub.com/content/book/978-0-8261-5674-7. Qualifying instructors may request access by emailing textbook@springerpub.com.

Available resources include:
- Instructor's Manual
  - Case Studies
  - Questions for Discussion
  - Teaching Corner Questions and Answers
- Test Bank
- Chapter-Based PowerPoint Presentations

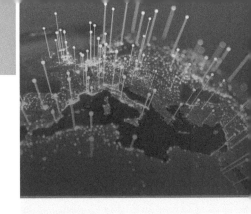

PART I

DISEASE EMERGENCE AND BASICS

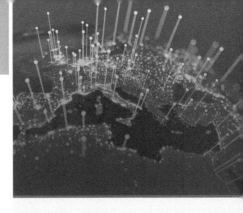

CHAPTER 1

DISEASE EMERGENCE AND RE-EMERGENCE

INTRODUCTION

An Emerging Pandemic

In December of 2019 the hints of something bad started circulating. Hospitals in a central Chinese city were overwhelmed with patients suffering from acute respiratory disease. By January 2020, we were watching images of apartment buildings full of people on lockdown singing to cheer themselves. In February, we heard of a 1,000-bed hospital constructed in a mere 10 days. Although an amazing feat of engineering, it was also frightful evidence of just how overwhelmed hospitals were. On March 11, 2020, COVID-19 was declared a global pandemic by the World Health Organization (WHO). We then watched this new disease explode across our countries, wondering which would be next and how bad it would be. Each of us was impacted by COVID-19; some of us lost a loved one, most of us locked down at some level, and many of us separated from our families. COVID-19 represents not just these losses but also is a reminder that we are not immune to infectious diseases. In this chapter, we discuss the continued threats that are infectious diseases, how we classify diseases, and the reasons we will continue to experience infectious diseases.

LEARNING OBJECTIVES

By the end of this chapter, readers will be able to:

- Define what infectious diseases are and describe what makes them unique from other causes of disease.
- List reasons for why we are seeing disease re-emergence.
- List the differences in major infectious disease classification systems.
- Describe how the relationships between an agent, host, and environment inform disease prevention.

WHAT ARE INFECTIOUS DISEASES?

You come home and are not feeling well. Over the day you develop symptoms of body aches, fatigue, a cough, and fever, and you are wondering whether this is a bad cold or something worse. When you call your doctor's office, they tell you to self-isolate and quickly go, fully masked, to get a COVID-19 test.

Fever is a classic sign that the body is fighting an infection; however, the other symptoms are common to both flu and emphysema. How do we identify a disease as infectious? What makes infectious diseases unique from other conditions that afflict humans?

Over the course of centuries, definitions and concepts of disease have changed. Hippocrates (490–370 BCE) wrote about the spread of disease by means of "airs, water, and places."[1] In ancient Rome, the Goddess Febris protected people from fever and malaria. People believed that disease was a curse upon a family or individual, and risk factors included morally wrong behavior. Case in point, *malaria*, which we now know to be caused by infection with the *Plasmodium* parasite, gets its name from the Italian term for "bad air," mal' aria.[2] The miasma theory stated that different disturbances, such as earthquakes and comets, charged the air with poisonous vapors known as "miasmas" that spread disease (Figure 1.1).

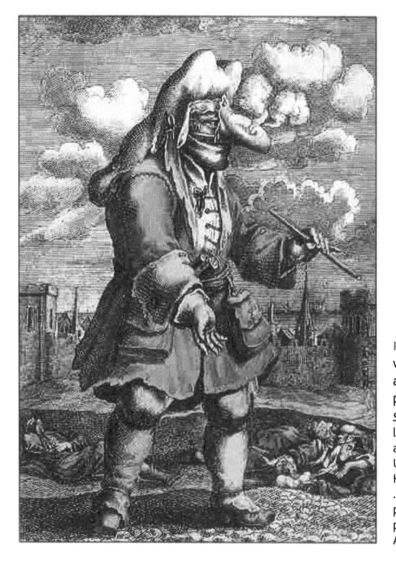

Figure 1.1 A doctor depicted wearing a mask to protect against "miasmas" during a plague outbreak in France.

Source: "A brief history of public health." Office of Teaching and Digital Learning. Boston University School of Public Health. https://sphweb.bumc.bu.edu/otlt/mph-modules/ph/publichealthhistory/publichealthhistory2.html. Accessed March 28, 2022.

THOUGHT QUESTION

Imagine yourself as an infectious disease epidemiologist before we knew what might cause these diseases. You think there must be something more than bad air but how do you convince your colleagues? How do you begin to draw on evidence for an alternative explanation?

Microbes are the oldest form of life on earth and outnumber all other life forms. There are 100 million times as many bacteria in the oceans (13×10^{28}) as there are stars in the known universe.[3] However, it was not until the microscope was developed by Anton van Leeuwenhoek in the 17th century that humans could finally visualize microorganisms. This allowed for observation of van Leeuwenhoek's **animalcules**, but it took the French chemist Louis Pasteur proposing a germ theory of disease for the broader theory that microorganisms cause disease to take root. However, these innovative ideas were not easily won. The pushback to these scientific approaches was vehement. For example, Antoine Béchamp, a chemist contemporary of Pasteur's, denied germ theory and instead posited that disease depended on "tiny molecular granulations" called microzymas, which only become pathogenic when a change in environmental balance or function made them so (Figure 1.2).[4]

animalcules: Microscopic animals (often protozoans), as observed by Leeuwenhoek for the first time under a microscope.

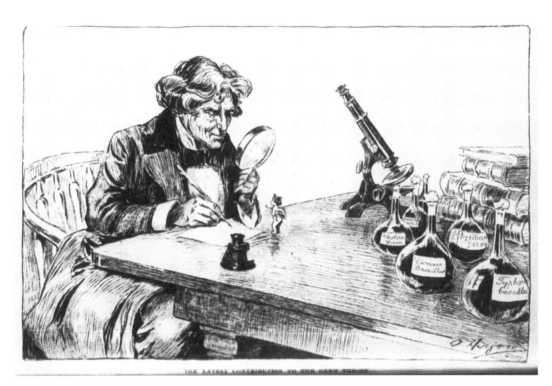

Figure 1.2 Opposition to the emerging world of bacteriology in the 1890s.
Source: "The latest contributions in the germ theory." National Library of Medicine.

In 1884, the German scientist Robert Koch envisioned four postulates to assess whether a particular microorganism causes a disease.[5] These postulates have been critical in establishing agreement that a particular pathogen is responsible for a disease and are as following:

1. The microorganism must be found in diseased but not healthy individuals;

2. The microorganism must be cultured from the diseased individual;

3. Inoculation of a healthy individual with the cultured microorganism must recapitulate the disease; and

4. The microorganism must be re-isolated from the inoculated, diseased individual and matched to the original microorganism.

If a disease passes all four postulates, it is categorically described as causal for a disease outcome and meets the criteria for an infectious disease.

asymptomatic: *a-* (without) symptoms. Individuals who are infected but do not show clinical symptoms of the disease. This is in contrast to symptomatic individuals.

symptomatic: Individuals infected who exhibit clinical symptoms of the disease.

carrier: An individual who is infected and able to spread an infection to others.

Since Koch, there has been some added nuance to these definitions. For example, **asymptomatic carriers** illustrate the importance of asymptomatic infection. In addition, genomic technologies have allowed for sequencing of pathogens to understand whether specific strains are responsible for disease outcomes (Figure 1.3). Nevertheless, there is broad agreement on the following:

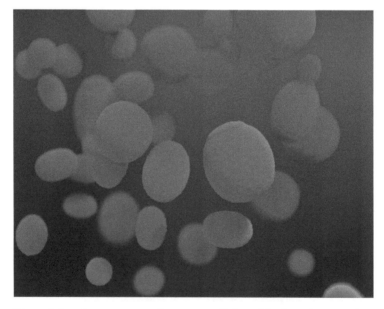

Figure 1.3 *Candida auris* is a fungus presenting a potential antibiotic resistance threat in the United States. In addition, some organisms may result in short-term, or acute, infection, whereas others are chronic; sometimes something that begins acutely ends up lasting for a long time.
Source: With permission from Stephanie Rossow/SCIENCE PHOTO LIBRARY.

- Infectious diseases are caused by microorganisms, such as viruses, bacteria, fungi, or parasites, or by infectious proteins called prions. These organisms, mostly microscopic in size, are often harmless or even helpful, but in some cases or certain situations may go on to cause disease.
- By the very nature of the term, infection refers to a process whereby these microorganisms enter the body and grow or multiply.
- Infectious diseases are transmitted to humans from other humans, animals, or the environment.
- Infectious diseases, each in their own unique way, usually follow recognizable patterns of symptoms, timing, and progression.
- Infectious diseases may evolve over time as new organisms emerge and human behavior and environments change.

THOUGHT QUESTION

Would you characterize cervical cancer as an infectious disease now that we know it is caused by human papillomavirus? Which of Koch's postulates are satisfied for cervical cancer?

HOW DOES EPIDEMIOLOGY FIT IN?

As we watched and waited to see if COVID-19 would transmit widely across the world, as we waited to hear if this spreading infection would be declared a pandemic, and even as we listened to how we could protect ourselves, epidemiologists were hard at work trying to answer questions of who, where, and how fast it would spread.

An epidemiologist searches for different patterns and distributions of diseases and works to identify the **etiology** of the observed disease. With training in statistics, biology, and public health, these indivduals work to identify how to control the disease from spreading or else to help prevent it from happening in the first place. As such, an epidemiologist takes a certain viewpoint to the world; in this viewpoint, the epidemiologist works as a medical disease detective, considers the evidence at hand to figure out what caused a disease, and, ideally, uses a toolkit to find out how a particular health problem was introduced and can be stopped.

The field of infectious disease epidemiology refers to the study of the incidence and spread of infectious diseases in populations over time. In particular, we will learn how a host, a pathogen, and the environment interact in a dynamic process that influences the course of infection. Of primary interest are questions related to cause and pathogenesis of disease, why people respond in diverse ways to a given pathogen or intervention, why certain subtypes of a pathogen predominate or transmit more frequently, and how to prevent ongoing transmission.

THOUGHT QUESTION

What did you just learn? List all the people who might be involved in identifying the etiology of a disease, such as physicians, nurses, and epidemiologists. Now list what their roles would be, paying close attention not only to what each might do, but how they differ from each other.

WHAT DOES AN INFECTIOUS EPIDEMIOLOGIST DO?

As it became increasingly apparent that COVID-19 was more than just an outbreak, citizens started asking the same questions epidemiologists ask every day. What is the cause of this disease? Who is at greatest risk for infection? Who is most at risk for adverse outcomes? How bad will it get? Epidemiologists were central to the identification of risk factors, for the emergency declaration, for modeling cases, and for estimating the impact of the vaccine.

Infectious disease epidemiologists are "shoe leather" epidemiologists. That is, they often go into the community to interact with individuals in the community, or with public officials, to get a better understanding of what is happening or causing a disease, and observe and sample the environment, including food, water, living patterns, and so on. The infectious disease epidemiologist is thus heavily involved in understanding where their data come from as well as related concepts, such as data reliability and quality. Possibly the most famous example of this is that of John Snow, who in 1854 linked an ongoing epidemic of cholera in London to water contamination.[6] Snow did so by mapping out both the deaths and the water supply for households served by two different water companies. Snow utilized descriptive epidemiology in examining the patterns and distribution of cholera deaths in London, as well as an experimental intervention, when he removed the Broad Street pump handle, which had water provided by just one of the water companies, and deaths plummeted.

Modern day epidemiologists are still disease detectives trying to uncover the etiology or causes of disease. They work in state and local health departments tracking and designing interventions to improve the health of their constituents. They may work in hospitals evaluating sanitation protocols and tracking hospital-acquired infections. Others still may work in academics designing and implementing various types of epidemiologic investigations to understand disease occurrence. Physically, they may work with the pathogens in laboratories, in the field collecting data and conducting outbreak investigations, or in offices focusing on data analysis.

Tools of the Trade

DISEASE MORBIDITY

Much like the scout with a Swiss Army knife, the infectious disease epidemiologist has their own versatile repository of tools.

The primary tool of the epidemiologist is pattern recognition. Epidemiology is a field focused on identifying patterns in morbidity, mortality, and risk factors. Counting the number of new and existing cases is one approach to evaluating morbidity. **Incidence proportion**, the risk of developing the disease, and **prevalence**, the existing burden of disease, are the starting place. Each measure an epidemiologist calculates reveals another piece of the disease puzzle.

$$\text{Incidence proportion} = \frac{\text{No. of new cases among exposed}}{\text{Exposed population during time period}}$$

$$\text{(Point) prevalence} = \frac{\text{Number of current cases among exposed}}{\text{Exposed population during time period}}$$

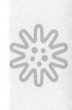

incidence proportion: A measure of the risk of developing the outcome of interest. It is calculated as the number of new cases in a given population at a given time period over the total population at risk for developing a disease during the same time period.

prevalence: A measure of the burden of disease in a population. It is calculated as the number of existing cases over the population able to get the disease during a given time period. It may be represented as a rate or a percentage.

DISEASE MORTALITY

Just as we might examine disease incidence in a population, we may be interested in characterizing deaths in a population. The **mortality rate** is the incidence of deaths in a population in a given time period:

$$\text{Mortality rate} = \frac{\text{Number of deaths}}{\text{Total population in a given year}}$$

The numerator reflects all deaths, while the denominator reflects those at risk of dying. Mortality rate can be a good surrogate for disease incidence rate if survival from the disease is low. Mortality rates can also be examined among specific causes, age groups, or populations.

When we are interested in identifying leading causes of death, we might use the **proportionate mortality ratio (PMR).** The PMR provides information on which causes of deaths might be most important compared to others.

$$\text{PMR} = \frac{\text{No. of deaths from a given cause in a given time period}}{\text{Total deaths in the same time period}} \times 100$$

The **case fatality rate (CFR)** (also known as case fatality ratio) is a proportion of the total cases which are fatal. It answers the question of how many people die of a disease out of the number of individuals who have been diagnosed with a disease in a given time period:

$$\text{CFR} = \frac{\text{No. of deaths due to disease X}}{\text{No. of cases of disease X}} \times 100$$

The CFR provides us with a metric of how deadly a particular disease is within a population. It is important to note that the number of deaths (the numerator) depends on the lag between infection and death and the number of cases (the denominator) will depend on how much testing/diagnosis occurs in the first place. Both PMR and the CFR are usually converted to a percentage by multiplying the answer by 100.

mortality rate: A measure of deaths in a population at a given time period.

proportionate mortality ratio (PMR): A measure of the proportion of deaths due to a given cause from all deaths in a population.

case fatality rate (CFR): A measure of disease severity considering the deaths due to a disease as a proportion of the total number of cases of that disease.

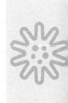

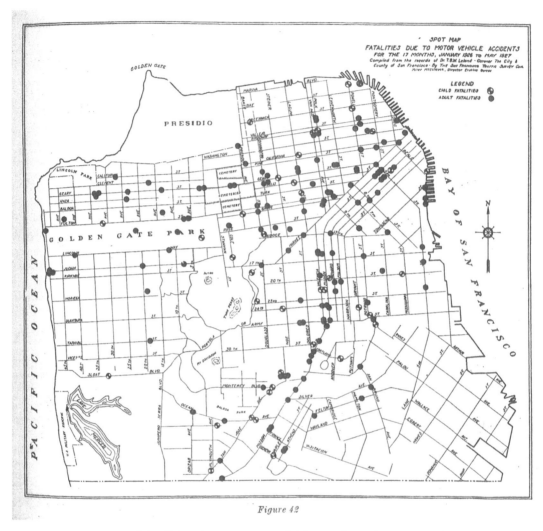

Figure 42

Figure 1.4 **Spot map of fatalities due to motor vehicle accidents in San Francisco, 1926–1927.**
Source: From *A Report on the Street Traffic Control Problem of San Francisco.*

DISEASE EXPOSURES

As mentioned earlier, mapping has been an essential approach to visualizing disease outbreaks, how they evolve over time, and relevant **exposures** and risk factors. One can start out by plotting individual cases to describe person, place, and time to better understand the possible mode of transmission and source of an outbreak. A spot map (Figure 1.4) is used to show where known cases live or congregate, and to assess where cases are clustered more densely or are scattered more widely. This kind of information can be used in tandem with other observations, such as how close cases are to a source of pollution, an unregulated water source, or an area with policy measures that might impact one's health. Mapping has evolved over time and is used extensively as part of a Geographic Information System (GIS). GIS systems allow for integration of layers of spatial information as well as various data fields. This allows for a multidimensional depiction of an environment as well as for integration of various data sources.

Table 1.1 **Examples of Key Epidemiologic Study Designs**

STUDY DESIGN	APPROACH	TYPE
Case report	Describes interesting clinical occurrences	Descriptive
Ecologic	Comparison of groups of people or communities instead of individuals	Observational
Cross-sectional	Data on exposure and outcome are collected at one point in time	Observational
Case-control	Identification of participants based on presence or absence of an outcome, with data about exposures collected retrospectively	Observational
Cohort	Identification of exposures of interest in a population, with follow-up until a disease or outcomes occurs	Observational
Randomized controlled trial	An experimental trial where participants are allocated randomly to an intervention or control group	Experimental

exposure: Any factor that may be associated with an outcome of interest. This may be the primary independent variable or risk factor of interest in an epidemiologic study.

germ theory: The science-backed explanation that infectious diseases arise from exposure to microorganisms and germs.

To understand the relationships between exposures and outcomes, epidemiology uses a number of different study designs. These designs typically take on a hierarchy from more hypothesis-generating to providing stronger evidence for causality (Table 1.1). Study designs may be **descriptive**, in that they do not have a specific hypothesis, or **analytic**, where a hypothesis is examined tying an exposure to an outcome. Analytic studies, in turn, are either **observational** or **experimental**. In contrast to experimental designs, which randomize participants to a study condition, observational studies do not do so; instead, the researcher observes the effect of a risk factor or intervention without trying to change exposure status.

Each design has its own strengths and limitations. The choice of design typically depends on the research question and hypothesis, the resources (infrastructure, budget, timing) available, the types of exposures and outcomes under study, and associated ethics with carrying out the study using a given design.

LABORATORY METHODS

In the 1860s Louis Pasteur demonstrated that spontaneous generation, which proposed that simple life arises spontaneously from nonliving matter, was not possible. He did so by boiling meat broth in a flask, heating the neck of the flask in a flame, and bending the flask in an S shape. This allowed air to enter the flask, whereas microorganisms would settle in the upper neck. No microorganisms grew; in fact, when Pasteur tilted the flask and the broth came into contact with the neck, it became cloudy, demonstrating both **germ theory** and the lack of credibility for the spontaneous generation theory.[7]

It is within the past 50 years that the branch known as molecular epidemiology, merging molecular biology into epidemiologic studies, has transformed the field of infectious diseases. Starting with the development of high throughput techniques that allow for large-scale analyses, these types of studies have provided invaluable insights into disease pathogenesis, causation, transmission, prevention, and therapy.[8] For example, Kaposi's sarcoma (KS) was hypothesized to be caused by an infectious agent, but culture-based techniques could not detect any infectious agent in KS patient specimens. In 1994, Chang et al. found a unique DNA sequence in more than 90% of KS patients who also had AIDS. The sequence, detected also in tissue of non-AIDS patients with KS, was similar to herpes viruses.[9] Commonly used techniques to examine microbes include pulse field gel electrophoresis (PFGE) and restriction fragment length polymorphism (RFLP) analysis. During COVID-19, polymerase chain reaction (PCR), which is used to amplify quantities of genomic material of an organism, became a household word and has allowed for close to real-time detection of individuals with SARS Coronavirus 2 (CoV-2), virus relatively quickly and accurately.

This field has evolved over time, such that it can be used to further subclassify organisms and detect even minuscule amounts of organisms in the human body. The types of data that can be examined have developed tremendously as well, with metagenomic information used to characterize changes over time in genes or transcript composition to better understand how pathogens interact with a host over the course of a disease.

THOUGHT QUESTION

What did you just learn? What epidemiologic tools do you imagine D. A. Henderson used in his smallpox eradication campaign? Consider the time period when smallpox was eradicated to restrict your list to tools available at the time.

WHY DO WE SEE CHANGES IN INFECTIOUS DISEASE TRENDS OVER TIME?

Even in the short time frame of the COVID-19 pandemic, we saw rapidly decreasing in-hospital mortality rates.[10] Initially, extremely high numbers of individuals hospitalized or rapid implementation of brand-new isolation and personal protection procedures may have adversely impacted patient outcomes in locations with very high rates of COVID-19. After some time, numbers decreased, and healthcare workers became more familiar with new procedures. For example, the use of supplemental oxygen at admission increased and use of mechanical ventilation decreased even though rates of ICU admissions changed only slightly. At the same time, best practices were noted, with increased use of noninvasive ventilation, and prone patient positioning potentially improved outcomes.

In addition to the devastation that COVID-19 has had globally in 2020 and 2021, the pandemic serves as a reminder of our continuing risk from infectious disease. In 1962 Sir McFarlane Burnett stated, "By the end of the Second World War it was possible to say that almost all of the major practical problems of dealing with infectious disease had been solved."[11] Yet even in the 21st century, infectious diseases are a leading cause of death worldwide and continue to represent significant burden in the United States (Figure 1.5). While pneumonia/flu are consistently in the top 10 leading causes of disease in the United States, with COVID-19 in 2020, an infectious disease was the third leading cause of death in the United States.

	1980	1990	2000	2010	2020
1	HD	HD	HD	HD	HD
2	Cancer	Cancer	Cancer	Cancer	Cancer
3	CVD	CVD	CVD	CLRD	COVID-19
4	Injury	Injury	CLRD	CVD	Injury
5	CLRD	CLRD	Injury	Injury	CVD
6	P/Flu	P/Flu	DM	AD	CLRD
7	DM	DM	P/Flu	DM	AD
8	KD	Suicide	AD	KD	DM
9	Atherosclerosis	KD	KD	P/Flu	P/Flu
10	Suicide	HIV	Septicemia	Suicide	KD

Figure 1.5 Leading causes of death in the United States at the onset of each decade. In blue are those diseases which are almost exclusively non-infectious, tan are those which are exclusively infectious, and the light colors are those for which there may also be infectious causes.

AD, Alzheimer's disease; CLRD, chronic lower respiratory disease; CVD, cardiovascular disease; DM, diabetes mellitus; HD, diseases of the heart; KD, kidney disease; P/Flu, pneumonia and influenza.

THOUGHT QUESTION

What are some explanations for why leading causes of disease change over time? What factors have contributed to a decrease in overall infectious disease mortality?

Disease Re-Emergence

Basic epidemiologic principles of sanitation, hygiene, and vaccination drove the burden of infectious disease down (Figure 1.6). In the 1960s and 1970s the medical disciplines in the United States turned their sights away from infectious diseases.[12] Medical students were encouraged to seek other specialties, and funding for infectious disease research

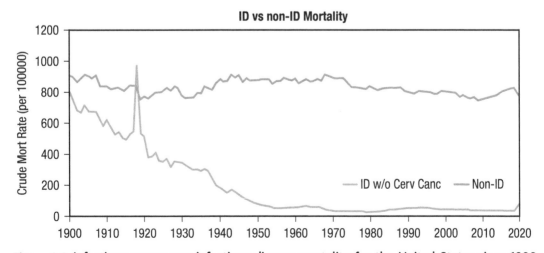

Figure 1.6 Infectious versus non-infectious disease mortality for the United States since 1900. Annual mortality data for this figure from the Centers for Disease Control and Prevention WONDER Database.

increased by just 20% when the whole budget for the main U.S. governmental funding agency for health, the National Institutes of Health, doubled.[13] Yet, as recent examples including COVID-19 and Zika have taught us, infectious diseases continue to cause significant morbidity and mortality. Increasingly, infections are being causally attributed to certain cancers and other chronic diseases, so the true burden is likely underestimated.

As science and the germ theory taught us, infectious disease does not spontaneously happen; rather, it requires that a host come into contact with the pathogen. Our world is changing in the way we interact and potentially expose ourselves. One of those changes is increasing population density. It is estimated that about 56% of the global population lives in urban areas compared with 30% in 1950, with the biggest change in Latin America (up by 40% to 81% now living in urban areas) and the highest percentage of urban dwellers currently in North America where 84% live in urban areas.[14] Poor housing, lack of adequate sanitation and water supply, and waste management in these urban areas may lead to increased zoonotic (particularly rodent-borne), vector-borne, or soil-transmitted helminth disease. Building and ventilation quality may create a risk for certain respiratory diseases. The density and resulting number of close contacts between inhabitants may promote the rapid spread of emerging infectious disease.

Related, the increased connectivity and mobility between people and populations means that pathogens can spread quickly between populations. Societal issues of war, displacement camps, migration, deforestation, and climate change force populations to be exposed to pathogens. These new interactions between hosts and the quick capacity to spread to additional susceptible hosts create a space for the emergence of disease. The pathogens themselves evolve as they pass through hosts and between hosts, changing the way they interact with the immune system. All of these create opportunities for diseases to emerge or to re-emerge and present new challenges to infectious disease control.

With the challenges come solutions. As with the *simple* steps of hygiene and handwashing that brought infectious disease incidence down to where it is now, strengthening public health systems supports resilience against emerging infectious disease. A modern public health system that uses evidence-based approaches, with robust data-sharing capacity, that collaborates across its own nation and internationally, and one with the human capacity to respond to and maintain a response to dual hazards is one that is resilient in the face of emerging infections.

THOUGHT QUESTION

What did you just learn? Use Figure 1.6 to mark and notice the effect of major public health advances on the trend. For example, penicillin was discovered in 1928 by Sir Alexander Fleming when he noticed the lack of mold on a neglected petri dish. The use of antibiotics became widespread during World War II (1940s). Find some additional dates on your own: measles, mumps, rubella vaccination. When did Moen invent the single tap water faucet?

HOW DO WE CLASSIFY DISEASES?

COVID-19 represented the third known "spillover" of an animal coronavirus to humans over the course of just two decades, resulting in major pandemics. Coronaviruses belong to the family Coronaviridae, with the COVID-19 virus designated as SARS-CoV-2. The other two newly emerged viruses were severe acute respiratory syndrome (SARS) and Middle East respiratory syndrome (MERS).

We now know COVID-19 is caused by a virus, specifically SARS-CoV-2, but how do we get from symptoms to causative agent? Like many scientific fields, epidemiologists seek to identify patterns through classification of what they see. When it comes to disease, these too are classified. Any infectious disease might be classified based on the **causative agent**. That is, is the pathogen a **virus**, **bacteria**, **fungus**, **parasite**, or **prion**? Classifying based on agent aids in identifying treatment. For example, antibiotics work against bacteria and antifungals work against fungal infection. Most viruses are either prevented by vaccination or the symptoms are treated until the host can clear the infection.

virus: Viruses are generally the smallest pathogens and are encapsulated DNA or RNA. They require a host (cellular machinery) to replicate. Examples include HIV (causative agent of AIDS) or SARS-CoV-2 (causative agent of COVID-19).

bacteria: Small, single-celled organisms that can be beneficial or detrimental. Examples include *Helicobacter pylori* (strongly associated with stomach cancer) and *Mycobacterium tuberculosis* (causative agent of tuberculosis).

fungus: Fungi represent their own kingdom. A few of the millions of fungi may infect hosts. Examples include *Candida spp.* (yeast infections) and *Coccidioides spp.* (causative agent of Valley fever).

parasites: An organism that lives in or on other organisms. Like a virus, parasites need hosts to survive, but unlike a virus, they do not require the host machinery to reproduce. Examples include *Taenia spp.* (tapeworms) and *Plasmodium spp.* (malaria).

prions: Transmissible proteins that induce abnormal folding of normal cellular proteins. Examples include Creutzfeld-Jakob disease and scrapie.

Another classification scheme is based on mode of transmission, or how the pathogen is transferred from source to host. Typically, these are divided into direct (skin-to-skin or over short distances) or indirect (airborne over longer distances, on surfaces or in water and food, or through an intermediary like a vector). This classification scheme pinpoints interventions, places to break the chain of transmission. For example, for sexually transmitted diseases, condoms provide a barrier between bodily fluids. For a food-borne disease, proper food handling and cooking can break the chain of transmission. Yet a third method of classification can focus on the reservoir or source of the pathogen. This approach, common to eco-epidemiology, focuses on whether the pathogen normally resides in humans, animals, soil, or water. As with a focus on mode of transmission, understanding where the pathogen is coming from can inform how to prevent exposure and thus break the chain of transmission.

Still, not all pathogens fit nicely into one of these categories. Prions were only identified in the 1980s by Dr. Stanley Prusiner when no other agent could be identified to explain scrapie, Creutzfelt-Jakob, or bovine spongiform encephalopathy.[15] Other diseases, like the plague, caused by the bacteria *Yersinia pestis,* may be transmitted by fleas (vector-borne disease) or through direct-contact pneumonic plague. Regardless of the classification scheme used, understanding leads to control.

THOUGHT QUESTION

How would you classify a disease such as SARS by each of the three classification systems presented in this chapter?

As noted in the text, depending on your discipline, you might characterize diseases differently. The more medical approach might be the agent (e.g., virus, bacteria) while the epidemiologist might go by routes of transmission (e.g., food-borne, vector-borne). There is not a right or wrong way; they are simply different approaches providing different methods of characterization.

The Epidemiologic Triad

COVID-19 is a viral disease that affects humans and is primarily acquired via respiratory transmission. But what does that knowledge tell us about how to protect ourselves? If we break down the opening sentence: a *viral* disease (agent) that affects *humans* (host) and is acquired through *respiratory exposure* (environment), we have the three points of the epidemiologic triad. The epidemiologic triad provides a framework for thinking about disease transmission but also for intervention (Figure 1.7). The vertices of the triangle are agent, host, and environment. Disease agents, be they bacteria, prions, viruses, or parasites, or be they non-infectious chemical or radiation agents, create

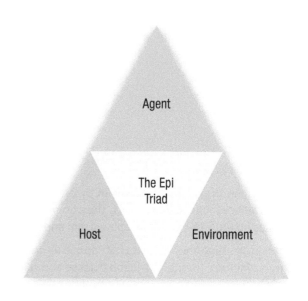

Figure 1.7 **The epidemiologic triad. A framework for disease transmission and intervention.**

exposure within the environment and have consequences for the host. Each of the sides represents the link between agent–host, host–environment, and environment–agent. Important for public health, they also represent places for intervention. By breaking the link between any pair, the triangle, the transmission cycle, also breaks. It is at these linkages that many epidemiologists focus their attention on research, policy, and implementation.

What characteristics of the host, agent, and environment might be conducive to transmission of measles? The common cold? Amoebiasis?

CASE STUDY

Dr. Donald Ainslie Henderson (known as D. A.) evokes instant recognition as the epidemiologist who led the campaign eradicating smallpox (Figure 1.8).[16] D.A. worked earlier as the director of disease surveillance for the Centers for Disease Control and Prevention (CDC) under the legendary Alexander Langmuir, the epidemiologist who founded the CDC's "disease detective" program. When Henderson began working for the WHO as chief medical officer in 1966, he began a campaign that attempted to identify every case of smallpox, and subsequently vaccinating every person exposed, a strategy known as ring vaccination. A special vaccine that was able to withstand high temperatures allowed for a successful roll-out across the world using a small cadre of dedicated workers. In what was an amazing feat of "shoe-leather epidemiology," Henderson promoted ring vaccination and surveillance, using active case finding and community mobilization until the last known case of wild smallpox infection was found in a hospital

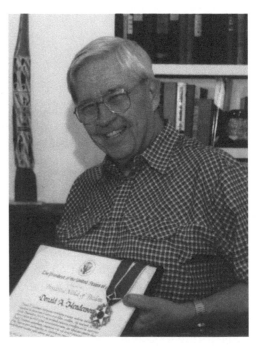

Figure 1.8 Dr. Henderson in 2002 after he received the Presidential Medal of Freedom from President George W. Bush.

cook in Somalia in 1977 and the disease was declared eradicated in 1980. To this day, smallpox remains the only human disease to have been eradicated.

CONCLUSION

Infectious disease epidemiologists face numerous challenges in their work. Beyond the heterogeneity of organisms and conditions mentioned previously, identification of appropriate frameworks and measures for studying diseases is very important. How does one study and make predictions regarding an asymptomatic infection? How does one decide on the target population of interest for a study? How does one handle new infectious disease outbreaks and agents and communicate findings with policy makers and the public? To successfully do this, epidemiologists engage with multiple disciplines from colleagues in basic science laboratories to government officials working to implement public health policy. In this chapter we have examined the work of infectious disease epidemiologists; assessed how to distinguish a disease with an infectious causative agent from one that does not have one; considered infectious disease trends and reasons for disease re-emergence; illustrated major infectious disease classification systems; and looked at the characteristics of the host, agent, and environment that might enable disease transmission.

TEACHING CORNER

DID YOU KNOW?

While most introductory to public health students can tell you a definition of incidence and prevalence, some struggle to see how they are related to one another. Trigger words help students discern between incidence (*risk*, *develop*, and *new* cases) and prevalence (*burden* of disease, *existing* cases). But how do incidence and prevalence relate to one another and what do they tell us about disease?

TRY THIS

In 2021, the incidence of COVID-19 was 1.9 times higher for American Indians and Alaska Natives (AI/AN) when compared to Non-Hispanic Whites (NHW). Death rates among AI/AN were 2.4 times that of NHW. Can you use this information to make a prediction about the prevalence of COVID-19 in AI/AN and NHW? One way to understand this is a "gum ball machine," where incidence fills the jar, and the only ways out are deaths and recovery/cure. The size of the arrow indicates the rate of flow (Figure 1.9).

Here, the AI/AN incidence rate is about twice that of NHW, while the case fatality rate is almost 2.4 times that of NHW. Assuming that the course of disease is otherwise similar, that is there is no difference in duration of disease, and recognizing that, in general, the incidence will be much greater than the CFR, we can assume that the prevalence of COVID-19 among AI/AN is higher.

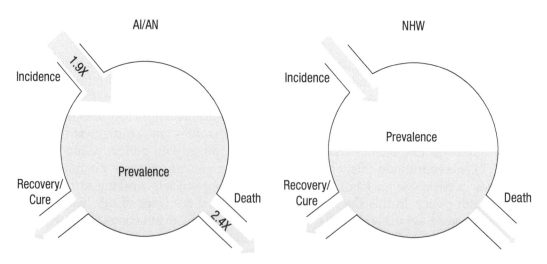

PREDICT WHAT PREVALENCE WILL LOOK LIKE, KNOWING INCIDENCE AND MORTALITY

Figure 1.9 The "gum ball machine" analogy for incidence and prevalence.
AI, American Indian; AN, Alaska Native; NHW, non-Hispanic White

TAKE IT A STEP FURTHER

Now that you're seeing how they relate, play around. *Flip it:* Keeping incidence at 1.9x NHW and mortality at 2.4x NHW, how could you make the prevalence equal? Let us imagine the prevalence was the same and we knew the incidence rate to be 1.9x NHW. What would have to be happening at either recovery or death? *Apply it:* What public health measures could you undertake to balance the prevalence? *Analyze it:* What does this potentially tell you about health disparities? What measures do you think you could engage in to reduce mortality? To reduce incidence?

The "gum ball" analogy is a common way to teach this concept. There are great resources online that provide animations to reiterate. One of our favorites is here: "Incidence and Prevalence: All You Need to Know" by MedMastery (www.youtube.com/watch?v=cTp_ONVVrh8).

QUESTIONS FOR FURTHER DISCUSSION

1. Food poisoning is considered an infectious disease because it is caused by a bacterium. But given that you cannot transmit the infection to others, why is it considered to be an infectious disease?

2. With decreasing trends in infectious disease mortality over time (although one could argue the COVID-19 pandemic bucks the trend), what are some other possible metrics to assess whether we have been successful in dealing with infectious diseases?

3. How would you propose to modify Koch's postulates to prion diseases?

 A robust set of instructor resources designed to supplement this text is located at http://connect.springerpub.com/content/book/978-0-8261-5674-7. Qualifying instructors may request access by emailing textbook@springerpub.com.

REFERENCES

1. Hippocrates.*Hippocrates on Airs, Waters, and Places. 'Ipparchou Ton 'Aratou Kai Eu'doxou Phainoménon 'exegéseos Biblia Tria.* Printed by Wyman & Sons; 1881.
2. Hempelmann E, Krafts K. Bad air, amulets and mosquitoes: 2,000 years of changing perspectives on malaria. *Malar J.* 2013;12:232. doi:10.1186/1475-2875-12-232. PMID: 23835014; PMCID: PMC3723432.
3. Microbiology by numbers. *Nat Rev Microbiol.* 2011;9:628. doi:10.1038/nrmicro2644
4. WB. Béchamp or Pasteur? A lost chapter in the history of biology. *Nature.* 1924;113:121. doi:10.1038/113121b0
5. Brock TD. *Robert Koch: A Life in Medicine and Bacteriology.* American Society of Microbiology Press; 1999.
6. Snow J. Cholera and the water supply in the south districts of London in 1854. *J Public Health Sanit Rev.* 1856;2(7):239–257. PMID: 30378891; PMCID: PMC6004154.
7. Levine R, Evers C. The slow death of spontaneous generation (1668–1859). https://blblack.sciences.ncsu.edu/bio183de/Black/cellintro/cellintro_reading/Spontaneous_Generation.html#:~:text=From%20the%20time%20of%20the,spontaneously%20from%20non%2Dliving%20matter
8. Haghdoost AA. Molecular epidemiology, concepts and domains. *J Kerman Univ Med Sci.* 2008; 15(1):97–104.

9. Chang Y, Cesarman E, Pessin MS, et al. Identification of herpesvirus-like DNA sequences in AIDS-associated Kaposi's sarcoma. *Science*. 1994;266(5192):1865–1869. doi: 10.1126/science.7997879

10. Roth GA, Emmons-Bell S, Alger HM, et al. Trends in patient characteristics and COVID-19 in-hospital mortality in the United States during the COVID-19 pandemic. *JAMA Netw Open*. 2021;4(5):e218828. doi:10.1001/jamanetworkopen.2021.8828

11. Brachman PS. Infectious diseases--past, present, and future. *Int J Epidemiol*. 2003;32(5):684–686. doi:10.1093/ije/dyg282. PMID: 14559728.

12. Spellberg B. Dr. William H. Stewart: mistaken or maligned? *Clin Infect Dis*. 2008;47(2):294. doi:10.1086/589579

13. Spellberg B, Taylor-Blake B. On the exoneration of Dr. William H. Stewart: debunking an urban legend. *Infect Dis Poverty*. 2013;2(1):3. doi:10.1186/2049-9957-2-3

14. Statista. Share of urban population worldwide in 2021, by continent. 2021. https://www.statista.com/statistics/270860/urbanization-by-continent/

15. Ayers JI, Prusiner SB. Prion protein—mediator of toxicity in multiple proteinopathies. *Nat Rev Neurol*. 2020;16(4):187–188. doi:10.1038/s41582-020-0332-8

16. Donald Ainslie (D.A.) Henderson, M.D., M.P.H. (1928–2016) Smallpox eradication: leadership and legacy. *J Infect Dis*. 2017;215(5):673–676. doi:10.1093/infdis/jiw640

CHAPTER 2

CONCEPTS OF DISEASE TRANSMISSION

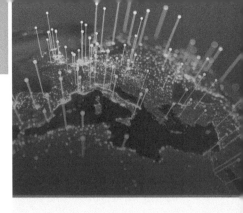

INTRODUCTION

Helicobacter pylori *infection occurs when the bacteria infect the stomach. After many years of living in the digestive tract, that can cause sores, peptic ulcers in the stomach lining or small intestine, and infection and eventually lead to stomach cancer. About two-thirds of the world's population has* H. pylori *in their bodies but it only progresses to infection in a small fraction. The infection usually persists for life unless treated by antibiotics. A few years ago in Colombia, a study team found that people of Amerindian descent carrying largely African strains of* H. pylori *were five times more likely to have gastric cancer or precancerous lesions than were coastal people of largely African descent who carried similar strains. Why this large difference? One thought is diet—coastal people eat more fruits, vegetables, and fish.*[1]

LEARNING OBJECTIVES

By the end of this chapter, readers will be able to:

- Distinguish between predominant modes of transmission.
- Define the chain of infection and identify the implications for public health control strategies.
- Describe the natural history of disease.
- Explain how infectious causes of cancer and other diseases blur the chronic/infectious divide.
- Show how we know if an exposure is associated with an outcome.

WHAT ARE DIFFERENT MODES OF INFECTIOUS DISEASE TRANSMISSION?

H. pylori *seems to infect mostly children, with a clustering of infection occurring within families. Infection is associated with congregate settings, low socioeconomic status, storage and consumption of certain foods, and poor sanitation. However, its mode of transmission is poorly understood, with no single pathway identified. To date, person-to-person transmission (both horizontally and vertically), as well as fecal-oral transmission, including contaminated water and food sources, have been implicated.*

Consider how markedly different diseases may be from each other in how they spread—whereas the common cold can be transmitted from touching contaminated objects, also known as **fomites**, flu likely spreads mainly through droplets made when people who are sick cough, sneeze, or talk, which are then inhaled by people nearby. The **mode of transmission** refers to the method that a pathogen uses to get from a starting point to a destination. Knowing the mode (of transmission) for a given disease can be useful for a number of reasons:

- The mode defines certain characteristics of the pathogen and the resulting disease.
- It allows us to target our response and interventions to predict and prevent a particular disease or other pathogens transmitted through similar routes.
- Knowing the mode of transmission allows us to conceptualize how a given disease may be at the interface of the epidemiologic triangle and the relationships between the host, the pathogen, and the environment.
- It can help us project and visualize the trajectory of the disease and its pattern of spread (through epidemic curves and other tools). As we will see, epidemic curves in turn can be used to determine the mode of transmission when unknown.

How do epidemiologists identify the mode of transmission? Inferring how a disease is spread based on behaviors among cases and their contacts is one approach. Sometimes contact tracing shows us commonalities among individuals and their environments and behaviors. Pathogen location, site of infection, age, and other characteristics of who is infected, and the biology of the transmission stages, are all additional clues to the transmission mode.

THOUGHT QUESTION

How do modes of transmission relate to our epidemiologic triad framework of agent, host, and environment?

Horizontal and Vertical Transmission

Various classifications exist for modes of transmission. One approach is to begin by distinguishing between horizontal and vertical transmission. In **horizontal transmission,** viruses are transmitted among individuals of the same generation or those not in a parent/offspring relationship, while **vertical transmission** occurs across generations, typically in reference to mothers and their offspring (Table 2.1).

Horizontal transmission can be either *direct*, through close personal contact, or *indirect*, through airborne transmission, fomites, or vectors. **Direct contact transmission** occurs through body contact with the tissues or fluids of an infected individual. Microorganisms are physically transferred from one person to another through mucous membranes such as the eyes or mouth, through open wounds, or through sexual contact. Varied pathogens fall under this category including methicillin-resistant *Staphyloccocus aureus* (MRSA), syphilis, rabies, and HIV.

Indirect contact transmission occurs when there is no direct human contact, but rather transmission occurs through contact with vectors, surfaces, or objects. Airborne transmission occurs when pathogens are transferred via very small particles or droplet

Table 2.1 Horizontal and Vertical Virus Transmission

MODE	ROUTE	EXAMPLES
Vertical	Transplacental	HIV, herpes, rubella
Vertical	Perinatal	Hepatitis B, HIV, herpes simplex virus, syphilis
Vertical	Postpartum	HIV
Horizontal direct	Sexual	HIV, syphilis
Horizontal direct	Droplet	Ebola
Horizontal indirect	Vector	Yellow fever, malaria
Horizontal indirect	Fomite	Giardiasis
Horizontal indirect	Vehicle	*E. coli*, shigellosis
Horizontal indirect	Airborne	Anthrax, hantavirus

nuclei once they are suspended in the air. This is a predominant mode of transmission for COVID-19 and measles. Fomites may be contaminated transfusion products or injections, as well as contaminated food, objects, or surfaces. Food and water may also be included in this category and are known as vehicles. Food can carry pathogens such as Salmonella. Vectors are arthropods, organisms that do not directly cause disease by themselves but by transmitting pathogens from one host to another. Examples of vectors are mosquitoes that transmit malaria, yellow fever, or West Nile virus (WNV); fleas that transmit plague; and ticks that transmit Lyme disease.

Vertical transmission involves infectious disease spread from the mother to child. Common terms include "transplacental," meaning transmission from mother to child through the placenta; "perinatal," meaning the period before, during, or slightly after birth; and "postpartum," meaning after birth. Transmission during any of these situations is vertical transmission.

fomites: Inanimate objects contaminated with some microorganism.

horizontal transmission: The transmission of an agent from one to another person of the same generation in the same population.

vertical transmission: Transmission of an agent from an individual to its offspring.

direct contact transmission: Transmission through physical contact between and infected person and a susceptible one.

indirect contact transmission: Transmission without direct contact. Contact occurs through contaminated surfaces or objects, or through a vector.

Many diseases spread through several different pathways. For example, HIV can be spread through direct sexual contact, indirectly through needles, or from mother to child. The mode of transmission can also depend on the physical composition of the infectious agent—for example, anthrax in its natural form isspread through direct contact with infected animals, contact with infected animal products (wool, hides), or eating contaminated meat. In weaponized form, it is transmitted into very small particles that can float through the air, becoming an airborne disease. Debates have occurred about the relative importance of different modes of transmission for a given pathogen. For example, in the case of avian influenza, experiments have shown how the virus can persist in the environment, emphasizing the importance of drinking water and fecal-oral transmission in addition to airborne transmission. Alternative transmission pathways have been explored for other pathogens, such as *H. pylori*.

THOUGHT QUESTION

How does the common cold get transmitted? How about the plague?

WHAT IS THE CHAIN OF INFECTION AND WHAT ARE IMPLICATIONS FOR PUBLIC HEALTH CONTROL STRATEGIES?

H. pylori is likely transmitted directly from person to person or through environmental contamination. High recurrence rates have been reported in many countries, likely due to re-exposure due to high prevalence in the community. Its path can be followed from the portal of entry, as the bacteria enters the body through the mouth, then moves through the digestive system and onto the stomach and small intestine. It may then be shed through saliva or feces and infect the next person.

We sometimes call the spread between individuals or between individuals and the environment the **chain of infection**. The sequencing of the chain provides a path, or route, taken using the chosen mode and includes the site of pathogen presentation, or portal of exit; a specific pathway used; and a destination where the pathogen enters a new host (Figure 2.1). The routes for one mode may be singular or several and tell us how the pathogen will leave one body and infect another. This information can suggest whether a particular pathogen is more limited or widespread in its transmission, which in turn

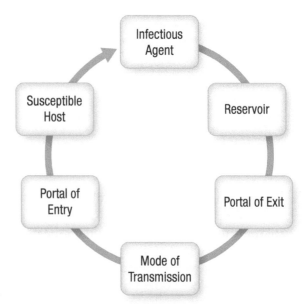

Figure 2.1 **The chain of infection.**

suggests how narrowly or broadly we define our disease control activities. For example, airborne pathogens mainly spread from one respiratory tract to another, while vector-borne pathogens can be transmitted by the vector to a susceptible host through the skin (e.g., from the vectors' feces infecting a cut, or from a vector bite directly into the blood stream).

An agent usually has a place in the environment where it lives until it contacts a host or vector. This is known as a **reservoir**. Reservoirs may include other humans, animals, or non-living places in the environment. Some viruses have no non-human reservoir: poliomyelitis and smallpox are prominent examples. In contrast, many fungal agents can live and multiply in the soil, such as those that cause Coccidioidomycosis, or valley fever, which causes infection when inhaled (Table 2.2). The natural reservoir of some diseases remains unclear. This is the case for the Ebola virus, often seen in bats, but without clear attribution to a particular species.

The reservoir typically harbors the infectious agent without injury to itself and serves as a source from which other individuals can be infected. The infectious agent primarily depends on the reservoir for its survival and may feed on it. It is from the reservoir that the infectious substance is then transmitted to a human or another susceptible host.

HEADS UP!

Medicine and epidemiology sometimes use words differently. Reservoir to a physician might mean the organ where the pathogen is commonly found (e.g., the stomach is a reservoir for *H. pylori*). But epidemiologists use reservoirs to be the naturally occurring source of infection. So, for epidemiologists, humans are *H. pylori* reservoirs, not just their stomachs. While we are at it: Medicine will use antibiotics to eradicate a bacterial infection, but epidemiologists reserve the term "eradicate" to refer to the global elimination of a disease (e.g., only when talking about the 1980 successful eradication of smallpox or the 2011 eradication of rinderpest).

A pathogen must leave its host through a **portal of exit** in order to subsequently infect others. The portal of exit usually corresponds to the primary organ the pathogen infects, such that respiratory pathogens will exit the respiratory tract when one coughs, sings, or sneezes, and cholera will exist in the feces. In the case of vertical transmission, bloodborne pathogens may exit by crossing the placenta from mother to fetus, as in rubella and syphilis. Once the pathogen leaves the host, it then uses its preferred mode of

Table 2.2 **Examples of Pathogens in Animal and Environmental Reservoirs**

Animal:	West Nile virus in migratory birds via mosquito vectors Lyme disease (*Borrelia burgdorferi*) in rodents via tick vectors *E. coli* O157:H7 in cattle via ingestion Cryptosporidiosis in calves
Environment:	Botulism—neurotoxin from *Clostridium botulinum* in soil Tetanus neurotoxin from *Clostridium tetani* in soil *Legionella* species in water *Mycobacterium avium* complex in soil and water Cocci in soil and dust *Aspergillus* fungal species everywhere Blastomycosis in soil and dust

transmission to enter another host through a **portal of entry**. This might be the mouth, nose, or skin. However, even if a pathogen enters a host, unless the host is susceptible, no infection may occur, or the infection may be very limited (e.g., in the case of an individual who is vaccinated).

reservoirs: Any person, animal, plant, soil, or substance in which an infectious agent normally lives and multiplies. These may naturally harbor the organism because it grows there, or the environment could become contaminated with a pathogen.

portal of entry: Sites through which infectious pathogens get into the body, often mucous membranes, injuries, or the respiratory, gastrointestinal, or genitourinary tracts.

portal of exit: The means, or body site, through which a pathogen exits from a (human) reservoir.

THOUGHT QUESTION

For what diseases are we primary reservoirs? Can you map out the chain of infection for MRSA? How about for enterohemorrhagic E. coli (EHEC; e.g., *E. coli* O157:H7), which through its release of shiga toxins results in severe human disease?

Implications for Public Health

Knowing the chain of infection allows us to more effectively determine the best public health response. Typically, we want to intervene to "break" the chain. A particular response might thus attempt to control or eliminate the pathogen at the transmission source, interrupt transmission, protect the portals of entry, or improve the ability of the susceptible host to defend itself (see Figure 2.1). An example of controlling at the source is treating with antibiotics to eliminate a bacterial infection. If the antibiotics work, then the chain is interrupted. With an environmental reservoir, one approach would be to decontaminate the soil to prevent pathogen escape or spread. Interrupting transmission can occur by isolating the infectious case, handwashing, modifying ventilation systems, spraying mosquitoes, and so on. Protecting portals of entry might occur through donning masks and gloves or use of bed nets and long shirts and pants in the case of vector-borne disease. Finally, increasing host defense to reduce susceptibility may occur through vaccination, prophylaxis, or herd immunity. Vaccination can promote the body's ability to protect itself against future infection, as can effective prophylactic drugs. Herd immunity, on the other hand, prevents the pathogen from encountering a susceptible host in the first place. If a large enough proportion of individuals in a population are no longer susceptible, then the few who are are likely to be protected since the chain of transmission has been interrupted by the non-susceptible individuals.

THOUGHT QUESTION

Why do you think smallpox was successfully eradicated? What are some necessary conditions for disease eradication?

WHAT IS THE NATURAL HISTORY OF DISEASE?

Although many individuals with H. pylori *colonization are asymptomatic, prolonged or more severe infection can result in the formation of ulcers or loss of glandular tissue, known as atrophy. Those with gastric ulcers may progress to astrophic gastritis, leading to intestinal metaplasia, dysplasia, and such conditions as non-cardia gastric cancer. This progression is known as the end result of a sequence of events in the gastric mucosa.[2]*

The **natural history of disease** refers to disease progression over time in an individual, assuming the person is not being treated. This means that no external intervention is applied that might change the pathway from health to disease (i.e., no prevention measures or treatment). Understanding this progression allows us to consider what factors could potentially alter this course of disease. It also provides a reference which allows us to understand how much interventions do or do not matter. For example, close to 90% of the decline in scarlet fever (a bright red rash covering the body caused by the same bacteria, group A streptococcus, that causes strep throat) mortality occurred prior to the introduction of antibiotics,[3] raising the question of what other public health infrastructure may already have been in place. In another example, untreated infection with HIV causes a spectrum of clinical problems beginning at the time of seroconversion (primary HIV) and terminating with AIDS and eventually death, which may not happen for 10 or more years after seroconversion.[4]

In order to get the disease, a number of factors have to occur over time. First, the individual must be susceptible. During this time some type of single exposure or accumulation of exposures must occur. For example, an individual is exposed to a microorganism. The pathogen usually will move to the preferred tissue or target organ and begin to multiply. The person then goes through a period of subclinical disease where the disease is not noticeable but pathological changes are occurring in the body even as the body responds, before going on to clinical, symptomatic phases until the disease has run its course, that is, the person is cured or recovers, remains chronically disabled, or has died (Figure 2.2).

It is possible to see how one could prevent an individual from becoming exposed (primary prevention), stop or reduce the exposure or else prevent the individual from progression (secondary prevention), or else improve treatment and recovery (tertiary prevention).

THOUGHT QUESTION

Is vaccination considered primary or secondary prevention?

Incubation and Latent Periods

If the disease process has begun, changes may occur within the body without an individual's awareness. The time from exposure to an infectious pathogen until first signs or symptoms of a clinical illness is known as the **incubation period.** During this time an individual might be asymptomatic but may still be infectious to others. The length of the incubation period helps to identify the pathogen and can help differentiate between types of pathogens. Conversely, if the pathogen is known, the infectious period can help

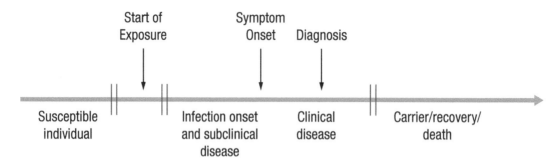

Figure 2.2 **The progression of disease. The horizontal arrow indicates time in an individual's life and their progression through disease stages. Double-red lines show possible points of prevention (*primary*, *secondary*, and *tertiary* prevention from left to right).**

identify the source or reservoir of the pathogen during an outbreak or epidemic and it may be possible to identify the source of the exposure. Furthermore, the incubation period can help identify the period of infectiousness and, importantly, identify individuals who might be at higher risk for infection. For example, the last weeks of a hepatitis A infection are also the most infectious. Tracing the contacts during this period can help identify people exposed to known cases and improve prognosis through early action to limit the progression of disease. Symptom onset can provide tell-tale signs to the type of exposure. Vomiting is likely to occur shortly after exposure to a disagreeable food but is unlikely to happen until some time later due to exposure from a heavy metal. Diseases have characteristic incubation periods, some short and some long. Paralytic shellfish poisoning caused by eating contaminated shellfish occurs just minutes after exposure. In contrast, the interval between HIV infection and development of AIDS can be as long as 10 to 15 years.

THOUGHT QUESTION

What are the incubation periods of Salmonella? Measles? COVID-19? What interventions would you use based on the natural history of each of these diseases?

The **latent period** specifically measures the time from infection until an individual becomes infectious themselves. The time when the individual is infectious is also known as the period of communicability and may overlap with the incubation period. The duration of the latent period is also characteristic of particular infections. Disease control becomes difficult when the latent period is shorter than the incubation period since an infected individual may transmit the pathogen to numerous contacts prior to identification of clinical disease and subsequent implementation of control interventions. This may happen with the flu, COVID-19, or measles (Figure 2.3).

When one person transmits an infection to another, then the time that elapses between the onset of symptoms in the primary (or index) case and onset of symptoms of the secondary case is called the **generation time**, referring to the time it takes for the first group of sick individuals to generate the next group.

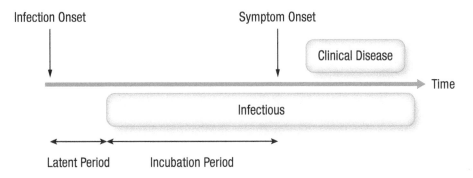

Figure 2.3 **Latent and incubation periods mapped out onto the course of disease.**

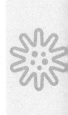

natural history of a disease: Natural course of a disease from the time immediately prior to its inception, progressing through its presymptomatic phase and different clinical stages to the point where it has ended and the patient is either cured, chronically disabled, or deceased without external intervention.[5]

incubation period: Time between exposure to an infectious agent and first signs or symptoms of a clinical illness.

latent period: Time from acquiring infection to the onset of infectiousness.

THOUGHT QUESTION

What happens if the latent period is longer than the incubation period? What are some examples of diseases that fit these criteria?

The Spectrum of Disease

For any exposed individual, several outcomes are possible as a disease progresses. This range is called the spectrum of disease. Possibilities include no infection, infection, disease, or serious infection, eventually ending in recovery, disability, or death. In some people, the exposure will result in infection. This is described by **infectivity**, the ease at which others are infected. In others, the infection will develop clinical disease. This is described by **pathogenicity**, the ability to cause disease. Finally, the disease may be mild, severe, or fatal. The severity of the disease is described by **virulence**. This progression depends on both the exposed person and the pathogen itself (host–microbe interaction; Figure 2.4).

Infectivity describes the proportion of exposed persons who become infected. They can be measured by the number infected divided by the number exposed in the population. Infectivity is affected by the portals of exit, the portals of entry, and an agent's ability to survive outside the host. As we will see, infectivity is a useful metric for comparing different infectious diseases. Measles, pertussis, and smallpox all exhibit high infectivity.

$$\text{Infectivity} = \left(\frac{\text{Number infected}}{\text{Total exposed population}}\right) \times 100$$

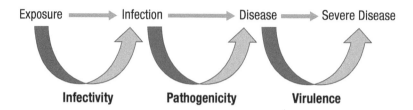

Figure 2.4 **Progression through the spectrum of disease.**

Pathogenicity refers to the proportion of infected people who develop clinical symptoms of the disease out of the total number of infected persons. In other words, this is the ability of an organism to cause disease (i.e., harm the host). Both rabies and chickenpox viruses are highly pathogenic, as there is a high likelihood that infection results in disease. However, this has no indication on the severity of disease—rabies is almost always fatal, while chickenpox is a relatively mild illness. On the other hand, polio virus is of low pathogenicity since most people infected with polio virus do not become ill at all. However, a small percentage of infected people become extremely ill, leading to paralysis or death. Without vaccination, this illness occurs frequently enough to cause severe epidemics.

$$\text{Pathogenicity} = \frac{\text{Symptomatic cases}}{\text{Number (infected) cases}} \times 100$$

Virulence refers to the degree of pathology caused by the organism. In other words, it is a measure of the severity of the disease a pathogen causes. It is measured by the number of individuals with severe disease or fatal cases, divided by the total number with disease and often multiplied by 100 to get a percent:

$$\text{Virulence} = \left(\frac{\text{Severe cases}}{\text{Total cases}} \right) \times 100$$

The extent of virulence is usually correlated with the ability of the pathogen to multiply within the host. Highly virulent pathogens include the Ebola virus, smallpox, pandemic flu, rabies, and polio. A microorganism with a low virulence is the rhinovirus, which causes the common cold.

infectivity: The likelihood a disease infects others, commonly examined using the proportion of exposed individuals who become infected.

pathogenicity: The likelihood of developing clinical disease, commonly examined through the proportion of infected individuals who develop disease.

virulence: The likelihood of developing severe disease, commonly examined through the proportion of diseased individuals who develop more severe or fatal outcomes.

THOUGHT QUESTION

Which diseases are the most infectious? Which are the least? How does that translate to our ability to control them?

HOW DO INFECTIOUS CAUSES OF CANCER AND OTHER DISEASES BLUR THE CHRONIC/INFECTIOUS DIVIDE?

The discovery that H. pylori *can induce gastric inflammation opened the door for treatment to eliminate it from the stomach with antibiotic treatment to reduce the incidence of peptic ulcers and stomach cancers. Previous studies found that up to 75% of the Alaska Native population are infected with* H. pylori, *and that they are 2 to 4 times more likely to develop stomach cancer than the white U.S. population.[6] Clinical actions may include a screening program for high-risk individuals; if infection is present, antibiotic treatment can be provided and broader community education for prevention and screening can be offered.*

As we consider the natural history of disease, it is plausible to consider how an infectious cause initiates or precipitates an eventual chronic disease outcome. Recent papers have found that at least 8% of the noncommunicable disease burden can be attributed to infectious risks globally.[7] Around 92%, or 2 million, new cancer cases are attributable to just four infectious agents: *H. pylori*, human papillomavirus (HPV), and hepatitis B and C viruses.[8] Studies associate HPV with 90% to 99.7% of malignant cervical cancer lesions, the second leading cause of cancer mortality in women worldwide.[9] Chronic Lyme arthritis, which was thought to be an immune disorder, is now attributed to *Borrelia burgdorferi* bacterial infections. This is contrasted with infectious diseases that themselves have become chronic diseases in many countries due to improved care or treatment, such as HIV.

So how can an infection cause chronic outcomes? One scenario is for the pathogen to produce progressively worse tissue damage, as in the case of hepatitis B and hepatocellular carcinoma (HCC), the most common type of primary liver cancer.[10] A second scenario is that the initial stages of the infection cause permanent disability, as in the case of polio paralysis. A third is that the chronic deficits are more indirect, such that infection increases risk of longer-term adverse outcomes, as may be the case with long COVID, technically known as post-acute sequelae SARS-CoV-2 infection (PASC). Duration and timing of infection all play an important role in determining these outcomes. Inflammation is a possible link between the exposure and the chronic disease, as are aberrant immune responses.

It is clear that complex interactions between human, microbe, and environment determine whether exposure, infection, and the development of chronic sequelae will take place. It is important to note that the effect of lifelong infections such as those caused by cytomegalovirus and hepatitis C virus is somewhat controversial.[11,12] Since humans have co-evolved with a number of microbes, there are numerous examples of populations in non-industrialized societies which exhibit very low rates of inflammation-related chronic diseases.[13]

In some cases, there are clear interventions that can disrupt the chain of transmission. Blood donor screening, along with programs to prevent hepatitis B and hepatitis C transmission, have been shown to reduce long-term outcomes of HCC and chronic liver disease. We also see how immunization against HPV is successfully reducing cervical cancer prevalence.

THOUGHT QUESTION

What is the evidence for an infectious cause for heart disease? For diabetes?

HOW DO WE KNOW IF AN EXPOSURE IS ASSOCIATED WITH AN OUTCOME?

Several studies have found a familial predisposition for gastric cancer. Most studies suggest that first-degree relatives of patients with gastric cancer are at higher risk. This risk has been quantified such that the relative risk for the development of gastric cancer in association with a positive family history is 2.35.[14] Similarly, the broader odds ratio between H. pylori *infection and the subsequent development of gastric cancer has been shown to be 2.36.[15] A reduction in the risk of gastric cancer has been found following the eradication of* H. pylori *infection, with an odds ratio of 0.67.[16]*

In order to understand risk factors for an infectious disease and for transmission, one can begin testing hypotheses. Epidemiologic studies typically collect information on factors associated with a disease and thus serve as an excellent source of data for answering these types of questions. The key feature of **analytic epidemiology** is the use of a comparison group to examine measures of association. Measures of association allow us to compare the risks of an outcome in two different groups, given that they have different exposures. A measure of association quantifies the relationship between exposure and disease among the two groups and allows us to observe whether the association is stronger in one group or the other.

Imagine that 200 people attend a wedding, which is of course catered. After the wedding 75 of the attendees become ill, leaving 125 who did not. Based on the symptoms present among those who got ill, the epidemiologist investigating this outbreak might look to the foods that were eaten, focusing here on what we'll call food "A." The epidemiologist then groups ill and non-ill individuals based on whether or not they ate food "A." In our example, 50 of the 75 ill individuals and 50 of the 125 non-ill individuals ate food "A." A great way to show this is to tabulate it in what epidemiologists call a 2x2 contingency table as follows:

EXPOSURE	ILL	NOT ILL	TOTAL
Ate food "A"	50	50	100
Did not eat food "A"	25	75	100
Total	75	125	200

The **risk ratio**, also known as the incidence proportion ratio or relative risk, is the ratio between the two risks observed in the exposed and unexposed groups. Mathematically, we would show it as:

$$\text{Risk ratio} = \frac{\text{Incidence among exposed}}{\text{Incidence among unexposed}} = \frac{\dfrac{\text{New cases among exposed}}{\text{Exposed population}}}{\dfrac{\text{New cases among unexposed}}{\text{Unexposed population}}}$$

In our example, the exposure is eating food "A" at the wedding and, reading across our table, 100 individuals did. Our risks, or incidence proportions, are 50/100 = 50% in our exposed group, and 25/100 = 25% in our unexposed group. Our risk ratio (RR) is 50%/25% = 2.0. We would then interpret this as expecting to see a two-fold greater incidence of illness (the outcome) among those who ate food "A" (i.e., the exposed guests) compared to the unexposed. If the risk in both groups is the same, then the RR will be equal to 1, the null value. An RR greater than 1.0 indicates an increased risk for the group in the numerator (the exposed group). An RR less than 1.0 indicates a decreased risk for the exposed group, indicating that the exposure may be protective. Note that the RR has no units because they cancel each other out in the numerator and denominator. The **risk difference** refers to the difference in risk between the two groups:

$$\text{Risk difference} = \text{Incidence among exposed} - \text{Incidence among unexposed} =$$

$$\frac{\text{New cases among exposed}}{\text{Exposed population}} - \frac{\text{New cases among unexposed}}{\text{Unexposed population}}$$

We can calculate a risk difference (RD) as 50%–25% = 25%. We might say then that the RD between the exposed and unexposed groups is 25%. An RD of zero indicates a null effect, as that means the risk in both is equal. The highest possible risk is 1 and the lowest –1, with a negative RD indicating that an exposure is protective.

The **odds ratio** provides us with a ratio of the odds of an outcome given exposure compared to the odds of an outcome for the unexposed:

$$\text{Odds ratio} = \frac{\dfrac{\text{Exposed cases}}{\text{Unexposed cases}}}{\dfrac{\text{Exposed controls}}{\text{Unexposed controls}}}$$

In our example, the odds of exposure among cases (those who are ill) are 50/25 = 2. The odds of exposure among controls are 50/75 = 0.67. The odds ratio would be reported as 2/0.67 = 3, or the odds of the outcome in the exposed group being 3 times higher than among the unexposed. Odds can be difficult to interpret but useful in situations when we cannot estimate risk directly (e.g., a case-control study design). If the odds in both groups are the same, the odds ratio = 1, the null value. In this example we see a strong positive association between being ill and consuming food "A."

analytic epidemiology: Studies that measure the association between a particular exposure and a disease, and aim to further examine known associations or hypothesized relationships.

odds ratio: The ratio of the odds of exposure among cases over the odds among non-exposed. It is the commonly calculated measure of effect for case control studies.

THOUGHT QUESTION

Under what circumstances does the odds ratio approximate the risk ratio? Can you name a disease where this approximation might be likely?

CASE STUDY

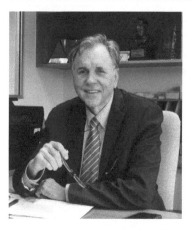

Figure 2.5 **Barry Marshall, 2021.** *Source*: http://commons.wikimedia .org.

During his gastroenterology rotation in 1981, Barry Marshall (Figure 2.5) met pathologist Dr. Robin Warren. Warren and Marshall began to study spiral bacteria present in the stomachs of a number of their patients suffering from ulcers and gastritis.[17] They discovered that peptic ulcers were due to the bacteria H. pylori, not stress or diet as previously thought. However, the wider medical community remained hard to convince. In an act of frustration, Marshall deliberately infected himself by drinking a solution filled with the bacterium, as part of a successful experiment to prove Koch's postulates. He then documented both the formation of his own stomach ulcers and their cure following treatment. In 2005 the two won the Nobel Prize in Physiology or Medicine for their discovery of the bacteria and its role in gastritis and peptic ulcer disease.

CONCLUSION

Infectious diseases have their own unique modes of transmission and natural histories. These disease progressions also mark important points for potential public health intervention. The spectrum of disease allows us to quantify several outcomes as a disease progresses, as well as how many individuals in a population may have these outcomes. Infectious diseases are heterogeneous, with recent evidence pointing to a major role in the etiology of chronic diseases. However, as of now, only two infectious pathogens, hepatitis B virus (HBV) and HPV, are addressed in the Non-Communicable Disease Global Monitoring Framework from the World Health Organization.[18] Analytical epidemiology provides a framework for assessing associations between exposures and disease outcomes and allows us to better understand risk factors for an infectious disease and for transmission.

END-OF-CHAPTER RESOURCES

TEACHING CORNER

DID YOU KNOW?

WNV is a mosquito-borne virus and is the leading cause of mosquito-borne disease in the United States. In 2020, over 650 cases of WNV were reported based on symptoms. It is spread to people through the bite of an infected mosquito. Mosquitoes often get the virus from birds. Nevertheless, the exposure is considered rare (less than one in 100 mosquitoes harbor the virus).

TRY THIS

About 80% of the people infected with WNV do not develop disease. Up to 20% of those infected will develop disease symptoms, such as fever, headaches, and malaise, for a few days to a few weeks. Of those who develop disease, about one in 150 will have severe neurologic symptoms. What is the infectivity, pathogenicity, and virulence of WNV?

TAKE IT A STEP FURTHER

Assuming that severe encephalitis and meningitis (neurologic conditions) occur in about seven per 100,000 Americans, and assuming they are not exposed to WNV, what is the relative risk of severe neurologic disease comparing WNV to the general population?

QUESTIONS FOR FURTHER DISCUSSION

1. A friend in your class who has a cold sneezes. Another friend sitting nearby breathes in and later develops a cold. What is the most likely mode of transmission? It later turns out the second friend also touched a number of fomites in the classroom. What is this mode of transmission? What are some possible fomites?

2. What is the chain of infection for a parasitic disease such as schistosomiasis? What is the natural history of the disease?

3. Do you think other diseases such as polio, HIV, or yellow fever could be eradicated from human populations? Why or why not?

A robust set of instructor resources designed to supplement this text is located at http://connect.springerpub.com/Content/book/978-0-8261-5674-7. Qualifying instructors may request access by emailing textbook@springerpub.com.

REFERENCES

1. Kodaman N, Pazos A, Schneider BG, et al. Human and *Helicobacter pylori* coevolution shapes the risk of gastric disease. *Proc Natl Acad Sci U S A*. 2014;111(4):1455–1460. doi:10.1073/pnas.1318093111

2. Correa P, Piazuelo MB. The gastric precancerous cascade. *J Dig Dis*. 2012;13(1):2–9. doi:10.1111/j.1751-2980.2011.00550.x

3. Silverman WA. *Human Experimentation*. Oxford University Press; 1985: Chapter 4.

4. Mindel A, Tenant-Flowers M. ABC of AIDS: natural history and management of early HIV infection. *BMJ*. 2001;332:1290–1293. doi:10.1136/bmj.322.7297.1290

5. de la Paz MP, Villaverde-Hueso A, Alonso V, et al. Rare diseases epidemiology research. *Adv Exp Med Biol*. 2010; 686:17–39. doi:10.1007/978-90-481-9485-8_2

6. Nolen LD, Vindigni SM, Parsonnet J; Symposium leaders. Combating gastric cancer in Alaska native people: an expert and community symposium. *Gastroenterology*. 2020;158(5):1197–1201. doi:10.1053/j.gastro.2019.11.299

7. Coates MM, Kintu A, Gupta N, et al. Burden of non-communicable diseases from infectious causes in 2017: a modelling study. *Lancet Glob Health*. 2020;8(12):e1489–e1498. doi:10.1016/S2214-109X(20)30358-2. Epub 2020 Oct 21.

8. Brown HE, Dennis LK, Lauro P, Jain P, Pelley E, Oren E. Emerging evidence for infectious causes of cancer in the United States. *Epidemiol Rev*. 2019;41(1):82–96. doi:10.1093/epirev/mxz003

9. Franco EL, Duarte-Franco E, Ferenczy A. Cervical cancer: epidemiology, prevention and the role of human papillomavirus infection. *CMAJ*. 2001;164:1017–1025. https://www.ncbi.nlm.nih.gov/pmc/articles/PMC80931

10. O'Connor SM, Taylor CE, Hughes JM. Emerging infectious determinants of chronic diseases. *Emerg Infect Dis*. 2006;12(7):1051–1057. doi:10.3201/eid1207.060037

11. Root-Bernstein R, Fairweather D. Complexities in the relationship between infection and autoimmunity. *Curr Allergy Asthma Rep*. 2014;14:407. doi:10.1007/s11882-013-0407-3

12. Virgin HW, Wherry EJ, Ahmed R. Redefining chronic viral infection. *Cell*. 2009;138:30–50. doi:10.1016/j.cell.2009.06.036

13. McDade TW. Early environments and the ecology of inflammation. *Proc. Natl Acad. Sci. USA*. 2012;109:17281–17288. doi:10.1073/pnas.1202244109

14. Yaghoobi M, McNabb-Baltar J, Bijarchi R, Hunt RH. What is the quantitative risk of gastric cancer in the first-degree relatives of patients? A meta-analysis. *World J Gastroenterol*. 2017;23(13):2435–2442. doi:10.3748/wjg.v23.i13.2435

15. Helicobacter and Cancer Collaborative Group. Gastric cancer and *Helicobacter pylori*: a combined analysis of 12 case control studies nested within prospective cohorts. *Gut*. 2001;49(3):347–353. doi:10.1136/gut.49.3.347

16. Fuccio L, Zagari RM, Minardi ME, Bazzoli F. Systematic review: *Helicobacter pylori* eradication for the prevention of gastric cancer. *Aliment Pharmacol Ther*. 2007;25(2):133–141. doi:10.1111/j.1365-2036.2006.03183.x

17. Hellstrom PM. This year's Nobel Prize to gastroenterology: Robin Warren and Barry Marshall awarded for their discovery of *Helicobacter pylori* as pathogen in the gastrointestinal tract. *World J Gastroenterol*. 2006;12(19):3126–3127. doi:10.3748/wjg.v12.i19.3126

18. NCD Global Monitoring Framework. Ensuring progress on noncommunicable diseases in countries. World Health Organization. https://www.who.int/teams/ncds/surveillance/monitoring-capacity/gmf

CHAPTER 3

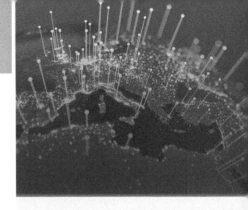

DISEASE TRANSMISSION DYNAMICS

INTRODUCTION

In 2000, the World Health Organization (WHO) declared that the United States had successfully eliminated measles due to strong vaccination. The term "elimination" is reserved for regions or countries with good surveillance that can document no local transmission of a disease for at least 12 months. However, early in 2015 the California Department of Public Health was notified of a suspected measles case in an unvaccinated 11-year-old who reported no out-of-state travel.[1] On the very same day, an additional six suspected cases were reported among California and Utah residents. A month later, a total of 125 cases had been reported from eight states. About 30% could be traced to the same exposure at a California theme park, another third of the cases were secondary exposures (i.e., exposed to those exposed individuals), and the exposure for the final third could not be determined. Only 18% had documentation of starting vaccination and 40% were too young to be vaccinated.

While the occasional outbreak is expected even in a country with elimination status, if transmission occurs for more than a year, elimination status is rescinded. In 2019, this almost happened in the United States. A total of 1,249 cases (the most reported in one year since pre-elimination) were reported from 22 outbreaks with cases in 31 states.[2] Most (89%) were unvaccinated or their vaccine status could not be established, and 10% of the cases were hospitalized. Two associated outbreaks in vaccine-resistant communities in New York accounted for 75% of the cases. Immunization campaigns, active surveillance, and intense community engagement quelled the transmission and the United States was able to retain its measles elimination status.

LEARNING OBJECTIVES

By the end of this chapter, readers will be able to:

- Classify distinct types of epidemics.
- Define the reproductive number and explain what it tells us about a disease.
- Describe how diseases are transmitted and how we quantify the mechanisms of transmission.

TYPES OF EPIDEMICS

Measles is a highly contagious viral disease. It is estimated that up to 90% of susceptible contacts will become infected when exposed to an infected individual.[3] Because measles is transmissible between humans, cases arise from cases, presenting after the incubation period. When visualized, a measles outbreak in a region where the disease had been eliminated might present as peaks of increasing size, an incubation period apart.

Epidemiology is a discipline focused on identifying patterns to improve health and well-being. While this is achieved through a variety of tools and techniques, many infectious disease techniques distill down to visualizing data and making comparisons with known patterns of transmission. Knowing the patterns to expect allows us to determine what is different and to then design additional studies and work with collaborators across different disciplines to investigate and test hypotheses. This first stage of describing the disease is classified as observational epidemiology. A disease that is known to occur in a given place and at a given frequency is **endemic** (Figure 3.1). When we see cases rise above the expected number of cases, the disease has become **epidemic** (see Figure 3.1). A term related to epidemic, but more limited in its geographic or temporal reach, is an **outbreak**. As we saw with influenza in 1918 and SarsCoV-2 in 2020, once a disease spreads and local transmission in excess of expectation occurs in many countries across the globe, the epidemic is classified as a **pandemic**. While typically we look for this deviation from normal when classifying disease, the unusual aggregation of health events in both space and time can be indicative of a **cluster**. The primary tool for an epidemiologist in classifying a disease and understanding transmission dynamics is to visualize the available data.

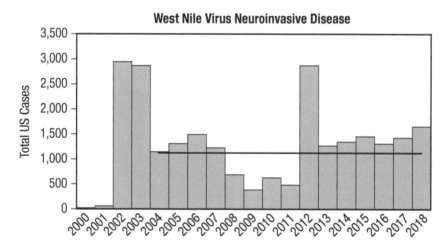

Figure 3.1 Histogram of the total number of West Nile virus neuroinvasive disease cases in the United States by year since 2000. The disease was only introduced into the United States in 1999, so the early years, even though the case counts are low, would be an epidemic phase. By 2004, however, the disease was well established across the United States (black line), though epidemic years occur.

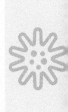

endemic: Usual or constant prevalence of a disease in a population within a geographic area.

epidemic: An increase, or higher than expected numbers, in the prevalence of a disease in a population within a geographic area. Distinguished from an outbreak in its greater geographic or temporal reach.

pandemic: An epidemic that is widespread or has global spread and impact and may infect a great number of people.

Visually organizing data into charts and graphs is the first and final step to understanding disease transmission. It is the last thing, because of the efficacy with which visualizations can convey data or information. It is also the first step, where real-time, or as close to real as possible, trends are plotted, and a general overview of the disease emerges. Looking at the data with a critical and quantitative eye, the epidemiologist can identify a lot about the disease, even before the causal agent is identified. This visual organization allows for hypotheses to be generated about the disease and can help to focus an ongoing disease investigation.

Epidemiology uses the same tools as other disciplines: bar graphs for discrete data, histograms for continuous data, line graphs for temporal data, and so on. Unique to epidemiology is the **epidemic curve**, or epi curve. The epidemic curve is a modified histogram that plots cases on the y-axis and time, usually in days, on the x-axis. Because the curve uses continuous data—that is, time—there are no gaps between entries unless no cases were reported in that period, consistent with the touching bins of a histogram. Like any figure, the axis labels and title should be informative such that the figure can stand alone.

Looking at the shape of the epidemic curve is informative as to the nature of the exposure (Figure 3.2). If there is a single point that is the source of the exposure then the cases have a mountain shape to them, which is, they go gradually up and then gradually down. The slope of the peak, how fast cases rise, has to do with the incubation period and the infectiousness of the pathogen. A foodborne disease from a picnic or banquet is a good example of a *point source* outbreak. Once the picnic is over and the food is cleared, there are no new exposures and cases stop. In contrast, a *propagating source* outbreak is one where cases lead to new cases and the epidemic builds. The epidemic curve for a propagating source exposure is one where there are multiple peaks, usually growing in size as each person may infect multiple additional people. Again, the time between peaks and the growth of the epidemic are dictated by the **incubation period** and the infectiousness, respectively. A *continuous source* outbreak, like cholera from the Broad Street pump, will grow and then plateau until the source is removed. Famously, removing the handle from the Broad Street pump, in the case of John Snow, finally stopped the exposure to a continuous source of contaminated water and stopped the transmission of disease. Another typical shape for an epidemic curve is an *intermittent source*, like water-borne exposures from run-off from an agricultural field. Here the gap between peaks is a combination of incubation periods and whatever is promoting the exposure itself. For example, rainfall might drive run-off to contaminate a spring, which is a water source for a community, exposing only those who collected water that day, who then become ill after the incubation period has elapsed. Because so much can be gleaned from just visualizing the data in this way, an epidemic curve is one of the most powerful tools to an epidemiologist.

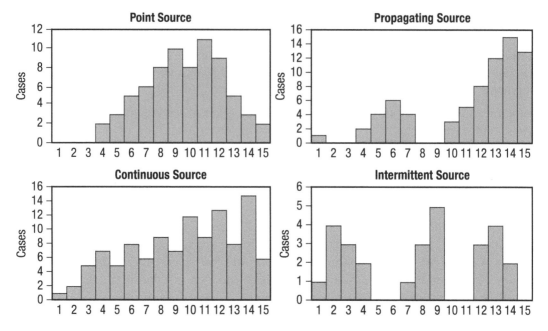

Figure 3.2 Four types of epidemic curves. When graphing an epidemic, the x-axis is time, usu-ally in days, and the y-axis is the number of cases. Each bar then represents the number of cases on a given day of the epidemic. The shape of the curve informs the probable source of an outbreak and can help identify incubation periods. To learn more about epi curves, have a look at this great website by the Public Health Agency of Canada: https://outbreaktools.ca/background/epidemic-curves/#basic.

Source: Data from Public Health Agency of Canada, National Collaborating Centre for Infectious Diseas-es/National Collaborating Centre for Environmental Health. Epidemic curves. https://outbreak tools.ca/background/epidemic-curves/#basic

epidemic curve: A graph where time is on the x-axis and number of cases is on the y-axis to show the progression of an epidemic. The shape of the curve informs the probable type of exposure.

incubation period: The time between exposure to an infected individual and the onset of symptoms.

THOUGHT QUESTION

Build your own epi curve using graph paper or a spreadsheet like Excel. You are responding to an outbreak of illness after a high-school soccer game. Two players were sick on the day of the game. Three more became ill the day after along with two spectators. The next day, two more spectators were ill. Despite actively calling and interviewing 80% of the participants and spectators, there were no more cases reported. Enter these data into a spreadsheet and plot an epi curve (be sure to set the gap between days to 0, and be sure to have the cells square, not rectangular). What does the shape of your curve tell you about the likely exposure?

QUANTIFYING DISEASE TRANSMISSION

Measles is among the most contagious human diseases. In a fully susceptible population, it is estimated that introducing one infected individual will lead to 12 to 18 new infections.[4] Those infected individuals will then lead to another 12 to 18 each, about 2 weeks later, and the cycle will continue until the pool of susceptible individuals is exhausted.

At the beginning of an outbreak, before there are any recovered individuals (either by immunization or by prior exposure), careful contact tracing can allow for the estimation of how contagious an infectious disease will be. **Contact tracing** is, as it sounds, the identification, or tracing, of individuals who may have been exposed through contact with a case. Through contact tracing, we not only get the number of secondary cases but also the number of exposures and can then calculate a rate because we have both a numerator (secondary cases) and a denominator (contacts). Specifically, when we calculate the number of secondary infections in a totally naive population, we are estimating how many secondary infections will arise as the result of a single case (Figure 3.3). This is known as the **basic reproduction number** and is written R_0. It captures three components of disease transmission: (1) the frequency of contact between susceptible and infected individuals, (2) the probability that that interaction will lead to transmission, and (3) how long an infected individual is infectious and able to infect susceptible individuals.

For measles, the R_0 is estimated to be between 12 and 18, depending on the population density and behavior. For comparison, the seasonal flu is between 0.9 and 2.1 depending on the year, population density, and behavior. When R_0 is close to 1, each infected person will infect one additional individual and the disease will neither grow nor die out; rather, it will remain stable. If it is greater than 1, then one case will lead to at least one more case and the disease will establish in a population and may cause an outbreak. If it is less than 1, then

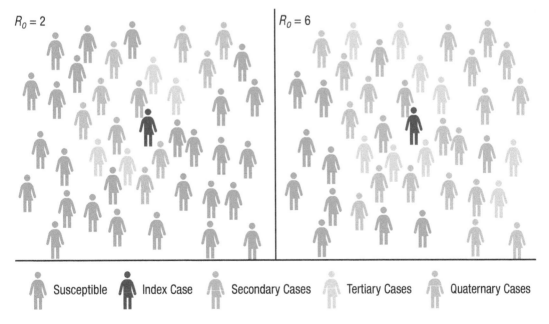

Figure 3.3 The reproductive number, a measure of the transmissibility of an infectious disease. In this figure we visually represent two different R_0 values as a hypothetical disease progresses through three generations.

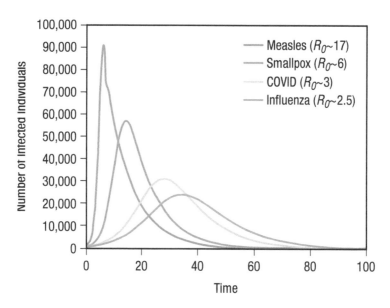

Figure 3.4 A comparison of reproduction numbers (R_0) for four infectious diseases: measles with an estimated R_0 of 17, smallpox with an estimated R_0 of 6, COVID ($R_0 \sim 3$), and influenza ($R_0 \sim 2.5$). *Source*: R_0 estimates based on Fine PE. Herd immunity: history, theory, practice. *Epidemiol Rev.* 1993;15:265–302. doi:10.1093/oxfordjournals.epirev.a036121

each case leads to less than one additional case, and it is likely that the disease will die out and not become established in this new population of exposed individuals. How quickly it grows or dies out is a function of how many additional cases result from an exposure.

Remembering that the basic reproduction number assumes a naïve population and that it is an estimate of disease transmission, we can predict the steepness of an epidemic curve. In a closed population, where individuals do not migrate in or out, diseases with a higher R_0 will have a steeper, faster curve (Figure 3.4). For example, the number of individuals infected by the more transmissible measles will quickly rise and peak higher than for less transmissible influenza. Bearing in mind that R_0 is not a measure of disease severity or of the corresponding treatment capacity, it is helpful in comparing across diseases by providing guidance when estimating the needed response and how quickly the cases will enter the healthcare system. To capture the full burden of disease, more than just R_0 is needed. Other useful measures include case fatality rate (CFR) as a measure of lethality or hospital data on severity of illness and treatment availability. Still, R_0 is a helpful tool to understand and compare transmission between disease occurring at various places and time periods.

Where Does the Reproduction Number Come From?

Descriptive epidemiology involves creating tables and graphs to summarize the data. The epidemiologist describes the cases with respect to person, place, and time. Demographic information like age, sex/gender, race, and ethnicity aids in identifying who may be at risk for becoming a case and may indicate how the disease is transmitted. Likewise, knowing where cases occur adds context to potential transmission and risk factors and can help to identify a point source or an urban/rural difference. Time includes the components of infections such as quantifying the duration of the epidemic, the duration of illness, and the incubation period, and aids in comparison between epidemics. Descriptive epidemiology is the critical process of reviewing the available data, comparing it with known information, and generating hypotheses about the health outcome that is being studied.

descriptive epidemiology: Epidemiology that describes person, place and time and often will summarize data in tables and graphs.

When the descriptive epidemiologist is documenting the numbers of cases, they are collecting an estimate for R_0. Mathematical modelers then use that information to refine and try to estimate the components of R_0 to gain insight to transmission. The first two components of R_0, namely the frequency of contact and probability of transmission occurring given the contact, are hard to explicitly measure. Frequency of contact needs to capture what the case is doing as well as what potential contacts are doing, but also is influenced by what a "contact" is. For example, a person shaking hands might be a contact for influenza, but is not a contact for HIV. Likewise, the probability of transmission is an inherent characteristic of the pathogen but is also influenced by the nature of the contact. For example, with SARS-CoV-2 the probability of transmission is influenced by whether the exposure is indoors or outdoors and how long the case and contact are in proximity. However, descriptive epidemiology is a useful source for estimating the third component of R_0, the duration of infection. Working with case data as well as with laboratory based assessments, epidemiologists can determine the length of time an individual is infected. It is then an iterative process of modeling informed by data as mathematicians and epidemiologists work together to refine the estimate.

While R_0 assumes a fully susceptible population, as the epidemic evolves and susceptible individuals are replaced by recovered ones, the number of subsequent infections will change. This requirement of a naïve population and the challenges in measuring some of its components can be unrealistic in an ongoing outbreak and has been considered by some to be a limitation of R_0.[5] To capture that an epidemic is a dynamic process, R_e, the **effective reproduction number**, can be calculated, still referring to the number of secondary infections but no longer assuming a fully susceptible population. Because the number of subsequent infections is dependent on both the innate transmissibility (how long an individual is infectious and how easily the pathogen can pass to another) as well at the contact rate (the per capita rate at which infectious and susceptible individuals come into contact), it is a situational estimate and changes as the epidemic evolves.[6] For example, the contact rate will change based on human behavior (for example, seasonal differences where people come together for holidays or go outdoors because of weather), which varies by location. Relatedly, as the epidemic progresses, the number of susceptible individuals decreases, hence the effective reproduction number ($R_e = R_0 \times S$). The basic reproduction number is useful for comparing diseases and for estimating the epidemic potential of a pathogen in a population, whereas the effective reproduction number evolves with the epidemic and is useful for understanding time-dependent trends in an epidemic.[7]

contact tracing: Also known as contact investigations, they provide a systematic process to identify people, known as contacts, who have been exposed to cases of an infectious disease.

basic reproduction number (R_0): The number of secondary infections that will arise from a single case in a fully susceptible population.

effective reproduction number $(R_e$, sometimes called $R_t)$: The number of secondary infections, this estimate changes over the course of an epidemic as the number of susceptible individuals, and therefore the contact between infectious and susceptible individuals, changes.

THOUGHT QUESTION

While these values are often discussed during an epidemic, they are estimates based on the data available. List public health interventions that would influence the reproduction number. How might these be different in different communities? Considering these, how would you explain R_0 to a reporter who is interviewing you during an outbreak?

MODELING DISEASE TRANSMISSION

In 2015, there was a reported measles outbreak in western Uganda. A probable case was defined as fever and generalized maculopapular rash with at least one of the following clinical symptoms: coryza, conjunctivitis, or cough. Individuals meeting the probable case definition who also had measles-specific IgM in serum samples were identified as confirmed cases. Cases were confirmed by reviewing medical records and comparing them with age-matched controls from the same village. A total of 213 probable cases were identified from April to August. Almost half of the cases had visited health centers during their exposure period, compared with only 12% of controls, indicating the crowded health clinics may have been a source of infection (OR = 6.1; 95% CI = 2.7%–14%). Vaccine coverage was estimated at 75% (95% CI: 67%–83%) among children in the affected communities. Read more about this outbreak at bmcinfectdis.biomedcentral.com/articles/10.1186/s12879-017-2941-4.

In any disease system, the pathway to disease is complex and full of interdependencies. As previously discussed, the nature of a contact matters. Other comorbidities of the individual and their prior exposures to similar pathogens can influence individual susceptibility. And importantly, the health-promoting interventions already in place can all influence disease dynamics. That complexity is beneficial from the lens of identifying ways to engage and break the transmission cycle, but also challenging to understand disease etiology or to estimate the potential effect of or cost effectiveness of various interventions. Mathematical models can address these challenges by first being built to simulate transmission dynamics and then manipulating them to test alternative control strategies, identify vaccination coverage goals, and estimate the ultimate size of an epidemic. Such models are often simplifications, and they are only as good as the parameter estimates that go into them. The quality of the parameter estimates often comes from the quality of the epidemiological study and the availability of descriptive epidemiologic data. As was famously attributed to statistician George Box, "All models are wrong, but some models are useful."[8] Models are simplifications, but they are usually smart simplifications, distilling transmission into those core parameters that can be estimated and which robustly

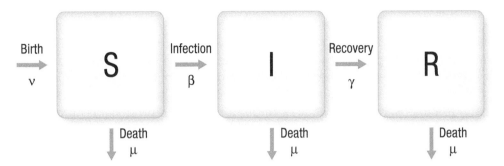

Figure 3.5 A simple SIR compartmental model, where susceptible individuals, S, become infected and move to infectious, I, and then to recovered, R. This version of the model is an open system, where there are births and deaths in the system.

characterize the disease. Importantly, they can be used to test a hypothesis on a time scale that we could not wait to play out during a lethal epidemic with so many pieces moving simultaneously.

At its simplest, disease transmission takes the form of susceptible individuals becoming infected and then recovering. This classical form is mathematically described by the SIR (susceptible-infected-recovered) compartmental model (Figure 3.5). Susceptible individuals become infected at a rate, β, which is dependent on how frequently they contact with infected individuals and how transmissible the agent is. They then recover at a rate, γ, which is the inverse of the duration of infectiousness.

Complexity can be added to this basic depiction to model increasingly complex systems. First, adding a birth rate (commonly denoted with nu, ν) and a death rate (commonly denoted with mu, μ) to this closed system, the model can incorporate endemic equilibrium with the infusion of new susceptible individuals. Adding parallel and interacting models can allow for multi-species systems like vector-borne disease where one SIR model for humans is linked to a related SI model for the vector. Similarly, by stacking SIR models and linking them, age-structured systems can be simulated to incorporate age-specific infection rates or recovery rates. Additional compartments can also be added to incorporate latent periods by adding, for example, an additional category for exposed but not yet infectious (e.g., an E in SEIR models) for diseases with acute and chronic stages and associated differing transmissibility (see, for example, SEIR models for tuberculosis).[9]

HEADS UP!

It's Greek to me! Epidemiologists be warned, the Greek letters used to identify the parameters for the SIR model, namely β, γ, ν, and μ, are technically arbitrary. In this book, we chose to represent them how we usually see them but be warned they might be written differently in other texts or papers you read.

How Do We Parameterize the SIR Model?

Even with this simplest model, to simulate disease we need to know how many susceptible, infected, and recovered individuals are in the population at the start (the initial values for S, I, and R) and we need to know how quickly they will move from each compartment, β and γ. Mathematical models will often assume a total population and then use fractions thereof to initialize the model, where at the beginning everyone but one infected person is susceptible, and set $S+I+R$ equal to the total population, N. The β and γ parameter are usually iteratively estimated from both the literature and from the modeling process. The recovery rate, γ or 1/ duration of infection, can be estimated from clinical data as it is the period when a person is shedding enough pathogen to potentially infect another. The transmission rate and its components of a contact rate and the probability of transmission are harder to empirically estimate, but can be estimated through fitting models to observed case data, or through the basic reproduction number, R_0 that can be estimated from the final epidemic size. Remember that three components of R_0 are the two components of β, namely, the frequency of contacting infected individuals and the probability that that interaction will lead to transmission and the duration of infectiousness, which is $1/\gamma$. So, β can be estimated from R_0, where

$$R_0 = \frac{\beta}{\gamma} \text{ or } \qquad \beta = R_0 \times \gamma$$

With the parameters of the model then estimated, a set of ordinary differential equations can be used to compute the evolution of an epidemic. This model can then be used to understand transmission dynamics, to test how well potential interventions work or identify the most effective interventions, and for cost-effectiveness analyses (Figure 3.6). When the intervention is mapped to the parameters in the SIR model, we can compare the effects on the R_0. The goal is identifying which interventions have the most significant effect on reducing disease transmission (see, for example, the use of SIR models to estimate the effects of influenza superspreaders).[10]

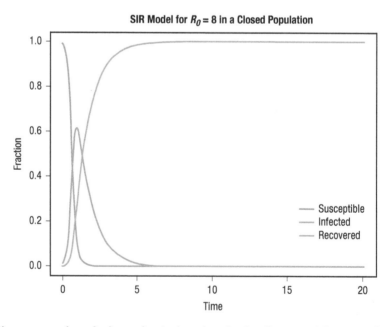

SIR Model for R_0 = 8 in a Closed Population

Figure 3.6 Three examples of a hypothetical outbreak of a disease with an R_0 of 8. Susceptible individuals are red, infected are green, and recovered are blue. The first example is a closed population (no births or deaths), whereas the second is the same disease but in an open system where births bring new susceptible individuals. The final is the same disease in an open system, but where 87% of the population is vaccinated. Notice that time is on the x-axis and fraction of the population affected is on the y-axis. (*continued*)

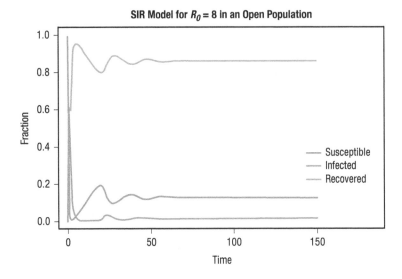

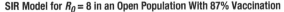

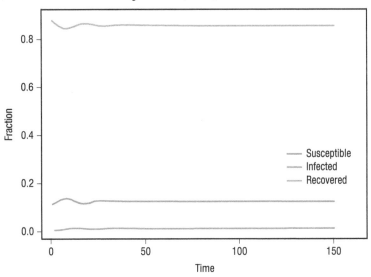

Figure 3.6 (*continued*)

THOUGHT QUESTION

Models are only as good as the data that go into them. Even the simplest SIR in a closed system model requires an estimate of the starting number of susceptible individuals, those infected and recovered (by prior infection or by immunization), as well as an estimate of the infection rate and the recovery rate. How would you go about identifying each of those parameters for an ongoing infection? What kind of questions would you ask? What data would you want to collect? Can you design an experiment to collect the data necessary?

CASE STUDY

In the late 1800s, British medical doctor Ronald Ross was working in India, which was experiencing a massive malaria outbreak (Figure 3.7). His work discovered the malaria parasite in mosquitoes, definitively showing that the malaria life cycle included a mosquito vector. Recall that in this period, the role of mosquitoes in disease transmission had yet to be established and germ theory was still somewhat in its infancy. Ross enjoyed math and wanted to mathematically describe the association between mosquito density and human disease so that he could test the impact of larval control on disease incidence. He realized he needed an expert and sought the help of Cambridge UK-trained mathematician Hilda Hudson. In 1917, together they published one of the first mathematical formulations of epidemiologic transmission. About 10 years later, two Scottish researchers, Anderson McKendrick, who had worked with Ross, and William Kermack refined the Ross model to account for the emerging understanding of disease complexity. The Kermack-McKendrick Theory allows for the prediction of the number of cases of infectious disease in a given population over time. It is considered the first SIR compartmental model for infectious disease transmission.

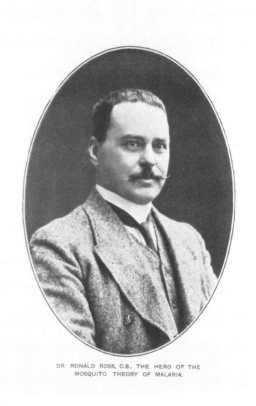

DR. RONALD ROSS, C.B., THE HERO OF THE MOSQUITO THEORY OF MALARIA.

Figure 3.7 Ronald Ross, hero of the Mosquito Theory of Malaria.
Source: National Library of Medicine Digital Collections. http://resource.nlm.nih.gov/101427700.

While these early formulations were certainly concerned with estimating the reproduction rate, it wasn't until the 1950s that zoologist George MacDonald explicitly described it. Finally, in the 1980s Roy Anderson and Robert May began framing this work in the way we think about it today. Their work pulled it back out of mathematics and into biology and their collaborations with large interdisciplinary teams were seminal in how we use infectious disease transmission models today. To read more about the evolution of the SIR model, have a look at the reviews by Mandal et al.,[11] Smith et al.,[12] and Heesterbeek and Roberts.[13]

CONCLUSION

Epidemiology has many tools to analyze infectious disease transmission dynamics. Even the simple graphing of cases over time hints at critical aspects of transmission—namely potential source types and incubation periods. More sophisticated modeling efforts like estimating the R_0 and using compartmental SIR models further our understanding and allow for the comparison of interventions and diseases across time and place.

Although we call these models simple, an immense amount of work goes into finding, cleaning, and compiling the data necessary to graph or parameterize these models. This is achieved by hard-working, interdisciplinary teams often involving epidemiologists working with mathematical modelers and ecologists on the estimation side; virologists, immunologists, and entomologists for laboratory experiments; and healthcare workers and public health providers for the disease data and interventions. Together, these are powerful tools that help us to better understand disease transmission dynamics and, thereby, open avenues for disease control.

TEACHING CORNER

DID YOU KNOW?

Disease modelers, epidemiologists, and policy makers work together to model infectious diseases and to decide what to do. The 2001 foot and mouth disease outbreak in the United Kingdom was one of the first times SIR models were used real-time to inform decision-making.[14] Foot and mouth disease is a highly transmissible livestock disease, with an estimated R_0 of 8.3, and while not itself lethal, it diminishes production and is a large economic burden.

TRY THIS

Using R (script in appendix) or a program like GeoGebra (https://www.geogebra .org/m/ga), build a simple, closed SIR model for foot and mouth disease. Here are some important transmission parameters to start with: Parameters: $\beta = 2.7$; duration of infection = 3.21. Play with the model. What happens when you change the duration of infection? What about when you lower and raise the transmissibility?

TAKE IT A STEP FURTHER

What can you do to flatten the curve? How would you translate that into a model? Duration of illness can be shortened (by culling). There is a vaccine. How would you incorporate those into the model? What does each do to your estimated infected?

QUESTIONS FOR FURTHER DISCUSSION

1. Distinguish between a bar graph, histogram, and epidemic curve.

2. Define and contrast R_0 and R_e.

3. Predict the epidemic curve (cases over time) for diseases with different reproduction numbers. For example, the R_0 for influenza, chickenpox, and smallpox are about 2.5, 9, and 6, respectively. Rank the transmissibility of each and then estimate the epidemic curves.

4. You are the hospital infection control epidemiologist at a 500-bed teaching hospital. You are faced with two infections. The first is a within-hospital *Clostridioides difficile* infection that is ravaging your intensive care ward. The second is a community wide norovirus infection. The R_0 of these two diseases is 0.5 to 2 for *C. diff* and 1.7 to 7 for norovirus. The CFRs are 6% to 30% for *C. diff* and 0.3% to 1.6% for norovirus. How would you allocate the limited resources you have to respond effectively to both outbreaks?

 A robust set of instructor resources designed to supplement this text is located at http://connect.springerpub.com/Content/book/978-0-8261-5674-7. Qualifying instructors may request access by emailing textbook@springerpub.com.

REFERENCES

1. Zipprich J, Winter K, Hacker J, Xia D, Watt J, Harriman K. Measles outbreak—California, December 2014-February 2015. *MMWR Morb Mortal Wkly Rep*. 2015;64(6):153–154. Erratum in: *MMWR Morb Mortal Wkly Rep*. 2015;64(7):196. https://www.ncbi.nlm.nih.gov/pmc/articles/PMC5779601

2. Patel M, Lee AD, Clemmons NS, et al. National update on measles cases and outbreaks—United States, January 1–October 1, 2019. *MMWR Morb Mortal Wkly Rep*. 2019;68:893–896. doi:10.15585/mmwr.mm6840e2external icon

3. Anderson RM, May RM. *Infectious Diseases of Humans: Dynamics and Control*. Oxford University Press; 1991.

4. Guerra FM, Bolotin S, Lim G, et al. The basic reproduction number (R_0) of measles: a systematic review. *Lancet Infect Dis*. 2017;17(12):e420–e428. doi:10.1016/S1473-3099(17)30307-9

5. Li J, Blakeley D, Smith RJ. The failure of R_0. *Comput Math Methods Med*. 2011;2011:527610. doi:10.1155/2011/527610

6. Delamater PL, Street EJ, Leslie TF, Yang YT, Jacobsen KH. Complexity of the basic reproduction number (R_0). *Emerg Infect Dis*. 2019;25(1):1–4. doi:10.3201/eid2501.171901

7. Nishiura H, Chowell G. The effective reproduction number as a prelude to statistical estimation of time-dependent epidemic trends. In: Chowell G., Hyman JM, Bettencourt LMA, Castillo-Chavez C, eds. *Mathematical and Statistical Estimation Approaches in Epidemiology*. Springer; 2009. doi:10.1007/978-90-481-2313-1_5

8. Box GEP. Science and statistics (PDF). *J Am Stat Assoc*. 1976;71(356):791–799. doi:10.1080/01621459.1976.10480949

9. Ozcaglar C, Shabbeer A, Vandenberg SL, Yener B, Bennett KP. Epidemiological models of *Mycobacterium tuberculosis* complex infections. *Math Biosci*. 2012;236(2):77–96. doi:10.1016/j.mbs.2012.02.003

10. Skene KJ, Paltiel AD, Shim E, Galvani AP. A marginal benefit approach for vaccinating influenza "superspreaders." *Med Decis Making*. 2014;34(4):536–549. doi:10.1177/0272989X14523502

11. Mandal S, Sarkar RR, Sinha S. Mathematical models of malaria - a review. *Malar J*. 2011;10:202. doi:10.1186/1475-2875-10-202

12. Smith DL, Battle KE, Hay SI, Barker CM, Scott TW, McKenzie FE. Ross, Macdonald, and a theory for the dynamics and control of mosquito-transmitted pathogens. *PLoS Pathog*. 2012;8(4):e1002588. doi:10.1371/journal.ppat.1002588

13. Heesterbeek JAP, Roberts MG. How mathematical epidemiology became a field of biology: a commentary on Anderson and May (1981) 'The population dynamics of microparasites and their invertebrate hosts'. *Phil Trans R Soc*. 2015;370(1666):20140307. doi:10.1098/rstb.2014.0307

14. Keeling MJ. Models of foot-and-mouth disease. *Proc Biol Sci*. 2005;272(1569):1195–1202. doi:10.1098/rspb.2004.3046

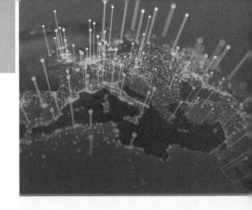

PART II

MODES OF
TRANSMISSION AND
TYPES OF DISEASES

CHAPTER 4

RESPIRATORY DISEASE

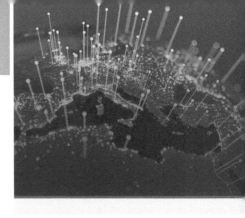

INTRODUCTION

Tuberculosis (TB), an infectious disease caused by a bacteria known as Mycobacterium tuberculosis, *is the world's leading cause of death from an infectious disease. TB bacteria are spread through the air from one person to another. Most of the time, the bacteria attack the lungs and kill cells; if untreated, TB can grow and spread into the rest of the body. Without proper medical therapy, one-third of patients with active TB die within 1 year of the diagnosis, and more than 50% during the first 5 years. However, not everyone infected with TB becomes sick. Individuals who are asymptomatic whose bodies are able to fight the bacteria to stop them from growing have latent infection. TB has been with us throughout our known human history, with evidence dating as far back as 8000 BCE and in Egyptian mummies to 2400 BCE. TB has been known variously as phthisis, consumption, the white death, and the white plague, due to the white pallor of those who were affected. The term "white" may also have referenced its association with youth and innocence. In 1882 Robert Koch used the term "tuberkulose," translated to English as tuberculosis, describing his discovery of the bacterium he called Tubercle bacillus, the first time an agent had been identified with this terrible disease.*

LEARNING OBJECTIVES

By the end of this chapter, readers will be able to:

- Discriminate between different types of respiratory transmission.
- List and describe standard precautionary measures.
- List preventive actions to stop respiratory transmission.
- Describe how the randomized controlled trial is used to study disease.

WHAT ARE DIFFERENT TYPES OF RESPIRATORY TRANSMISSION?

In the mid-1950s, Richard L. Riley, a lung physiologist, and his mentor, William F. Wells, identified a new mode of transmission for TB, a major cause of morbidity and mortality. The two constructed an air-tight ventilation system on top of the Baltimore Veterans Affairs Hospital, which connected 150 guinea pigs in an exposure chamber to a TB ward below. The guinea pigs were exposed to air from TB patients for 4 years. Over the course of the study, an average of three guinea pigs contracted TB each month, while in a control chamber where air ducts were exposed to TB-killing UV light, none were infected. While quantifying a dose-response relationship between exposure and infection, this experiment provided the first proof that TB was an airborne disease. Indeed, this was proof that even a single infected droplet could be carried through air currents and aerosolized until it reached the guinea pigs.

Our lungs are constantly subjected to exposure to particles, chemicals, and infectious organisms in the air around us, making them susceptible to infection and injury. Respiratory diseases are leading causes of death and disability in the world. Pneumonia kills millions of people annually and is a leading cause of death among children under 5 years old. Over 10 million people develop TB and 1.4 million die from it each year, making it the most common lethal infectious disease. In 2016, lower respiratory infections alone caused over 600,000 deaths in children younger than 5 years, over 1 million in adults older than 70 years, and almost 2.5 million deaths in people of all ages, worldwide (Figure 4.1).[1,2]

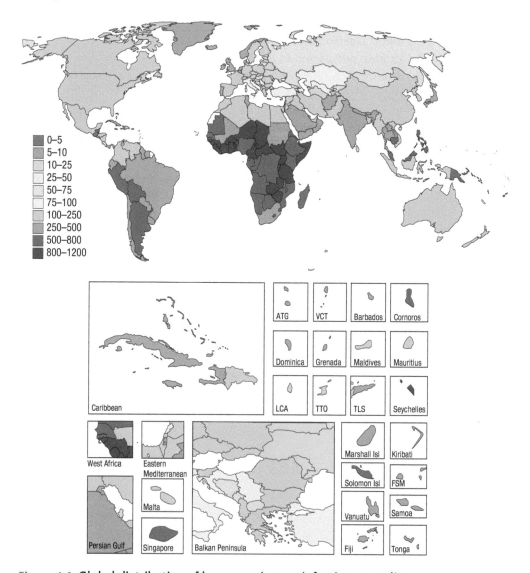

Figure 4.1 Global distribution of lower respiratory infection mortality.

ATG, Antigua and Barbuda; FSM, Federated States of Micronesia; LCA, Saint Lucia; TLS, Timor-Leste; TTO, Trinidad and Tobago; VCT, Saint Vincent and the Grenadines.

Infection defines the entrance and development of an agent inside a host (e.g., a human). In contrast, **colonization** implies that an individual has a sufficiently high concentration of organisms at a site where they can be detected, yet that the organism is causing no signs or symptoms. Colonization may occur in any part of the respiratory tract. A carrier is a person who is colonized with an organism and may transmit the organism to other people.

For example, approximately one-third of adults are persistently colonized with *Staphylococcus aureus*, with the highest concentration of organisms in the respiratory tract being in the nasopharynx (Table 4.1).[3]

Knowing what organisms infect which part of the respiratory system requires clinical knowledge. For example, while many organisms can be present in the pharynx, bacterial pharyngitis in the developed world is usually due to beta-hemolytic streptococci.

colonization: The presence of organisms on a body surface (like on the skin, mouth, intestines, or airway) without causing disease in the person.

THOUGHT QUESTION

What is the predominant colonization site for fungi such as Candida? For *Mycobacterium tuberculosis*? Can you link the colonization site to the observed symptoms?

Modes of Transmission

Multiple modes of transmission are possible when considering respiratory transmission. These include contact, droplet, and airborne transmission. What these all have in common is the respiratory tract as the portal of entry and exit for the agent. Probability of transmission often depends on factors such as the infectiousness of the person with disease, the duration and frequency of exposure, and the environment in which exposure

Table 4.1 Colonization Sites for Selected Organisms

DETECTION SITE	POSSIBLE ORGANISM	RESULTING DISEASE
Upper respiratory tract	Group A streptococcus bacteria Influenza virus Rhinovirus	Strep throat Influenza (upper and lower) Common cold
Lower respiratory tract	Hantavirus *Corynebacterium diphtheriae* toxin *Bordetella pertussis* bacteria Various bacteria: *Mycoplasma pneumoniae, Streptococcus pneumoniae, Haemophilus influenzae, Moraxella catarrhalis*, and *Bordetella pertussis* Various bacteria: *Streptococcus pneumoniae, Staphylococcus aureus, Group A streptococcus, Klebsiella pneumoniae, Haemophilus influenzae, Moraxella catarrhalis* SARS coronavirus	Hantavirus Diptheria Pertussis Bronchitis Pneumonia SARS

SARS, severe acute respiratory syndrome.

occurred (e.g., population density). **Superspreading** events, where one individual transmits disease to many others, often occur in close-contact settings such as households or schools.[4]

superspreader: A phenomenon where few people account for the majority of disease transmission, through behavior, biology, or the environment.

CONTACT TRANSMISSION

Some respiratory diseases are transmitted by direct contact with contaminated hands, doorknobs, or shared items. These include agents responsible for the common cold, respiratory syncytial virus (RSV), and parainfluenza, which are common childhood infections.

DROPLET TRANSMISSION

In this category are agents that land directly on the mucosal lining of the nose, mouth, or eyes of nearby persons or can be inhaled. These are usually:

- either 5 micron or larger droplets, and
- propelled no more than 3 feet from the infected person in any direction.

There are numerous diseases that transmit via these routes (Table 4.2).

Some other characteristics of droplet transmission are that the droplets in the air are relatively heavy with moisture, so they do not remain suspended in air for long periods of time (Figure 4.2).

AIRBORNE TRANSMISSION

This route refers to infections generated when an ill person sneezes, coughs, or speaks. For some types of infections (such as chickenpox or measles), a person can be infectious even before the onset of symptoms. With airborne transmission, aerosols become smaller by evaporation, with small aerosols (10 microns or fewer) remaining suspended for longer periods, and given their size, if inhaled, they travel deep into the lungs. **Droplet nuclei** are droplets less than 5 microns (μm) in diameter. Moisture surrounding nuclei evaporates, leaving small-particle residue of 5 microns or less that contains infectious microorganisms.

droplet nuclei: Droplets less than 5 microns (μm) in diameter and often implicated in airborne transmission due to their tiny size.

Table 4.2 Infectious Diseases Transmitted Through Droplet Transmission

BACTERIAL INFECTIONS	VIRAL INFECTIONS
Diphtheria, pertussis, pneumonic plague, hemophilus influenzae, meningococci, pneumococcal infections (invasive, resistant), mycoplasma pneumoniae, streptopharyngitis (strep throat), scarlet fever	Adenovirus, influenza, mumps, parvovirus, rubella, pertussis, common cold, SARS

Note that some agents can be spread via droplet and airborne transmission (e.g., SARS or varicella).

SARS, severe acute respiratory syndrome.

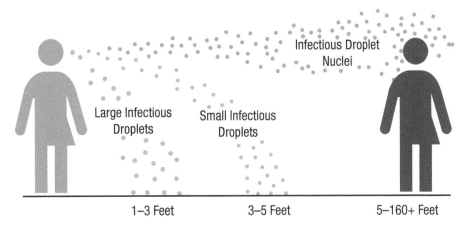

Figure 4.2 **Illustration of droplet transmission.**

Some examples of airborne disease include TB, measles, varicella, smallpox, SARS, SARS-CoV-2, and avian influenza. Since droplet nuclei are small, they can be carried over a long range by air currents or turbulences, but long-range infection risk is modulated by dilution, removal by ventilation, the actual amount of infectious agents at the source, biological decay, and the infectious dose.

THOUGHT QUESTION

Should we be more concerned about coughers or sneezers? Be sure to justify your answer using the terminology introduced above.

WHAT ARE STANDARD PRECAUTIONARY MEASURES?

Extensively drug-resistant (XDR) tuberculosis, which is the most severe form of drug resistance, limits treatment options, resulting in death rates of 50% to 80%. While drug resistance often occurs due to acquired resistance, because of inadequate treatment or adherence, direct infection is possible as well. In South Africa, the XDR epidemic has continued since 2006. Unfortunately, one reason has been because transmission chains have not been interrupted in hospital settings. In a study where the majority of participants had been hospitalized, 69% of XDR cases were attributable to inpatient transmission and 84% clustered according to their strain type with another patient. Hospitals may not be designed to limit infections, lack appropriate infection-control programs, and do not provide follow-up for outpatients as needed.[5]

Standard precautions are a group of infection prevention practices that apply to all patients in a clinical setting, not just those with an infection. These are based on the principle that the following can contain transmissible infectious agents:

- blood and body fluids
- secretions
- excretions (except sweat)
- non-intact skin
- mucous membranes

Implementation of Standard Precautions is the primary strategy for the prevention of healthcare-associated transmission of infectious agents among patients and healthcare personnel (Figure 4.3).[6] Standard Precautions are based on the principle that all blood, body fluids, secretions, excretions except sweat, non-intact skin, and mucous membranes may contain transmissible infectious agents.

standard precautions: The minimum infection prevention practices that apply to all patient care, regardless of suspected or confirmed infection status of the patient, in any setting where healthcare is delivered.

The Centers for Disease Control and Prevention (CDC) describe a hierarchy of infection prevention and control measures ranked in order from overall effectiveness in controlling disease in a population (protecting most of the people to protecting only the wearer). These work their way from complete removal of the hazard, through replacing the hazard, ensuring that an individual is away from the hazard, changing individual work patterns or behavior to minimize risk, through protecting individuals in direct contact with a hazard.

The most effective measure is to eliminate potential exposures. For example, patients with mild influenza-like illness can be asked to stay home, or a policy can be implemented to not allow ill visitors. **Engineering controls** do not require an individual employee to implement the control. For example, partitions can be installed in triage areas and other public spaces to reduce exposures by shielding personnel and other patients, or negative pressure rooms can be used for aerosol-generating procedures. **Administrative controls** are work practices and policies that prevent exposures. Their effectiveness is dependent on consistent implementation. Examples include vaccination; masks for

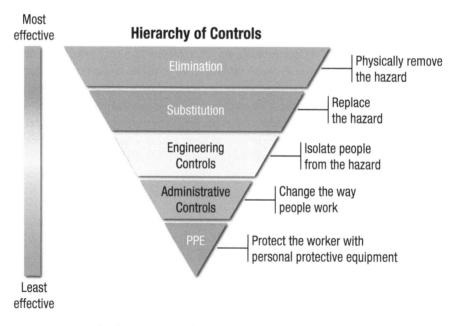

Figure 4.3 Standard Precautions for infection control.

Source: National Institute for Occupational Safety and Health (NIOSH), Centers for Disease Control and Prevention. https://www.cdc.gov/niosh/topics/hierarchy/default.html

symptomatic patients; and promoting respiratory hygiene and cough etiquette. Personal protective equipment (PPE) is a last line of defense for individuals against hazards that cannot otherwise be eliminated or controlled. PPE will not be effective if adherence is incomplete or when exposures to infectious patients or ill coworkers are unrecognized.

contact precautions: Precautions intended to prevent the spread of infectious agents that are transmitted by direct or indirect contact.

droplet precautions: Precautions intended to prevent the spread of infectious agents that are transmitted by respiratory secretions or mucous membrane contact.

Contact precautions may be applied when excessive wound drainage, fecal incontinence, or other body discharges increase the potential for environmental contamination. Single-patient rooms might be used, healthcare personnel might be asked to wear gowns and gloves, and PPE may be used upon entry to a room.

Droplet precautions prevent spread through secretions at short distances. Remember that droplets do not travel far (Table 4.2), and special ventilation systems are not required to implement droplet precautions. Precautions are intended to prevent the spread of infectious agents transmitted by respiratory secretions or mucous membrane contact.

To implement droplet precautions, single-patient rooms are preferred, as was the case with contact precautions. However, if this is not feasible and multi-patient rooms must be used, at least 3 feet of separation is recommended between patient beds; drawing the curtain between beds is also recommended. Healthcare personnel should wear a mask upon entering a patient's room and discard this PPE before exiting the room. Patients under droplet precautions that are being transferred out of the room should wear a mask if they are able to tolerate it and follow respiratory hygiene and cough etiquette.

Airborne precautions prevent transmission of respiratory agents over long distances. An Airborne Infection Isolation Room, or AIIR, is the preferred placement for patients under airborne precautions. These rooms are single-patient rooms and have special ventilation systems installed. AIIRs are monitored for negative pressure relative to the surrounding area; 12 air exchanges per hour for new construction and renovation and six air exchanges per hour for existing facilities (a measure of the refreshing of air in the room).[7] Air is exhausted directly to the outside or recirculated through high-efficiency particulate air (HEPA) filtration before return. Also important for airborne precautions is that healthcare personnel should don a fit-tested N95 mask before entry into the isolation room.

airborne precautions: Preventing transmission of infectious agents that remain infectious in air over long distances.

THOUGHT QUESTION

Discuss the benefits and limitations of administrative versus engineering controls. In which situation might you preferentially do one over the other (understanding of course that both are critical)?

WHAT ARE SOME PREVENTIVE ACTIONS TO STOP RESPIRATORY TRANSMISSION?

A cluster of TB cases was recognized in Seattle among four young East-African immigrants with histories of incarceration and illicit drug use.[5] Patients were interviewed to learn their contacts, activities, and locations frequented while they were contagious. Friends were defined as contacts of patients who spent time within a close-knit network of young men who exhibited similar marijuana-using behavior. Other contacts were defined as the families and relatives of patients and those who were named but were not closely associated with this network. Contacts received a TB evaluation. Ten additional patients were found. Isolates from all patients had matching TB genotypes, indicating that all the individuals were likely in the same transmission chain. While contagious, patients stayed in various locations, including cars, for most of the day.

Infectious diseases persist unless an infectious case meets someone susceptible before they have recovered. Respiratory infections, transmitted through the previously described modes, spread through physical and social contact, with these **contact patterns** determining who is at highest risk for infection and how a disease spreads. These patterns help us to understand the disease transmission process, who is at highest risk of contracting infection or disease, as well as how to propose effective control strategies. For respiratory illnesses in particular, contact patterns are key factors in determining transmission. Social mixing patterns across different population groups, often within and between age groups or households, affect the likelihood of transmission (Figure 4.4). For example, there are often more pronounced social contacts among school-aged children as compared to contacts between adults. For measles, for example, approximately 30% to 50% of transmission events occur within the same age group.[8]

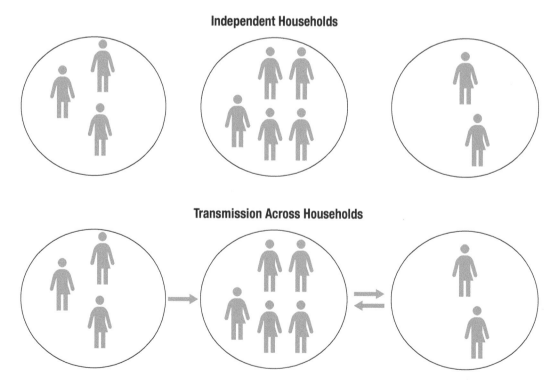

Figure 4.4 **Transmission between and across households.**

contact patterns: Patterns of contacts, such as those between different groups of people (such as age groups) and in different social settings.

Two main mixing patterns are usually considered. The first, homogeneous mixing, assumes that the population is fully mixed such that each individual has an equal chance of contacting any other member of the population. Mathematical models of transmission often include the pattern of mixing among the population, along with other factors such as the susceptibility within the population, the virulence of the infection, the probability of transmission per contact, and the changes in behavior in the affected population in response to an epidemic. The homogeneous mixing assumption may be incorrect, however, due to real-life interactions among people across space. For example, pertussis studies have shown that infection-acquired immunity wanes after 4 to 20 years and protective immunity after vaccination wanes after 4 to 12 years, resulting in age-dependent differences in susceptibility that must be taken into account when developing models.[9]

Contact Network Structure

Network structure better allows for heterogeneous mixing as previously noted and describes a contact network of a population, using mathematical graphical models to show disease spread, with nodes representing individuals, and links (or edges) corresponding to the relationships among people. The agent can spread from one node to the other node through the links (edges) between them. These models assume that an individual acts according to their proposed network structure, but this may not always be true (e.g., people contact strangers or others outside their network).

These graphs have several key measures, such as their size (node number, N), density (number of edges present), probability of nodes being connected (p), and degree (sum of connections to others and from others, k). If connections between people can be modeled as random graphs, we can look at some example networks, all of which have exactly 12 nodes. However, other than that the configurations are quite different (Figure 4.5).

If k is less than 1, we see only small, isolated clusters, with small diameters (the maximum edge length) and short average edges; when k is equal to 1, diameter peaks and edge averages are long, but when k is greater than 1, almost all nodes are connected and edge

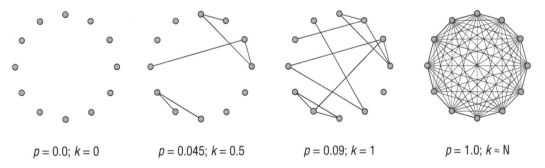

| $p = 0.0; k = 0$ | $p = 0.045; k = 0.5$ | $p = 0.09; k = 1$ | $p = 1.0; k \approx N$ |

Figure 4.5 Representation of contacts. People are represented as yellow circles (nodes) while connections are represented with lines (edges). In this example we see a number of different contact networks.

averages shorten again. Since most people know many other people, an argument has been made that the latter model more accurately reflects disease transmission processes, in a "small world" phenomenon where we are easily connected to others. This may explain why for a particularly contagious respiratory disease we might observe a high R_0.[10]

Contact Investigations

Contact investigations, or contact tracing, provide a systematic process to identify people, known as contacts, who have been exposed to cases of an infectious disease. These **contacts** can then be assessed for infection and disease and provided appropriate care (which may include quarantine) and treatment. In the case of an airborne disease such as TB, contacts might include household members, friends, coworkers, and other individuals who have spent a lot of time together with the case (Figure 4.6). Contact investigations help to interrupt the chain of transmission of a disease, to prevent new outbreaks, and to ensure that individuals are properly and appropriately treated, so that there is no disease progression or recurrence. For TB, on average, 10 contacts are identified for a single case, with approximately 20% to 30% of household contacts infected with latent TB and 1% diagnosed with active TB disease.[11] Typically, a contact investigation is carried out by state and local health departments, which have legal responsibility to investigate cases and to carry out and evaluate investigations.

THOUGHT QUESTION

In what three environmental settings do you think the index patient should be asked about priority contacts? Can you imagine circumstances where a person might not want to disclose contacts? What is a health department's obligation to require disclosure?

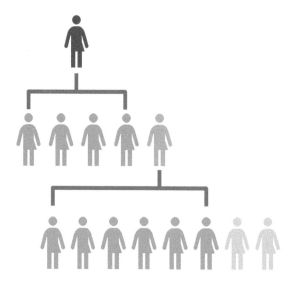

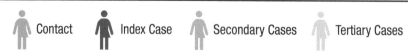

Figure 4.6 **Contact investigation revealing a transmission chain.**

contacts: Persons exposed to an organism by sharing air space with a person with (potentially) infectious disease. Contacts can include family members, roommates or housemates, friends, coworkers, classmates, and others classified as priority or non-priority.

HOW IS THE RANDOMIZED CONTROLLED TRIAL USED TO STUDY DISEASE?

George Comstock had just completed his doctorate in public health at Johns Hopkins University when the U.S. Public Health Service (PHS) decided to send him to Alaska to work with nurses who were treating TB. Comstock was already an established TB researcher, having led a study from 1947 to 1950 of the bacillus Calmette-Guerin (BCG) vaccine among schoolchildren in Georgia and Alabama. That study found that BCG was not particularly effective when TB prevalence was low and had led officials to decide not to use it in the United States. Comstock discovered a high prevalence of TB with one in 30 Alaskan adults in TB hospitals. The Alaskan project, a large, randomized trial which took place near the town of Bethel, showed that isoniazid was an effective prophylactic against TB, with a 69% decline in incidence after 1 year. The entire study, which took 6 years, found that 5 years after stopping isoniazid, study participants still had a 60% lower incidence of TB.[12]

The randomized controlled trial (RCT) is distinct from observational designs in that the exposure is manipulated by the investigator or epidemiologist. This means that as part of an **experiment**, there is some change made to an exposure or participant status, with an end goal of improving health. In contrast to observational study designs, the RCT can be classified as an intervention study, an "...experiment in which subjects are randomly allocated into groups, usually called test and control groups, to receive or not to receive a preventive or therapeutic procedure or intervention."[13 (p. 206)]

experiment: A series of observations performed prospectively under control of the researcher.

To understand an RCT, we can break the word into its component parts: *randomized*, that is, the manner by which individuals get assigned to treatment (or control) is purely by chance, with no possible way for individuals to influence or predict assignment. Thus, the groups are composed of otherwise similar people; *controlled*, such that the outcomes in a treatment group(s) are compared to the outcomes in a control population that doesn't receive the treatment; and *trial*, in reference to the experiment where the causal treatment (exposure) can be tried on a test population (Figure 4.7).

While clinical trials have been in use in some form or other since at least the 1700s, it is only in the past century that they have been used as the "gold standard" and are considered the most rigorous design in human research. This rigor is due to a number of reasons:

• They allow us to "prove" that an intervention does what it is hypothesized to do, using a control group.

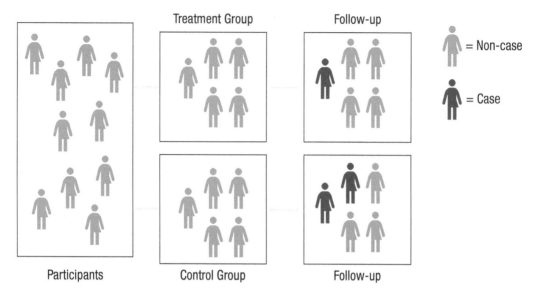

Figure 4.7 **Schematic of a randomized controlled trial (RCT). Notice that there are no cases in the participant group at the onset of the study. Individuals are assigned into treatment or control and then both groups followed over time to compare the development of disease.**

- In the controlled setting of RCTs, there are fewer issues with variability of disease and other unknowns (which in an observational study prevent our ability to confirm an effect).
- They allow us to get closer to actual etiologic inference, that is, an understanding of whether A causes B.

HEADS UP!

The proof is in the pudding! When epidemiologists and other scientists discuss something causing something else, they are very careful with their wording. One variable must lead to change in another for it to truly have a causal effect. Thus, when we talk about "proving" something, a high bar must be met. Ideally this can be done by creating comparable conditions among groups so that we can isolate the impact of one variable on the other. The RCT in particular also allows us to test causal hypotheses precisely because of its use of a comparison group to establish an association, knowledge that the exposure takes place prior to the outcome, and controlling for other explanations through the randomization process. Short of these conditions, we might talk about an association, but not causation!

In order to maintain this rigor, RCTs are often very narrowly defined and may not be generalizable beyond a specific study question and population being addressed. In addition, some exposures cannot be randomized ethically. For example, we cannot randomize individuals to smoke or not smoke in order to evaluate the health effects of smoking.

Analysis of data from RCTs is similar to that of a cohort study, where we can directly compare the risks of developing disease incidence by calculating the relative risk.

$$\text{Relative risk} = \frac{\text{Incidence among exposed}}{\text{Incidence among unexposed}} = \frac{\dfrac{\text{New cases among exposed}}{\text{Exposed population}}}{\dfrac{\text{New cases among unexposed}}{\text{Unexposed population}}}$$

The relative risk is intuitively interpreted as the ratio of the risk of developing disease among those exposed to the risk of developing disease among those not exposed.

One key difference from the cohort study is that given treatment assignment (randomization) in the RCT, we might want to know whether individuals actually took (complied with) the treatment, and how that influences our health outcomes. For example, if your professor randomly selects half of your class to go study at home, you can still decide whether or not to study regardless of your assignment. Typically, in an RCT, when we analyze the data, we examine the data based on the assignment (or intention) in order to preserve the benefits of randomization, in what is called **intention to treat** analysis. This ignores compliance. If we were only interested in analyzing those who followed treatment assignment, we would use a **per protocol** analysis that would break randomization, thus creating additional concerns that are present in a non-RCT design.

CASE STUDY

The Lakota TB and Health Association began during a TB outbreak among the Cheyenne River Sioux tribe. Amazingly, the founders were four Lakota grandmothers who banded together to tackle the outbreak. They shared their Indigenous knowledge and compassion to take care of those who were sick. Four of the grandmothers—Phoebe Downing at Standing Rock, Eunice Larrabee at Cheyenne River, Alfreda Janis-Bergin at Pine Ridge, and Irene Groneau at Sisseton-Wahpeton—banded together to track down a notorious person who was spreading active TB across the reservations. The Lakota Grandmas also served as a focal point for local tribal health committees that were advisory to the Indian Health Service, and were able to take on controversial issues, like mental health and alcoholism, and even birth control.[14]

CONCLUSION

Respiratory diseases can take on multiple modes of transmission, including contact, droplet, and airborne. Key methods for preventing respiratory transmission in community and clinical settings may include hand hygiene, prompt isolation precautions, and vaccination. Importantly, in hospital settings, administrative and engineering controls, in addition to individual measures such as use of PPE, can minimize transmission. Contact patterns allow epidemiologists to investigate the transmission of respiratory diseases through implementation of contact investigations. Contact investigations help to interrupt the chain of transmission of a disease and ensure appropriate follow-up based on an exposure. The RCT is a powerful study design that can be used to conduct experiments in respiratory and other diseases and to understand whether new interventions or approaches are more effective than others.

END-OF-CHAPTER RESOURCES

TEACHING CORNER

DID YOU KNOW?

While antibiotics were still being developed, a childhood vaccine for TB was being developed as well. This vaccine, known as bacille Calmette-Guerin, or BCG, was introduced in order to reduce the severity of TB disease, and ended up being most effective (to date) at preventing disseminated disease among infants and small children in countries where TB is common. Two early BCG clinical trials were conducted in New York City.[15]

TRY THIS

The first trial was impressive, with public health physicians assigned groups of at-risk newborns and told to randomly vaccinate half of them. The risk of dying before their first birthday was reduced among vaccinated babies; in the vaccinated group, three individuals died out of 445 cases, while in the control group 18 died out of 545 included. Can you calculate the relative risk of death among the vaccinated compared to control groups? What does this tell you about whether the BCG vaccine was effective or not?

TAKE IT A STEP FURTHER

In the second trial, instead of physicians randomly selecting babies, lots were drawn to select babies into the vaccination group, but this time the risk of dying before their first birthday was identical between vaccinated and nonvaccinated babies.[16] Results between the two trials were compared, and it turned out that when physicians made the decision to vaccinate some babies but not others, they were more likely to vaccinate babies who were headed for wealthier, less crowded households whose family members had less severe TB. The BCG-vaccinated babies thus were likely to have better outcomes even before they were vaccinated. Nonetheless, over time we have indeed seen that in studies using randomization the BCG is likely to provide a protective effect of over 60% against disease and over 70% against death.[16]

In which direction do you think the biased results changed the relative risk of death? How could you re-run this study to reduce the potential bias?

QUESTIONS FOR FURTHER DISCUSSION

1. Imagine a cluster of TB cases show up in your clinic waiting room. How would you ensure proper infection control measures, starting with precautions, PPE, and even room type and placement?

2. In a study to evaluate the efficacy of a new treatment for the common cold, 1,000 children 2 to 18 years old with newly diagnosed viral colds were recruited from pediatrician offices. Of these, 500 were randomly assigned to receive the new antiviral therapy and 500 were assigned to a control group. After 5 days, 250 of the study group had no

cold symptoms, while only 100 of the control group had no cold symptoms. What is the relative risk of curing the common cold for the study group compared to the control group? How would you interpret the result?

3. What are some approaches to decreasing respiratory transmission in the absence of mitigation strategies such as PPE?

 A robust set of instructor resources designed to supplement this text is located at http://connect.springerpub.com/Content/book/978-0-8261-5674-7. Qualifying instructors may request access by emailing textbook@springerpub.com.

REFERENCES

1. GBD 2016 Lower Respiratory Infections Collaborators. Estimates of the global, regional, and national morbidity, mortality, and aetiologies of lower respiratory infections in 195 countries, 1990–2016: a systematic analysis for the Global Burden of Disease Study 2016. *Lancet Infect Dis.* 2018;18(11):1191–1210. doi:10.1016/S1473-3099(18)30310-4
2. Doebbeling BN, Breneman DL, Neu HC, et al. Elimination of *Staphylococcus aureus* nasal carriage in health care workers: analysis of six clinical trials with calcium mupirocin ointment. *Clin Infect Dis.* 1993;17:466–474. doi:10.1093/clinids/17.3.466
3. Shah NS, Auld SC, Brust JC, et al. Transmission of extensively drug-resistant tuberculosis in South Africa. *N Engl J Med.* 2017;376(3):243–253. doi:10.1056/NEJMoa1604544
4. Lewis D. Superspreading drives the COVID pandemic - and could help to tame it. *Nature.* 2021;590(7847):544–546. doi:10.1038/d41586-021-00460-x
5. Oeltmann JE, Oren E, Haddad MB, et al. Tuberculosis outbreak in marijuana users, Seattle, Washington, 2004. *Emerg Infect Dis.* 2006;12(7):1156–1159. doi:10.3201/eid1207.051436
6. Centers for Disease Control and Prevention. Standard precautions. https://www.cdc.gov/oral-health/infectioncontrol/summary-infection-prevention-practices/standard-precautions.html
7. American Society of Heating, Refrigerating and Air-Conditioning Engineers. Improved ventilation system for removal of airborne contamination in airborne infectious isolation rooms. https://www.ashrae.org/technical-resources/ashrae-journal/featured-articles/improved-ventilation-system-for-removal-of-airborne-contamination-in-airborne-infectious-isolation-rooms
8. Gastañaduy PA, Funk S, Lopman BA, et al. Factors Associated With Measles Transmission in the United States During the Postelimination Era. https://www.ncbi.nlm.nih.gov/pmc/articles/PMC6865326/
9. Domenech de Cellès M, Rohani P, King AA. Duration of immunity and effectiveness of diphtheria-tetanus–acellular pertussis vaccines in children. *JAMA Pediatr.* 2019;173(6):588–594. doi:10.1001/jamapediatrics.2019.0711
10. Carnegie NB. Effects of contact network structure on epidemic transmission trees: implications for data required to estimate network structure. *Stat Med.* 2018;37(2):236–248. doi:10.1002/sim.7259
11. Fox GJ, Barry SE, Britton WJ, Marks GB. Contact investigation for tuberculosis: a systematic review and meta-analysis. *Eur Respir J.* 2013;41(1):140–156. doi:10.1183/09031936.00070812. Epub 2012 Aug 30.
12. Oransky I. George W Comstock. *The Lancet.* 2007;370(9592):1028. doi:10.1016/S0140-6736(07)61464-0
13. Porta M. *A Dictionary of Epidemiology*. 5th ed. Oxford University Press; 2009.
14. Centers for Disease Control and Prevention. American Indian & Alaska Native contributions to public health. https://www.cdc.gov/tribal/tribes-organizations-health/contributions/index.html
15. Levine MI, Sackett MF. Results of BCG vaccination in New York City. *Am Rev Tuberc.* 1946;53:517–532. doi:10.1164/art.1946.53.6.517
16. Brewer TF. Preventing tuberculosis with bacillus Calmette-Guérin vaccine: a meta-analysis of the literature. *Clin Infect Dis.* 2000;31(suppl 3):S64–S67. doi:10.1086/314072

CHAPTER 5

ZOONOTIC AND VECTOR-BORNE DISEASES

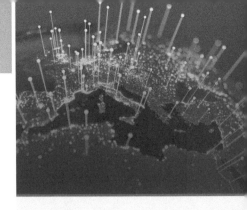

INTRODUCTION

It starts like so many other diseases: headache, fever, fatigue, loss of appetite. For most people, symptoms resolve in 3 to 4 days. However, in about 15% of those infected, the disease progresses to the namesake jaundice due to liver damage; abdominal pain; bleeding from the eyes, nose, and mouth; and gastrointestinal bleeding with subsequent black vomit (vomiting blood). Of those, the case fatality rate (CFR) is 20% to 50%.

It is a disease that turned the tides of wars as well as influenced the Louisiana Purchase and the construction of the Panama Canal. It wasn't until 1900 that the theory of Cuban epidemiologist Carlos Finlay was confirmed by Walter Reed's Yellow Fever Commission of transmission by mosquito vectors. About 30 years later, in 1927, the yellow fever virus was isolated, and within 10 years, a vaccine (17D) was developed which is still in use today. Yellow fever control is achieved through a combination of vector control and vaccination, yet occasionally major outbreaks still occur.

LEARNING OBJECTIVES

By the end of this chapter, readers will be able to:

- Describe how zoonotic and vector-borne diseases (VBDs) are different from other infectious diseases.
- Deconstruct what it takes to vector a disease.
- Articulate how zoonotic disease and VBD control approaches are similar to other disease control efforts, as well as how they are different.
- Defend why and how zoonotic diseases and VBDs rely on eco-epidemiologic methods.

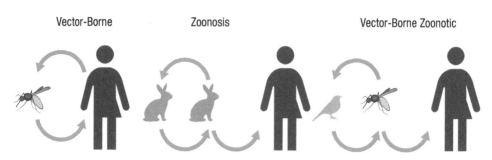

Figure 5.1 Schematic representation of vector-borne, zoonotic, and vector-borne zoonotic diseases, showing host, intermediaries, and vectors.

HOW ARE VECTOR-BORNE AND ZOONOTIC DISEASES DIFFERENT?

Approximately three quarters (75%) of emerging and re-emerging infectious diseases are zoonotic.[1] **Zoonotic diseases** are diseases of non-human animals, which can be transmitted to humans (Figure 5.1). Hantavirus pulmonary syndrome and rabies are examples of zoonotic diseases. These diseases are maintained in animals, and humans may contract the disease when coming into contact with infected animals or animal tissue/bodily fluid. Often but not always, the human host is incidental and not an integral part of the transmission cycle.

When the zoonotic disease requires a vector to maintain transmission, it is called a **vector-borne zoonotic disease** (VBZD; see Figure 5.1). Tularemia or plague are examples where the pathogen is maintained in an animal cycle and can be contracted from direct contact with the host but are also transmitted to humans through the bite of an infected arthropod.

Vector-borne diseases (VBDs) are those in which the pathogen is transmitted between hosts by an intermediary or vector (see Figure 5.1). Vectors are blood-feeding arthropods, including mosquitoes, fleas, ticks, lice, midges, and certain blood feeding bugs and flies. Vectors may successfully transmit viruses, as in the case of yellow fever, and also bacteria, like plague, and parasites, most famously malaria. When the transmission cycle requires only the vector and human hosts, it is called vector-borne anthroponoses, but more commonly just VBD. Regardless of VBD or VBZD for VBDs, the vector plays an integral role in the transmission and maintenance of the disease. It is part of the pathway and must itself become infected, not just relying on mechanical transmission.

zoonotic diseases: Diseases of non-human animals, which can be transmitted to humans.

vector-borne diseases: Diseases where the pathogen is transmitted between hosts by an intermediary or vector. Vectors are blood-feeding arthropods, including mosquitoes, fleas, ticks, lice, midges, and certain blood-feeding bugs and flies.

vector-borne zoonotic diseases: Diseases of non-human animals that require an intermediary to transmit to humans.

Life Cycles

While it varies by vector, most vectors go through life stages, namely egg, larvae, pupae, and adult. For many, the immature, egg to pupa, stages require a different environment than the adults. Mosquitoes, for example, require water for immature stages to survive. Most complete the life cycle within a season, but others may complete their life cycle over multiple seasons or years. Blood feeding is most common among adult females and associated with egg production. But some vectors—many tick species, for example—take blood meals at multiple life stages and both males and females blood feed.

Knowing about the host feeding preferences and the life stages is informative to vector control and to breaking the disease transmission cycle. Lyme disease is transmitted by the deer tick, *Ixodes scapularis*, in the northeastern United States. Larvae of this species typically feed on *Peromyscus leucopus*, the white-footed mouse, and pick up the spirochete, *Borrelia burgdorferi*, which is the causative agent. Nymphs and adults may feed on other mammals including white-tailed deer and humans, thus transmitting the bacterium. The abundance of mice, deer, and ticks as well as how humans interact with their landscape influences the prevalence of Lyme disease (Figure 5.2).[2]

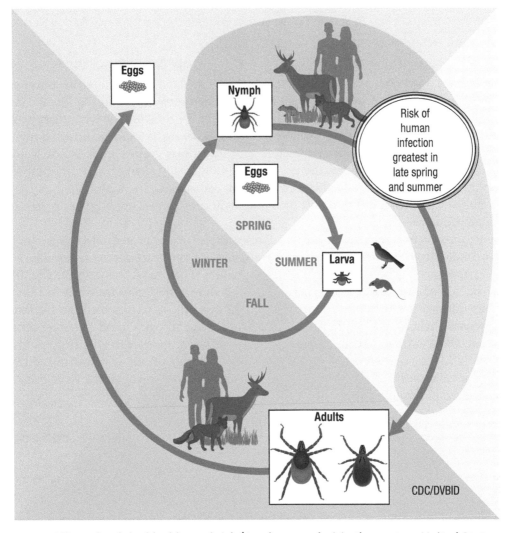

Figure 5.2 **Life cycle of the blacklegged tick (*Ixodes scapularis* in the eastern United States and *Ixodes pacificus* in the western United States), the primary Lyme disease vectors. These ticks feed on multiple hosts and need a new host for each life stage (larval, nymph, and adult).**
Source: Centers for Disease Control and Prevention. Lyme disease: lifecycle of black legged ticks. November 15, 2011. https://www.cdc.gov/lyme/transmission/blacklegged.html

THOUGHT QUESTION

Using the definitions presented, when a house fly lands on your hamburger and transfers *Salmonella typhi,* **which you then ingest, is the fly a vector of typhoid fever?**

HOSTS, RESERVOIRS, VECTORS, AND CARRIERS: WHERE DOES INFECTION START?

In order to definitively show the Aedes aegypti *transmits the yellow fever virus, members of the Walter Reed Yellow Fever Commission solicited volunteers to allow themselves to be bitten by mosquitoes. To disprove that fomites were responsible, another group of volunteers slept with the soiled bedding of yellow fever victims. Only those exposed to the bite of a mosquito became ill with yellow fever.*

Vertical and Horizontal Transmission

Yellow fever is a great example for a chapter on zoonotic diseases and VBDs because it exists in both a **sylvatic** and an urban cycle. In the sylvatic cycle, the virus is transmitted between non-human primates (e.g., monkeys) and mosquitoes in the forest canopy. Humans may contract the virus when they are bitten by mosquitoes when they visit or work in the jungle. However, the cycle can continue so long as there are infected non-human primates infecting competent vectors and infectious vectors infecting susceptible non-human primates. Similarly, the urban cycle involves humans and a different set of urban-adapted mosquitoes. In this VBD system, transmission is maintained as long as enough hosts are being infected and the competent mosquitoes are biting and acquiring or transmitting the virus.

Like raccoons for rabies in the eastern United States, rodents and hantavirus, non-human primates in the sylvatic yellow fever transmission cycle, are yellow fever **reservoirs**. That is, they are the natural source of the infection. They may be symptomatic, like a rabid skunk, or not, like a hantavirus-infected rodent. They may transmit to humans, but it is not necessary. Most zoonoses are maintained in reservoirs through **horizontal transmission** where infected individuals transmit the pathogen to other susceptible individuals. While some may have a **vertical transmission** (mother to offspring) pathway, this rarely is the maintenance pathway. Zika virus, for example, was transmitted from mother to child with detrimental effects like microcephaly. However, the virus transmission stopped at the child.

reservoir: Where the agent normally resides, be it humans, other animals, or the environment.

horizontal transmission: The passage of an agent from one individual to another of the same "generation."

vertical transmission: The passage of an agent from mother to offspring.

Vectorial Capacity

Vectors like non-human animals add another layer of complexity to understanding disease transmission. One way to break down and understand VBD is through vectorial capacity. Vectorial capacity is the average number of potentially infectious bites a single host will receive on a single day by all vectors.[3] It is typically written as C or VC, where

$$VC = \frac{ma^2 V p^n}{-lnp}$$

Here ma is the human-biting rate composed of both m, the density of vectors compared to hosts, and a, the host-biting habit or probability that the vector feeds on a human host. Vectorial capacity is contingent upon the mosquito species of question being the sort that is competent to acquire and transmit the pathogen, V, and importantly that it must survive (with a probability, p) the incubation period, n. How long an adult mosquito survives is estimated as $1/-\ln(p)$. The host-biting habit, a, appears twice—once for the mosquito to imbibe on an infectious blood meal and again to bite and transmit to a susceptible host.

VC brings together the critical components of the transmission cycles to guide the epidemiology of VBDs in a way that is intuitive and measurable. How many vectors are there, m, and are they biting humans, a? How long does it take for the vector to become infectious, n, and what is the probability it survives at least that long, p? Is it even a competent vector—the right species that can become infected, V.

Beautifully, though it was first conceptualized to understand malaria, it can be adapted to other mosquito-borne disease systems and other non-mosquito vector systems as well.[4] While this formula is helpful in estimating the transmission potential for a given VBD, it also serves as a framework for thinking about and understanding VBD transmission (Figure 5.3). In these next sections we take each component, describe it, and explain how it is measured in practice.

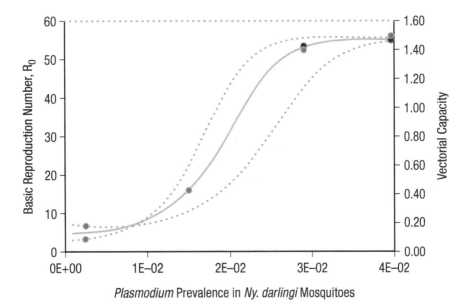

Figure 5.3 The association between vectorial capacity and the basic reproduction number.
Source: Adapted from Sallum MAM, Conn JE, Bergo ES, et al. Vector competence, vectorial capacity of *Nyssorhynchus darlingi* and the basic reproduction number of *Plasmodium vivax* in agricultural settlements in the Amazonian Region of Brazil. *Malar J.* 2019;18:117. doi:10.1186/s12936-019-2753-7.

Vector, vector, what's your sector? Did you notice? The formula sort of has two "Vs" in it: *VC* (or *C*), which is vectorial capacity. Vectorial capacity is what we're interested in, whether or not a disease will be spread by a given vector in a given place. The other *V* tucked in there is vector competence. Vector competence is a measure of whether a given mosquito species (or sometimes even a specific population of a species in a specific location) is able to become infected and transmit the pathogen.

MEASURING VECTOR DENSITY, M

In order to become infected by a VBD, there have to be enough vectors becoming infected and biting hosts. Vector density is a measure of the number of vectors that can be collected in a given period. Usually, it is a measure of host-seeking adults, but vector density may be measured as the number of immature or adult vectors.

Immature Stage Surveys

For mosquitoes, larval surveys include estimating the percent of houses in an area that are infected with larvae or pupae, known as the house index. Alternatively, vector density may be measured as the number of water-holding containers on a property that are infested, the container index, as well as a related index, Breteau index, which is the number of positive containers per 100 houses inspected. While these measure larva or pupa, the pupa index is the number of pupae per 100 houses inspected.

Larval and nymphal tick stages can be collected using a flag or drag where a cloth is dragged through vegetation. Host-seeking ticks will attach and can be collected from the cloth. Each method of collecting vectors paints a different picture of the abundance and richness of vectors one might encounter, known as the **entomologic risk**.

entomologic risk: Probability of encountering a disease vector.

Adult Surveys

Adult surveys give a better measure of risk for transmission as they are usually at the life stage at which they bite and therefore a stage likely to pass the infection. Dry ice or other sources of carbon dioxide may be used to mimic host exhalation and preferentially selects for different species and stages. Mosquito traps often employ carbon dioxide and a light to collect adults, but gravid females may be selected for through water-baited traps which provide an egg-laying opportunity. Color and color contrast may also aid in trapping. For example, tsetse flies, the vectors for *African trypanosomiasis*, are preferentially attracted to blue and black alternating colors. Ground-dwelling and crawling vectors like fleas and ticks are often collected by dragging a cloth to which they attach. The type of trap and the use of attractant influences the species collected, which in turn influences the perceived abundance and diversity of vectors present (Figure 5.4). Consistency and accurate descriptions of the trapping methods allows for comparisons between years and locations and provides comparable estimates of vector density. The greater the vector density, the greater the probability of a bite to either an infected or susceptible host.

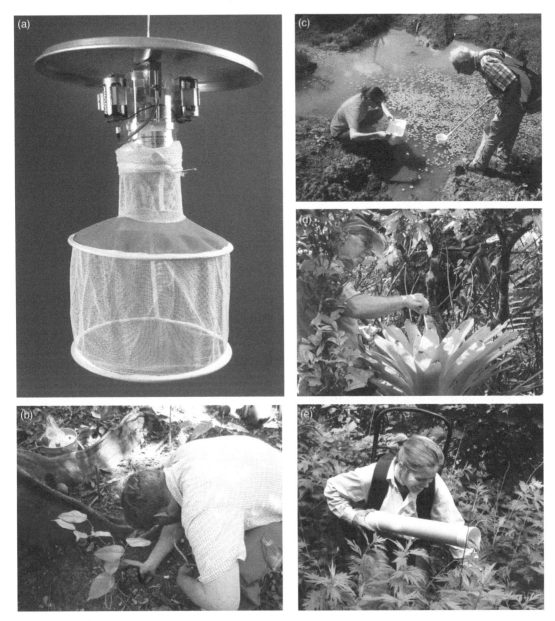

Figure 5.4 **Examples of trapping for mosquitoes.** (a) A miniature light trap for trapping host-seeking adult mosquitoes, (b) syphoning crab holes for mosquitoes, (c) dipping for immature mosquitoes in pooled water, (d) pipetting bromeliads for immature mosquitoes, and (e) backpack aspirator for resting adults.

THOUGHT QUESTION

Think about it: Take each of these indices and imagine how it might tell a different story about the risk of encountering a potentially infectious vector. Consider the labor it takes to complete each estimate. Might some be easier than others? Is there a balance to strike between the information you get from an index and the time it takes to estimate it? Dye, 1986 provides a nice review of the challenges measuring the components of vectorial capacity.[5]

MEASURING HOST-BITING HABIT

For some vectors, certain trap types will preferentially select for those with a blood meal. For mosquitoes, this can be by creating a resting place or through using/creating an immature habitat for egg laying. Other vectors may be collected on-host (e.g., ticks, fleas, and lice) or in host burrows (e.g., fleas and lice). If the vector collected has evidence of having taken a blood meal, the source of that blood meal can be identified using molecular techniques. As technology has evolved, scientists are increasingly precise in describing what hosts vectors are feeding on. Through DNA barcoding, even residual blood meals can be detected and analyzed.[6] Where blood meal analysis was once used to only identify what genus had been fed upon from fresh blood meals, now species can be identified, and even multiple species in one blood meal, even to the point of some real-time in-field capacity.[7]

Blood meal work has helped to identify those mosquitoes that likely transmit the disease to humans because they are able to transmit the pathogen and preferentially select human hosts. It also helps identify those mosquitoes that are part of maintaining the disease in non-human hosts but not transmitting to humans because, while they may be able to acquire and transmit, they typically feed on non-human hosts.

THOUGHT QUESTION

Everyone loves to hate mosquitoes, and with good cause; they are the world's deadliest animals. But did you know they are crime fighters, too? In 2008, an astute Finnish police officer noticed a recently fed mosquito in an abandoned car. The car later turned out to be stolen and the blood meal a DNA match to the suspected car thief. Can you imagine other situations (maybe less crime and more VBD research) where knowing the source of a mosquito's last meal might be useful information? To read more about the Crime Fighting Finnish Mosquitoes have a look here: http://news.bbc.co.uk/2/hi/europe/7795725.stm.

MEASURING SURVIVAL

How long a vector survives is critically important, especially when there is no vertical transmission. This is because a vector must first take an infected blood meal, then survive long enough to itself be able to transmit the pathogen. Survival varies by life stage and can be affected by temperature, precipitation, and humidity.[8] Temperature and precipitation can influence the availability of a moist habitat for immature stages to successfully complete their life cycle. Humidity may impact adult vectors in terms of survival or host-seeking behavior, for example, ticks will change questing behavior depending on the humidity.

Survival can be easily measured in the laboratory by placing mosquitoes into incubators with set temperatures and humidity levels. Mimicking real world conditions of fluctuating temperatures and humidity levels starts to make estimating vector life histories a little more complicated.[9] The real world with predators and other hazards is even more complex, but through a combination of methods and statistics, p, the probability of surviving, can be estimated for given conditions.

VECTOR COMPETENCE AND THE EXTRINSIC INCUBATION PERIOD

Vector competence is the ability of a vector to (1) acquire, (2) maintain, (3) become infected, and (4) transmit the agent (Figure 5.5). The time it takes to complete this cycle—that is, for the vector to become infectious—is the **extrinsic incubation period (EIP)**. This is the time from imbibing an infected blood meal until the vector is infected and can

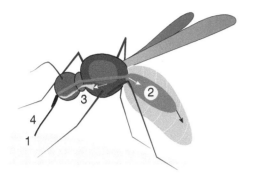

Figure 5.5 The extrinsic incubation period. The extrinsic incubation period is the time it takes for a vector (1) to imbibe an infectious blood meal, (2) for the agent to escape any innate immunity of the vector (e.g., the midgut barrier), and (3) for the pathogen to then travel to the salivary glands or rectum of the vector, so that it can (4) then be transmitted to the host in a subsequent host contact.

successfully transmit the pathogen. It is a process that is largely considered to be influenced by both the infectious dose as well as temperature.

extrinsic incubation period: The time for a vector to become infectious (able to transmit) after becoming infected.

THOUGHT QUESTION

Feeling comfortable with vectorial capacity yet? Play with it: http://idshowcase.lshtm.ac.uk/id503/ID503/M3S1/ID503_M3S1_050_010.html

HOW DO WE PREVENT THE SPREAD OF VECTOR-BORNE AND ZOONOTIC DISEASES?

In 1938, the live-attenuated 17D yellow fever vaccine developed through the collaborative work of Max Theiler, Hugh Smith, and Eugen Haagen at the Rockefeller Foundation was licensed for use. In 1951, Theiler was awarded a Nobel Prize for his work on this vaccine, and it currently is the only time the prize has been awarded for a vaccine.[10] More than 850 million doses of 17D have been administered and it remains in use today. It is considered 100% effective, well tolerated, and affordable, providing lifelong immunity from just one dose.[11] Certain countries require proof of vaccination to visit.

Often with VBD, we dive deeply into the vector's capacity to transmit the disease and to the environmental factors that influence the distribution of these diseases. This may be in part because these are typically quantifiable and modifiable in experiments. However, we must also consider the human actions that influence disease susceptibility. Early in describing a potential vector–host–environment association within a community or population, we may rely on a cross-sectional study design. **Cross-sectional** studies are a class of observational study where, after defining the population to be studied, information is collected from individuals about both their exposures and outcomes. This information is generally collected at the same time, so a typical survey asking participants about both risk factors and disease falls under this classification. Preventive practices and vaccination status may also be included as questions. Participants with or without a risk factor or exposure are compared to determine who has the selected disease or outcome of interest as well as the overall prevalence of the outcome. Exposure and outcome information are

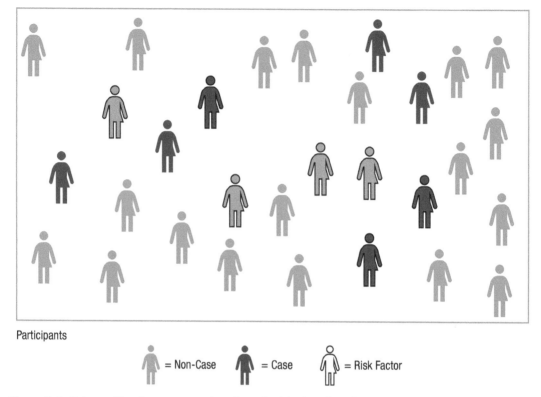

Participants

🚶 = Non-Case   🚶 = Case   🚶 = Risk Factor

Figure 5.6 Schematic of a cross-sectional study. Notice that the participants are recruited into the study based on inclusion and exclusion criteria. Next, disease and risk factor status are assessed, usually simultaneously. The cross-sectional study is a relatively quick way to collect data. It is commonly used in descriptive epidemiology to estimate the prevalence of exposures and outcomes in a population sample.

usually collected at the same time, so we do not have temporality nor incidence, and odds ratios are typically calculated (Figure 5.6).

Cross-sectional studies can be conducted quite quickly and inexpensively compared to prospective studies and can help in generating hypotheses for longer, more robust designs. However, a key drawback is the inability to disentangle the temporality of exposure and outcome, so there is no attempt to infer causality. One approach is to run multiple cross-sectional surveys over time to examine trends in a population. There may also be biases in terms of who is included in the study and being able to generalize to a broader population.

THOUGHT QUESTION

Since the prevalence of an outcome depends on the incidence of the disease as well as how long the disease lasts (and if someone survives or not), when might cross-sectional data collection not be an optimal study design?

Inoculations

Like other infectious diseases, inoculations are an important tool to prevent disease transmission. The yellow fever vaccine is an example of a successful inoculation against a VBD (yellow fever) that is still widely used today in endemic areas and among travelers to those areas. In contrast, a Lyme disease vaccine that showed 80% efficacy for preventing disease in humans was developed but then discontinued due to lack of demand; this stands as an example of the needs for vaccine communication.[12]

Universal inoculations are also underway for certain diseases. For example, rather than targeting the agent that causes disease, there are efforts underway to develop inoculation against the vector. For example, there is a candidate vaccine against proteins in mosquito saliva.[13,14] And, while the human vaccine for Lyme disease was discontinued, there is work in progress on a broader "anti-tick" vaccine.[15] These vaccines will be "universal" because they work against the vectors rather than the specific diseases they carry and rely on the host's immunity to quickly respond to the bite of the vector and prevent against multiple pathogens the vector might carry.

Another exciting form of inoculation is infecting mosquitoes with *Wolbachia* bacteria, which works either by suppressing mosquito abundance or by inhibiting the mosquito's capacity to subsequently transmit the virus.[16] *Wolbachia* is a naturally occurring insect bacteria, though it does not naturally infect mosquitoes. After many attempts, it was successfully inoculated into *Aedes aegypti* mosquitoes. Once the mosquito is infected, it transmits the bacteria to subsequent surviving offspring. Importantly, *Aedes aegypti* infected with *Wolbachia* are less competent vectors. Trials of releasing *Wolbachia*-infected mosquitoes as a means to control dengue are underway.

Regardless of the inoculation in question, these work by reducing vector competence—the ability of the vector to acquire or transmit the pathogen. Fewer infectious humans because they are vaccinated reduces the chance a vector will become infected, whereas *Wolbachia* infection reduces the chance a vector will transmit the pathogen.

Integrated Pest Management

While inoculations typically focus on the hosts, reducing the density of vector per host is the focus of integrated pest management (IPM). IPM came out of agricultural pest control with an aim to use effective and environmentally sustainable techniques not to eradicate all pests, but rather to keep pests below an **economic injury level**, that is, the lowest possible level where the pest causes damage equal to the cost of pest management. The strategies move from least toxic preventive methods through to chemical interventions (Figure 5.7). The effective use of multiple strategies has been adopted for other applications as well.

economic injury level: The lowest level of insects (the injury) where the loss productivity equals the cost for insect management.

IPM manages vectors through integrated use of cultural, biological, mechanical, and chemical strategies.[17] *Cultural strategies* include changing how crops are watered from flood irrigation to more transient targeted irrigation, rotating crops where pests must continually adapt, and changing the planting or other activity season not to coincide with vector peaks. This could reduce the host/vector density, m, by removing habitat for the vectors to grow their populations or by reducing the human-biting habit, a, by shifting the coincidence of vector peaks and human activity. *Mechanical strategies* include physical barriers or removal trapping of vectors. Bed nets and window screens can create a physical barrier between hosts and vectors, influencing human-biting rates, ma. Removal trapping similarly reduces the vector/host interaction, m. *Biological strategies* include cultivating natural predators

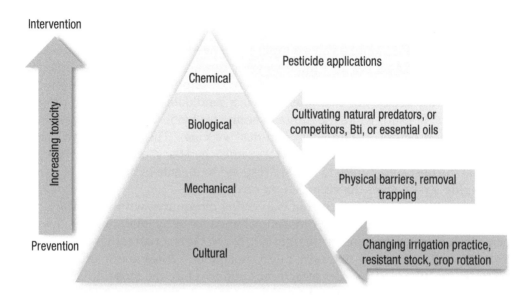

Figure 5.7 Integrative pest management (IPM) goes from prevention to intervention through the use of cultural, mechanical, biological, and chemical pest management methods. Bti, *Bacillus thuringiensis israelensis.*

Source: Adapted from Roth M. Varroa mites: new guide outlines integrated pest management options [Figure 4: Varroa mite IPM pyramid]. *Entomology Today.* 2020. https://entomologytoday.org/2020/02/07/varroa-mites-new-guide-outlines-integrated-pest-management-options/varroa-ipm-pyramid

of vectors or non-vectors that compete for the same ecological space. This again reduces the host/vector density. Another biological control strategy is the application of *Bacillus thuringiensis israelensis* (Bti) onto water surfaces where mosquitoes breed. Bti is a naturally occurring soil bacteria that produces toxins that specifically target and kill mosquitoes and black fly larvae, thus reducing vector populations, *m*. Finally, *chemical strategies* such as the use of pesticides can further reduce the density of vectors per host.

THOUGHT QUESTION

You are a rice farmer in a malaria endemic area. How would you use IPM to control malaria vectors? Be sure to list an action for each of the four strategies and use the internet to ensure your strategies are applicable to malaria vectors. How will climate change affect your farming (and specifically pest burden) and how might you need to respond?

ARE THESE ENVIRONMENTAL DISEASES?

Like many other VBDs, the mosquitoes that vector the yellow fever virus to humans are tightly associated with certain environments that allow for sufficient abundance of vectors and for humans to be exposed. So, are all VBD quintessential One Health?

Sylvatic yellow fever only exists in environments where humans interact with the wild reservoir. If the environment is not suitable to maintain sufficient reservoir hosts, or if humans do not encroach, the transmission cycle will be broken. While humans and other animals have been interacting since the first humans, the intensity to which humans now do is heightened due to the conversion of natural habitat for agriculture, transport, and settlement; illegal animal trade like exotic pets and bushmeat; and tourism to explore exotic locations.[18]

Most VBDs are driven by the environment in a way distinct from other infectious diseases. This is because the distribution of most vectors is constrained by climatologic and environmental conditions. Plague risk is associated with elevation in the Southwest United States, presumably linked to available habitat suitable for rodent hosts at those elevations. Dengue is an urban, tropical disease where humidity and thermal tolerances of the vectors dictate their survival and thus their function in disease transmission. Temperature drives the speed at which development occurs, and thereby how quickly populations can build. For many vectors precipitation creates that habitat necessary for immature life stages. It begs the question, then: Are these environmental diseases?

Changing Climate

Because of the strong association between many types of vectors and the environment, changing climate will likely influence the distribution of these diseases. This includes incursion of vectors into new areas that might not have been suitable. Areas that are marginally suitable might become more suitable as warmer temperatures lead to longer vector seasons and greater vector densities.

Forms of zoonosis, both sylvatic and domestic, are similarly affected by climate. Climate and climate change, as well as human-made changes to the landscape, influence the presence and abundance of animal hosts and also interactions with human hosts. Domestic animal zoonoses are still influenced by this interaction though it is somewhat buff-

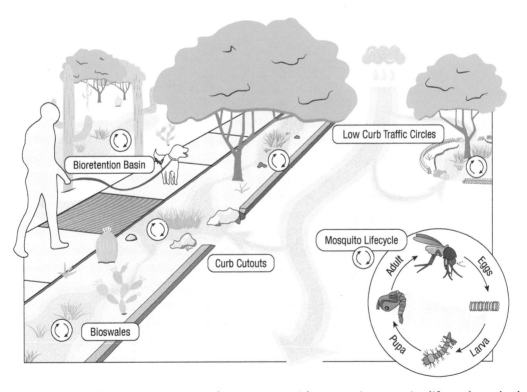

Figure 5.8 Examples of urban green infrastructure with a generic mosquito life cycle embedded. When stormwater or run-off collects and does not infiltrate for longer periods, it may become a source for mosquito emergence.

Source: Courtesy of Erika Lynn Schmidt.

ered by human control over the animal's environment. Changes in animal husbandry in response to climate will change the exposure of domestic animals and may also impact stress to the animals. While it is likely that the changes due to climate change will differ locally, in general the expectation is for increased disease transmission under warming and more extreme conditions.

As communities seek to be more sustainable and resilient against a warming climate with more extreme weather events, they are turning to installation of greenways and rainwater harvesting to balance water flow, mitigate heat, conserve water for urban landscapes, and sometimes even enhance local food production.[19,20] However, when green infrastructure falls into disrepair or was not properly designed and constructed in the first place, it may be maladaptive. That is, rather than supporting resilience it may inadvertently increase the vulnerability of the community. An example of one such maladaptation is when stormwater run-off collects and pools long enough for mosquitoes to complete their aquatic life cycle (Figure 5.8). This is yet another example where vector control can only be achieved with the concerted cross-sectoral collaboration.

Quintessential One Health

This interface between animals, humans, and the environment is quintessential One Health (Figure 5.9). Understanding and preventing zoonotic diseases and VBDs require a holistic view that improves health by considering the interactions of humans, animals, and environment through a collaborative and multidisciplinary approach. While this idea of One Health has been around as long as zoonoses have been studied, actively engaging with a One Health framework crosses disciplinary boundaries and facilitates new discoveries.[21]

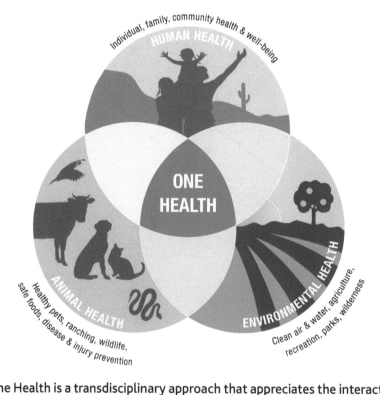

Figure 5.9 **One Health is a transdisciplinary approach that appreciates the interaction between animal and human health, in the environment which they share.**
Source: Courtesy of Paul Akmajian.

CASE STUDY

Carlos Finlay was born in Cuba in 1833 (Figure 5.10). His experience with infectious diseases was firsthand, suffering both cholera and typhoid fever. He studied in France and in the United States, graduating from Jefferson Medical College in Philadelphia in 1855. Interestingly, this was the year of yet another major United States yellow fever outbreak which devastated neighboring Virginia. Dr. Finlay returned to Cuba after his studies, setting up a general medicine and ophthalmology practice in Havana. However, a researcher at heart, in his free time he investigated the origins of disease, including yellow fever.

At this time in history, the idea that mosquitoes might be disease vectors was not yet established. In 1881 he presented and then published his proposal that humans were infected with yellow fever virus through the bite of an infected mosquito. Finlay faced ridicule and opposition. However, the impact of yellow fever was too large to be ignored and a cause needed to be found.

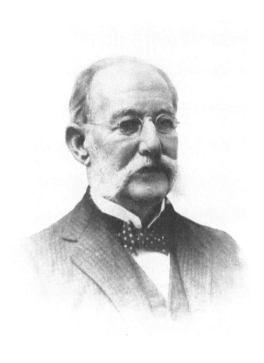

Figure 5.10 Carlos Finlay (1833–1915). Finlay discovered that mosquitoes transmitted yellow fever.

For nearly 20 years, he worked to prove his theory that mosquitoes transmitted diseases. In 1900, the Walter Reed Yellow Fever Commission, working with Finlay, finally confirmed Dr. Finlay's work. He was nominated seven times for the Nobel Prize.

CONCLUSION

Emerging pathogens are overwhelmingly zoonotic. How humans engage with the resources on the planet influences the risk of contracting a zoonotic disease or VBD. Lifestyles, be they forced migration or choosing to live in mega cities, or consumption of bushmeat and exotic travel, open up channels for exposure to novel hosts and pathogens. Relatedly, the changing climate will influence the abundance and distribution of non-human hosts and of vectors changing the distribution of the diseases they transmit. Science and epidemiology work to estimate where those interactions are likely to occur and to quickly identify them once they do. The One Health approach leads to a more robust understanding of the interactions that may lead to disease transmission and opens the ingenuity of potential solutions.

TEACHING CORNER

DID YOU KNOW?

The transmission cycles of many zoonotic diseases and VBDs can be extremely complex. They typically involve multiple animal hosts and dozens of competent vectors and occur across a variety of habitat types. Understanding a disease involves both simplifying it to understand the basics, but also embracing the complexity to identify sources for disease prevention.

TRY THIS

Take a specific disease and map out the transmission cycle. Use the transmission cycles developed by the Centers for Disease Control and Prevention (CDC) or build your own based on what you know. Keep them simple on the first iteration. Figure 5.11 shows a couple of examples.

Given these simplified transmissions, *identify* how you could break the transmission cycle to prevent disease. Now, *complexify!!* That is, add the detail that makes these simple transmission cycles more accurate by adding images of the alternate hosts or vectors. For example, rabies is transmitted to humans not only by domestic animals but also wild canids, cats, bats, raccoons, and skunks. Chikungunya is transmitted by multiple mosquito species which may differ in competency, and which may compete with each other.

TAKE IT A STEP FURTHER

These transmission cycles consider only the interaction of the host and the reservoir. Use a One Health approach to consider the greater ecosystem these diseases exist in. Now list additional ways to break the transmission cycle. How does that expand the range of potential sources to engage and reduce disease and promote health?

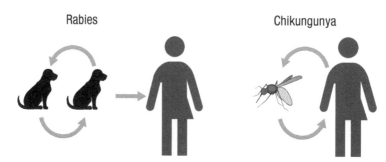

Figure 5.11 **Sample transmission cycles. Try building your own based on what you know.**

QUESTIONS FOR FURTHER DISCUSSION

1. Pick two different VBDs and compare their life cycles. Identify where they are similar (would the same intervention work for either?) and where they are different (what special interventions might be necessary).

2. Reconcile for yourself why we still worry about VBDs. In some cases, since we seem to have such an understanding and control, do we even need a chapter on VBZD?

3. Using the components of the vectorial capacity formula, describe how increasing temperatures due to climate change will impact VBD.

$$VC = \frac{ma^2Vp^n}{-lnp}$$

4. List and define the components of IPM. Using a VBD of your choice, design an IPM strategy.

A robust set of instructor resources designed to supplement this text is located at http://connect.springerpub.com/Content/book/978-0-8261-5674-7. Qualifying instructors may request access by emailing **textbook@springerpub.com**.

REFERENCES

1 Jones K, Patel N, Levy M, et al. Global trends in emerging infectious diseases. *Nature.* 2008;451:990–993. doi:10.1038/nature06536

2 Barbour AG, Fish D. The biological and social phenomenon of Lyme disease. *Science.* 1993;260(5114):1610–1616. doi:10.1126/science.8503006

3 Fine PEM. Epidemiological principles of vector-mediated transmission. In: McKelvey JJ, Eldridge BF, Maramorosch K, eds. *Vectors of Disease Agents. Interactions With Plants, Animals, and Man.* Praeger Publishers; 1981:77–91.

4 Brady OJ, Godfray HCJ, Tatem AJ, et al. Vectorial capacity and vector control: reconsidering sensitivity to parameters for malaria elimination. *Trans R Soc Trop Med Hyg.* 2016;110(2):107–117. doi:10.1093/trstmh/trv113

5 Dye C. Vectorial capacity: must we measure all its components? *Parasitol Today.* 1986;2(8):203–209. doi:10.1016/0169-4758(86)90082-7

6 Gariepy TD, Lindsay R, Ogden N, Gregory TR. Identifying the last supper: utility of the DNA barcode library for bloodmeal identification in ticks. *Mol Ecol Resour.* 2012;12(4):646–652. doi:10.1111/j.1755-0998.2012.03140.x

7 Borland EM, Kading RC. Modernizing the toolkit for arthropod bloodmeal identification. *Insects.* 2021;12(1):37. doi:10.3390/insects12010037

8 Lega J, Brown HE, Barrera R. *Aedes aegypti* abundance model improved with relative humidity and precipitation-driven egg hatching. *J Med Entomol.* 2017;54(5):1375–1384. doi:10.1093/jme/tjx077

9 Chen S, Fleischer SJ, Saunders MC, Thomas MB. The influence of diurnal temperature variation on degree-day accumulation and insect life history. *PLoS One.* 2015;10(3):e0120772. doi:10.1371/journal.pone.0120772

10 Norrby E. Yellow fever and Max Theiler: the only Nobel Prize for a virus vaccine. *J Exp Med.* 2007;204(12):2779–2784. doi:10.1084/jem.20072290

11 Elvidge S. Developing the 17D yellow fever vaccine. *Nature Portfolio.* September 28, 2020. https://www.nature.com/articles/d42859-020-00012-9

12 Nigrovic LE, Thompson KM. The Lyme vaccine: a cautionary tale. *Epidemiol Infect.* 2007;135(1):1–8. doi:10.1017/S0950268806007096

13 Manning JE, Oliveira F, Coutinho-Abreu IV, et al. Safety and immunogenicity of a mosquito saliva peptide-based vaccine: a randomised, placebo-controlled, double-blind, phase 1 trial. *Lancet.* 2020;395:P1998–2007. doi:10.1016/S0140-6736(20)31048-5

14 National Institutes of Health. Universal mosquito vaccine tested. *NIH Research Matters.* June 23, 2020. https://www.nih.gov/news-events/nih-research-matters/universal-mosquito-vaccine-tested

15 Bobe JR, Jutras BL, Horn EJ, et al. Recent progress in Lyme disease and remaining challenges. *Front Med.* 2021;8:1276. doi:10.3389/fmed.2021.666554

16 Slatko BE, Luck AN, Dobson SL, Foster JM. *Wolbachia* endosymbionts and human disease control. *Mol Biochem Parasitol.* 2014;195(2):88–95. doi:10.1016/j.molbiopara.2014.07.004

17 Lewis WJ, van Lenteren JC, Phatak SC, Tumlinson JH. A total system approach to sustainable pest management. *Proc Natl Acad Sci U S A.* 1997;94(23):12243–12248. doi:10.1073/pnas.94.23.12243

18 Devaux CA, Mediannikov O, Medkour H, Raoult D. Infectious disease risk across the growing human-non human primate interface: a review of the evidence. *Front Public Health.* 2019;7:305. doi:10.3389/fpubh.2019.00305

19 Boelee E, Yohannes M, Poda JN, et al. Options for water storage and rainwater harvesting to improve health and resilience against climate change in Africa. *Reg Environ Chang.* 2013;13:509–519. doi:10.1007/s10113-012-0287-4

20 Demuzere M, Orru K, Heidrich O, et al. Mitigating and adapting to climate change: multi-functional and multi-scale assessment of green urban infrastructure. *J Environ Manage.* 2014;146:107–115. doi:10.1016/j.jenvman.2014.07.025

21 Atlas RM. One Health: its origins and future. In: Mackenzie J, Jeggo M, Daszak P, Richt J, eds. *One Health: The Human-Animal-Environment Interfaces in Emerging Infectious Diseases.* Springer; 2012. doi:10.1007/82_2012_223

CHAPTER 6

SEXUALLY TRANSMITTED INFECTIONS

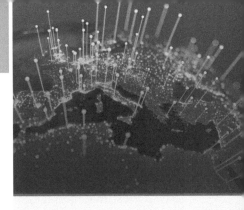

INTRODUCTION

Gonorrhea, aka the clap, is one of the oldest sexually transmitted diseases, traced as far back as a 2600 BCE description by Chinese emperor Huang Ti. The name tells us of its symptoms: gono for seed and rhea for flow as described by Galen (131–200 CE) to explain the discharge that resembles semen. Even "the clap" is believed to come from an old English word, "clappan," which means beating or throbbing, thought to describe the painful sensation during urination. But the causative agent was not identified until 1879 by Albert Neisser. Currently, it is one of the most well-known, most common, and, with rising rates of resistance, maybe most vexing sexually transmitted infections. Read more about the history of this fascinating infection at https://jsstd.org/gonorrhea-historical-outlook.

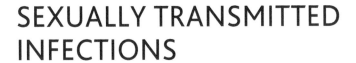

LEARNING OBJECTIVES

By the end of this chapter, readers will be able to:

- Describe the effect of sexually transmitted infections (STIs) on health.
- List challenges to reducing the burden of STIs.
- Describe how we identify the key risk factors and affected populations.
- Explain why strong research methodologies are important to the study of STIs.

OVERVIEW OF SEXUALLY TRANSMITTED INFECTIONS

Sexually transmitted infections (STIs) are infections that are transmitted between individuals through anal, oral, or vaginal sex. Occasionally they are also transmitted through intimate physical contact or via other modes of transmission—for example, STIs which enter the bloodstream and then are transmitted through injection drug use or blood transfusions. Globally, treatable infections such as trichomoniasis (near 150 million new cases annually), chlamydia (near 130 million new cases), gonorrhea (near 80 million new cases), and syphilis (near 7 million new cases) are leading causes of new infections, while an estimated 417 million people are living with genital herpes (herpes simplex type 2) and 291 million women are infected with human papillomavirus (HPV).[1]

sexually transmitted infection (STI): A viral or bacterial infection usually transmitted from person to person during vaginal, anal, or oral intercourse or genital touching.

The effects of STIs are far greater than most of us imagine (Figure 6.1). On any given day, it is estimated that one of five people in the United States—that is, nearly 68 million people—has an STI.[2] Among these, nearly half of the new cases (26 million new cases in 2018) were among those aged 15 to 24 years.[2] For the United States alone, medical costs for testing and treating STIs is $16 billion, $13.7 billion of which is attributed to HIV; another $1 billion for chlamydia, gonorrhea, and syphilis together; and $755 million attributed to infection with HPV.[2]

Symptoms of STIs include vaginal discharge, urethral discharge or burning in men, genital ulcers, or abdominal pain. However, these infections do not always result in clinical disease, complicating detection and treatment. It is estimated that around 70% to 75% of women with *Chlamydia trachomatis* infections are asymptomatic.[3] That does not mean that they are not infectious; asymptomatic individuals can still transmit pathogens.

For some STIs, the immune system may successfully clear the infection before it progresses to disease, or the symptoms can be so mild that the individual does not seek treatment. This means that STIs may go undetected, with negative consequences especially among women and their babies.[4] Importantly, untreated infections may move from the lower reproductive tract and cause more severe disease, such as pelvic inflammatory disease (PID), where the uterus, fallopian tubes, ovaries, or other pelvic structures become infected and inflamed, or else cause tubo-ovarian abscesses, ectopic pregnancy, or infertility. For this reason, an important public health message is for sexually active individuals to be tested, even if they are not experiencing symptoms.

Beyond the immediate effects of being infected, STIs can have serious long-term consequences on health. They may increase the risk of other infections; for example, individuals with herpes, gonorrhea, and syphilis show increased risk for contracting HIV. Pregnant women infected with an STI may pass the infection to their fetus with potential fetal loss or low birth weight or, when the infection is transmitted during birth, eye and lung damage may occur to the infant. The risk of STI and other bacterial infections to an infant's

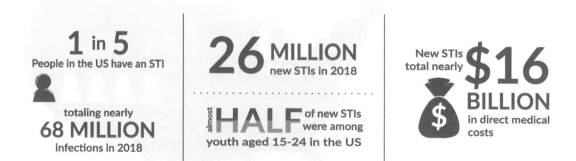

Figure 6.1 Overview of the burden of sexually transmitted infections (STIs) in the United States.
Source: Centers for Disease Control and Prevention. Sexually transmitted infections prevalence, incidence, and cost estimates in the United States. n.d. https://www.cdc.gov/std/statistics/prevalence-incidence-cost-2020.htm

eyes during the birth process is why most infants in the United States are treated with antibiotic eye ointment at delivery. Further, STIs like HPV and hepatitis B are causally associated with cancers, cervical and hepatocellular carcinoma, respectively. Finally, gonorrhea or chlamydia infections in women may lead to PID and infertility.

HEADS UP!

STI, STD, ST... Stop, What?

STIs are sexually transmitted infections, whereas STDs are sexually transmitted diseases. The difference is in the last letter: an infection versus a disease. While they are sometimes used interchangeably, they are distinct. All STDs start out as an STI, but not all STIs progress to an STD. There is some reason to use the more accurate STI when referring to an infection because it is the infection that is transmitted and is thus the target of preventive measures. A non-diseased individual can still be infectious.

THOUGHT QUESTION

How do you think the asymptomatic manifestation of many STIs creates unique challenges for STI control?

REDUCING THE BURDEN OF SEXUALLY TRANSMITTED INFECTIONS

While early treatment for gonorrhea included injection of mercury into the urethra, the real advances in treatment came with the introduction of sulfonamides in the late 1930s and again with the widespread use of penicillin in 1940. However, within a few short years of introduction, treatment failures arose for both sulfonamides and penicillin due to drug resistance.

Many STIs are preventable and treatable infections. Condoms protect against STIs by creating a physical barrier. When used correctly and consistently, they provide one of the most effective methods to prevent infection of most STIs, although they do not prevent syphilis or genital herpes, which present with extra-genital ulcers. Two viral STIs, HPV and hepatitis B, both of which are causally associated with cancers, have highly effective vaccines. The HPV vaccine, which is highly effective against nine types of HPV, including those most causally associated with cervical cancer, has been associated with a 90% reduction in cervical cancer among vaccinated.[5] Chronic infection with hepatitis B is associated with an increased risk of liver cancer; however, the vaccine is 98% to 100% effective at preventing infection. Vaccine development for other STIs is ongoing. PrEP, or pre-exposure prophylaxis, taken daily is 99% effective at reducing the risk of sexually transmitted HIV and 74% effective at reducing the risk of HIV from injection drug use.[6] Despite these significant treatment and prevention advances, why do STIs remain a significant public health challenge (Figure 6.2)?

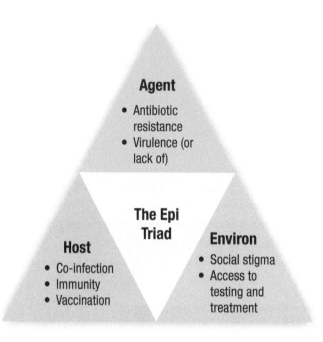

Figure 6.2 **The epidemiologic triad of challenges to STI control.**

Barriers to Care

In addition to the lack of symptoms or confusing symptoms that may delay care, another issue that limits care-seeking for STDs is **social stigma**. Social stigmas around STIs are a considerable barrier to care-seeking behavior even when services are available. The stigmatization of STIs makes individuals feel less valued. This stigma is particularly prevalent among college students, who will avoid testing despite most campuses providing services, and sexual minority populations, who face physical and symbolic violence beyond STI status.[7,8] These social stigmas create barriers to appropriate care-seeking behavior, reducing the likelihood a sexually active individual will be screened, and thus an infection will be detected and subsequently treated. Stigma may also decrease the likelihood that individuals will inform partners of their STI status or provide medication to their partners. In one study among male African American youth in San Francisco, for every increase in score on a validated stigma scale, the odds of providing medication to a partner decreased.[9]

social stigma: The judging or condemning of individuals based on their social characteristics, in this case having an infection.

Part of renaming STDs as STIs was an effort to address stigma. Moving from language about disease—which might have negative connotations—toward language that frames them as infections conveys the treatable nature and thus allows a less negative perception. Breaking down social stigma starts with engaging in informed, nonjudgmental conversations about healthy, safe sex. Empowering individuals to ask their partners to use a condom or dental dam is not just about *faithfulness* but about protection against these preventable infections. When newly diagnosed with an STI, talking with a medical provider or seeking advice from a clinic specifically providing for STI care can be helpful not only in getting correct treatment, but also in helping to manage the feelings around the diagnosis and any concerns over informing partners of the diagnosis.

Antibiotic Resistance

Another threat to the effective treatment of STIs is the growing rate of antibiotic resistance. Most notably, gonorrhea, caused by the bacteria *Neisseria gonorrhoeae*, has developed resistance to almost every antibiotic that is used to treat it, with only one class of antibiotics, cephalosporins, available to treat it (Figure 6.3). There are an estimated 550,000 new drug-resistant *Neisseria gonorrhoeae* infections each year, which is about half of all gonorrhea infections reported. In men, it commonly presents as urethritis (swelling of the urethra). In women, it presents as cervicitis (swelling of the cervix), which is usually asymptomatic, but can progress to pelvic inflammatory disease and infertility. This bacterium's ability to acquire and retain antimicrobial resistance genes, along with injudicious use of antibiotics, has facilitated the emergence of resistance.[10]

The antimicrobial resistance situation is sufficiently dire that the World Health Organization (WHO) and the United States Centers for Disease Control and Prevention (CDC) have specifically called for research into alternative treatment options and enhanced surveillance.[11,12] One program specifically designed around resistant strains of gonorrhea is the CDC's "Strengthening the United States Response to Resistant Gonorrhea" (SURRG) program. This program has established partnerships between communities, cities, and states to improve detection and response capacity.

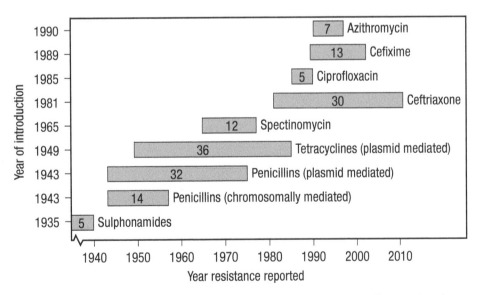

Figure 6.3 The history of antimicrobial resistance for *Neisseria gonorrhoeae*. On the x-axis is time in years. The length of the bar is the number of years from when the antibiotic was introduced until resistance was reported.

Source: Goire N, Lahra M, Chen M, et al. Molecular approaches to enhance surveillance of gonococcal antimicrobial resistance. *Nat Rev Microbiol*. 2014;12:223–229. doi:10.1038/nrmicro3217

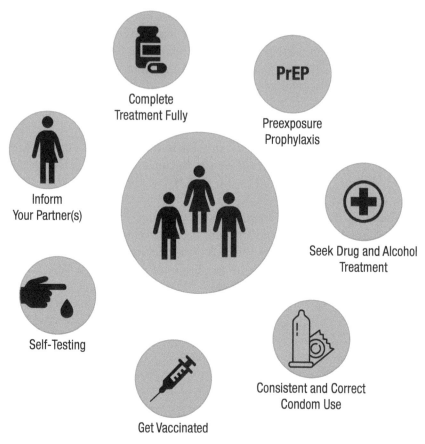

Figure 6.4 Interventions that individuals can take to reduce the transmission of STI. If they are at risk for HIV, PrEP can reduce the likelihood that an exposure becomes an infection. Getting the care needed for drug or alcohol abuse can reduce the likelihood of engaging in risky behaviors. Consistent and correct condom use protects against most STIs, and vaccination further protects against some viral infections. Knowing STI status through testing and sharing the status with partners can support access to treatment. Finally, completing and complying fully with treatment will support clearing the infection and reduce further antibiotic resistance.

Source: World Health Organization. *Self-care interventions for sexual and reproductive health*. https://www.who.int/images/default-source/infographics/self-care-interventions/self-care-srh.jpg?sfvrsn=f5108e1f_7

While drug-resistant gonorrhea is one of the more commonly cited resistant STIs, other pathogens are also showing increasing trends of resistance. In 2016, the WHO updated their treatment guidelines for chlamydia, gonorrhea, and syphilis in response to antibiotic resistance. While recurrence of chlamydia, caused by infection with *Chlamydia trachomatis*, was believed to be due to new re-infections, there is evidence that these recurrences may be due to treatment failure.[13] While the antibiotic resistance rates for chlamydia are not as high as with gonorrhea, it is a highly prevalent infection, so the number of resistant cases is high. Syphilis is further complicated by a shortage in the first-line treatment option, benzathine penicillin G, which has a small profit margin, high production cost, and with an active ingredient that is produced in only three factories.[14] These trends are reminders of the importance of not relying only on antibiotics, but also on promoting safe sexual behavior, including consistent and correct condom use (Figure 6.4). These trends also key in on the importance of breaking barriers to screening and testing to ensure those who need to be treated have access.

Given gonorrhea may present no symptoms, how do you think that compounds the issues of antibiotic resistance?

COINFECTIONS: SEXUALLY TRANSMITTED DISEASES AND OTHER DISEASES

Alone, infection with gonorrhea is bad enough. The asymptomatic nature of some infections further compounds our ability to treat the infection and reduce the disease burden. However, gonorrhea is also associated with increased acquisition and transmission of HIV.[15]

With the investment in research and drug development for the treatment of STIs there was concern over a paradox, sometimes called "treatment optimism," where effective treatment for one STI might lead to the rise of other STIs.[16] This refers to the perception that with effective treatment, prevention may be less important because subsequent disease will be more easily treatable. As a result, individuals may not assess the risk of infection as high and reduce their use of other prevention methods such as barrier prevention.[14] However, when systematically evaluating this concept, it appears that in many cases the riskier behavior changes pre-date the development of treatments, reminding us again of the importance of scientific advances into the treatment of disease.

Undetected infections, especially with certain STIs which often manifest with ulcers, like herpes and syphilis, or with inflammation, like gonorrhea and chlamydia, can increase the risk of being infected with other STIs, including HIV. The association goes beyond the behaviors that increase the risk of contracting an STI, such that the manifestation of the infection—swelling, sores, or breaks in the skin—may allow pathogens to pass more easily. In particular, individuals who have HIV and urethritis or a genital ulcer may be at increased likelihood of shedding HIV. This association can also be clinically relevant to detection; namely, coinfection with anogenital warts can be helpful for the detection of asymptomatic infections.[17]

Timely and adequate treatment is key to reducing the burden of STIs. The COVID-19 pandemic provided an interesting example of the effects of social behavior and delayed testing on STI. In spring 2020, health resources around the world shifted staff and funding resources to deal with the public health emergency of the COVID-19 pandemic. Although at the very beginning months of the pandemic changes in social behavior, including isolation and quarantine, did result in a drop of reported cases, STD rates subsequently surged.[18] Reduced screening, delayed detection, and redirected treatment resources likely influenced this surge.

What is the "treatment paradox" and does it outweigh the benefit of treatment?

IDENTIFYING RISK FACTORS AND KEY POPULATIONS

From Roman soldiers fighting with Julius Caesar (100–40 BCE) to the Crimean War (1854–1856 CE) to World War I when gonorrhea, along with syphilis, accounted for 10% of sick reports, gonorrhea has been associated with war.[19] This association continues today, with rates among the military higher than their civilian counterparts, although they also have higher screening rates.[20]

Sexual health is not equitable. Marginalized populations, such as sex workers, **men who have sex with men (MSM)**, injection drug users, and incarcerated populations, have the highest rates of STI. These disparities in reported rates of STD are not explained by sexual behavior, but rather by the lack of adequate access to health services and the interconnectedness of sexual networks. Rates of STD are higher among racial and ethnic minorities in the United States when compared to Whites. These disparities are driven by social conditions like poverty, economics, employment, and education level. Women suffer more frequent infections and more serious complications due to STI than men. This is due to biological differences (larger mucosal surface area, microabrasions during sex, and the greater presence of HIV in semen compared with vaginal secretions), cultural differences (norms where men have more partners or where women face abuse if they refuse sex), and economic differences (limited access to female-controlled prevention methods).[21] Youth (aged 15–24) account for half of all new STI diagnoses.[2] One of the issues is that adolescents may believe that condoms are just for use before the female partner starts using the pill, rather than recognizing them as the most effective prevention method against STIs among those who are sexually active.[22] Another issue includes concerns over confidentiality prohibiting care-seeking behavior.[23]

MSM: Men who have sex with men.

Each population has its own challenges and risk factors; however, for most STIs and most at-risk populations, the primary issues distill down to access: access to information, access to testing, and access to treatment. These services must also be offered confidentially. Addressing the global incidence of STIs must include adequately providing appropriate services to those in need. Improving medical provider knowledge, as well as gender-inclusive and trauma-guided healthcare, may increase care-seeking behavior.

Cohort Study

A cohort study design can be used to identify the key risk factors for the development of an STI among different populations. Unlike the case-control study which starts with diseased or non-diseased individuals, the **cohort study** starts with two communities or groups, one exposed and one not, to compare the development of disease between the two (Figure 6.5). If the groups are well selected such that there are limited differences except the exposure, differences in incidence may be due to that exposure. Because a cohort study is one that starts with exposed and non-exposed groups and follows them over time, cohort studies are incidence studies (able to collect data on new infections or disease), and we can compare the risks of developing disease by calculating the relative risk (RR).

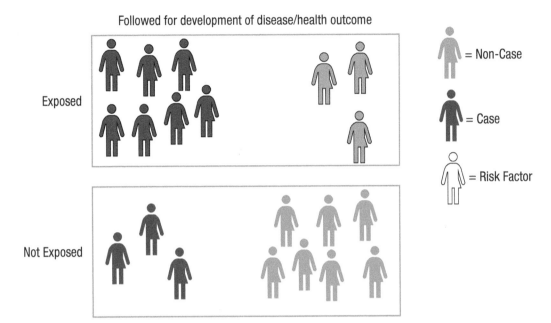

Figure 6.5 Schematic of a cohort study. Notice that individuals meeting the inclusion criteria are recruited into the study based on the exposure or risk factor status of the individual. Individuals are then followed over time to identify the development of the health outcomes of interest. Because of the follow-up, cohort studies are typically more expensive to conduct. However, a well-implemented cohort study generates useful data and can be used to support causal studies. Because we can calculate incidence, the measure of association that can be calculated is a relative risk (RR).

$$\text{Relative risk} = \frac{\text{Incidence among exposed}}{\text{Incidence among unexposed}} = \frac{\dfrac{\text{New cases among exposed}}{\text{Exposed population}}}{\dfrac{\text{New cases among unexposed}}{\text{Unexposed population}}}$$

The RR is intuitively interpreted as the ratio of the risk of developing disease among those exposed compared to the risk of developing disease among those not exposed. As with the odds ratio (OR), if the RR is 1, there is no difference in risk of developing disease and the exposure does not explain the outcome. If it is greater than 1, the risk of disease is greater among those exposed, and if it is less than 1, the exposure likely protects against the outcome.

The Longitudinal Survey of Adolescent Health Wave III (Add Health) is an example of a nationally representative cohort study with over 20,000 adolescents aged 7 to 12 who were interviewed five times as they were followed from adolescence into adulthood.[24] While a cohort study may be expensive and labor-intensive to perform because it follows individuals over time, the temporal component where exposures are documented prior to the outcome allows for a more rigorous assessment of an association.

cohort study: An incidence study where two groups, exposed and not exposed, are followed over time to compare the risk of developing a disease. The RR is the commonly calculated measure of effect.

THOUGHT QUESTION

We have learned about the case-control study and cohort study. Under which circum-stances do you think the cohort would be better suited and under which circumstances would the case-control be a better match? Be sure to think through the frequency of the outcome (is it an extremely rare disease such that it would take a long time to see enough cases for any statistical power), as well as the time you'd need for each study (and asso-ciated cost).

RIGOROUS STUDY DESIGNS

In 2012 and 2014, after a few years of decreases, gonorrhea rates jumped in Utah. While infection was more common in men than women, the rate of increase was larger among women and, while sexual behavior was not recorded for all patients, MSM rates also decreased over this period. Together these findings indicate an expansion of transmission into new sexual networks.[25]

Sexual behavior is usually a private activity and, as we have discussed, an activity and (potential) infection that carries social stigma. This may make the collection of precise but unbiased data challenging.[26] Large-scale behavioral level surveys may generate enough data for robust estimates of given behaviors but may not be sufficient to assess the mar-ginalized populations at higher risk of STI. Smaller, subgroup-specific surveys may reach these harder to reach populations but are typically costly and time consuming.

Partner and network studies are common to many person-to-person transmitted in-fections. These network analyses are critical to the control of STIs, but so far focus pri-marily on **Social network analysis (SNA)** to address prevention (Figure 6.6). Key exam-ples are SNA, **social network interventions (SNI)**, and **snowball sampling**. All of these methods use the social connectedness between individuals to recruit participants into a study or to push information into a network. Typically, SNA delineates the existing connections between individuals in a network and is commonly used to identify how a disease spreads within a network. Snowball sampling similarly uses connections, but as a means to recruit additional people within the network without explicitly identifying the connections. SNI, on the other hand, uses these formed social networks to dissemi-nate information about STI prevention, recruitment for testing and treatment, and sup-porting treatment adherence.[27] Specifically for sexual health interventions, SNI has been shown as more effective compared with other types of interventions 6 to 12 months after starting.[28]

social network analysis (SNA): A methodology to map and analyze the connections between individuals within groups.

social network intervention (SNI): A methodology to use social networks in order to influence healthy behavior.

snowball sampling: A methodology by which individuals recruited into a study are asked to recruit additional participants, thereby *snowballing* the effect of the sampling.

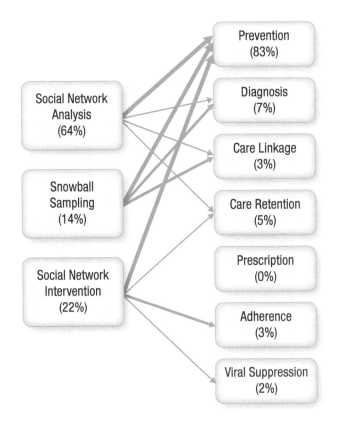

Figure 6.6 **Results from a me-ta-analysis of 58 papers performed to assess methodology and common health applications for each social network-based strategy along the HIV care continuum. The left side indicates the methodologies while the right side are the outcomes. The thickness of the arrows indicates the frequency of connection: thickest is 81% to 88% of papers, medium thickness indicates 13% to 15% of the papers, and the thinnest is less than 10%.**
Source: Data from Ghosh D, Krishnan A, Gibson B, Brown SE, Latkin CA, Altice FL. Social network strategies to address HIV prevention and treatment continuum of care among at-risk and HIV-infected substance users: a systematic scoping review. *AIDS Behav.* 2017;21(4):1183–1207. doi:10.1007/s10461-016-1413-y

As with other infectious diseases, the reproduction number, R_0, is an effective way to describe the population-level spread of an STI. When estimating the number of new cases of a STI generated by an infected individual in a fully susceptible population for STIs, the mean rate of partner change is also considered. Thus, for STIs R_0 is calculated as:

$$R_0 = \beta c D,$$

where β is the transmission rate, namely the frequency of contacting infected individuals and the probability that that interaction will lead to transmission, and D is the duration of infectiousness (also written as $1/\gamma$, the inverse of recovery). For STIs, the additional term c is included, the mean rate of partner change—and again we are faced with issues around social stigma in accurate reporting. The reproduction number is still interpreted as when R_0 is less than *1 the disease dies out, when R_0 equals 1 the disease is stable, and when R_0 is greater than 1 the disease spreads. R_0* is usually estimated at the population level; however, estimating the rate of partner change can be successfully implemented through surveys of STD patients and the previously mentioned tools, including SNA and cohort studies.[29]

Bias

While many study designs will be subject to biases (Figure 6.7), the social norms around STI research may make it particularly prone to two types of bias. **Participation bias** is a form of **selection bias**, where the characteristics of those who agree to participate are different from those who do not agree to participate. For example, only certain individuals may feel comfortable enough participating in surveys about their sex lives. **Social**

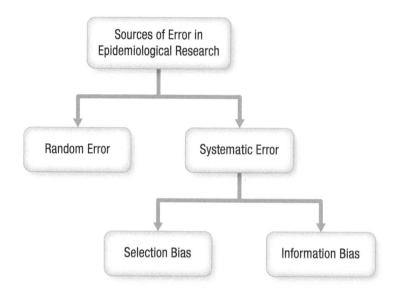

Figure 6.7 **Schematic of the potential sources of error in epidemiological research.**

desirability bias is a form of **information bias**, where the data collected may be biased when participants respond based on how they think the answers reflect on them as individuals. Participants may not feel comfortable responding truthfully to sensitive questions. Biases are a risk to internal validity of a study, that is, finding associations between the risk factors and outcome that are not real or missing actual associations. Information bias can lead to the over- or underestimation of an association, while selection bias will also influence external validity, that is, the ability to extrapolate from the sample to the source population (generalizability).

Study design and use of statistics help to address potential errors in research. Statistical inference is used to address whether the findings are due to random error or a true association. In contrast, biases are removed or limited through a careful focus on how the data are collected. Participation bias and social desirability biases are significant sources of error in estimating sexual behavioral risk factors. Interviewer training or computer-assisted self-interviewing can reduce some response bias by reducing the participant's feelings about being judged on their responses, supporting anonymous reporting, or removing the interviewer altogether. Offering reminders and providing information that the results are anonymous and confidential and ensuring that answers and questions are presented as neutral can also help to reduce social desirability bias.[30] Separately interviewing and comparing partner information and checking for consistency in answers both across partners and within an individual's responses also can be used to validate the data collected.

participation bias: A systematic error that occurs when the characteristics of those who agree to participate are different from those who do not.

selection bias: A systematic error that occurs when the individuals selected for the sample do not accurately represent the source population.

information bias: A systematic error in the way that information is collected.

social desirability bias: A systematic error that occurs when individuals answer questions in a way that may reflect more favorably on them.

THOUGHT QUESTION

If you were designing a study to identify risk factors associated with adolescent STI, what special actions would you do to reduce bias in your study?

CASE STUDY

During the 1950s, family planning was equated with loose morals and promiscuity. Unmarried women and youth had limited access to contraception, STI testing and treatment, or welcoming clinics to go to for services. Even married women often had limited control over their own contraception choices.

In response, family planning clinics started to fill this role by expanding services to all those who wanted access. One leading figure was Helen Brook. Brook was born in 1907 in London, United Kingdom. Driven by the knowledge that women should be able to make their own choices about their sexual health, she started informational sessions to educate young people about family planning options. By 1964, she opened the first Brook Advisory Centre in London. In these centers, clinicans, counselors, and social workers provided for the sexual health needs of young, unmarried individuals in a supportive environment. These centers are still in existence today providing free, confidential advice to more than 1.3 million under 25 across the United Kingdom (Brook.org.uk).[31] Some have argued that the listening approach used by the staff at the Brook Advisory Centres has had broader implications on how young adults in the United Kingdom view their sexuality, normalizing sexual behaviors.[32]

In 1995 Brook was awarded the Most Excellent Order of the British Empire (CBE) for her work in family planning and she has been recognized as one of the seven women with the largest influence on women's lives over seven decades by the BBC Radio Four's Woman's Hour.

CONCLUSION

Because STIs may be asymptomatic and thus under-reported and because of the stigma that remains about human sexuality, the true burden of STIs is hard to estimate. Addressing STIs includes strengthening STI surveillance, including that of antibiotic resistance, as well as ensuring access to information and services and better and less expensive technologies for diagnosing STIs.[33] While any medical facility should be supportive to their population, improving medical provider knowledge, as well as gender-inclusive and trauma-guided healthcare, are particularly important for STI work. One underutilized strategy in STI prevention, testing, and treatment is the use of existing social networks to not only collect data, but to disseminate information about STI prevention, testing, and treatment.

TEACHING CORNER

DID YOU KNOW?

About half of new STIs occur among adolescents. Figure 6.8 shows that by 15 years old, only 22% of adolescents have had sexual intercourse. However, by 18 years old, this is almost 3 times as high, 65%. That is, about two-thirds have had sex, compared to less than one-quarter just 3 years earlier. That also means that this is a critical time period to engage in order to prevent STI. However, being not yet 18, parental consent will be necessary and may result in a selection bias—parents not allowing their kids to participate. Approaching this group would require special training and a supportive/nonjudgmental environment.

TRY THIS

Design a cohort study for adolescents to assess the effect of high school sex education on the development of an STI. Why is a cohort study an appropriate study design for adolescent STIs? What biases are you concerned about for your cohort study and how will you address them?

TAKE IT A STEP FURTHER

In your hypothetical cohort study, you recruited high school freshmen who are sexually active but screen negative to any STI into your study from two different high schools (250 from each high school). One high school has a robust sex education program while

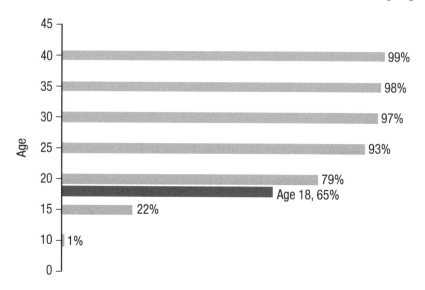

Figure 6.8 Age at onset of sexual activity.

Source: Data from Keller LH. Reducing STI cases: young people deserve better sexual health information and services. April 2, 2020. https://www.guttmacher.org/gpr/2020/04/reducing-sti-cases-young-people-deserve-better-sexual-health-information-and-services

the other focuses only on abstinence. The students are followed over the 4 years of high school and the first infection with chlamydia is recorded. Over the 4 years you follow the students you have zero drop out, and 100 students in the abstinence-only high school are diagnosed with chlamydia compared with 25 in the robust sex-ed program. Complete a 2x2 contingency table and calculate the appropriate measure of effect. Interpret the results in both "epi -speak" as well as how you might explain it during a media interview.

QUESTIONS FOR FURTHER DISCUSSION

1. List four serious consequences of infection with STI beyond the initial infection itself.

2. List and describe three barriers to reducing the burden of STI.

3. Describe how improving STI surveillance will improve STI treatment. Be sure to include the influence of social stigma and asymptomatic infection.

4. Distinguish between information and selection bias and list one way to reduce each.

A robust set of instructor resources designed to supplement this text is located at http://connect.springerpub.com/Content/book/978-0-8261-5674-7. Qualifying instructors may request access by emailing textbook@springerpub.com.

REFERENCES

1. World Health Organization. *Global health sector strategy on sexually transmitted infections, 2016–2021.* October 3, 2016. https://www.who.int/publications/i/item/WHO-RHR-16.09
2. Kreisel KM, Spicknall IH, Gargano JW, et al. Sexually transmitted infections among US women and men: prevalence and incidence estimates, 2018. *Sex Transm Dis.* 2021;48(4):208–214. doi:10.1097/OLQ.0000000000001355
3. Patel CG, Trivedi S, Tao G. The proportion of young women tested for chlamydia who had urogenital symptoms in physician offices. *Sex Transm Dis.* 2018;45(9):e72–e74. doi:10.1097/OLQ.0000000000000858
4. Gerbase AC, Rowley JT, Mertens TE. Global epidemiology of sexually transmitted diseases. *Lancet.* 1998;351:S2–S4. doi:10.1016/S0140-6736(98)90001-0
5. Lei J, Ploner A, Elfström KM, et al. HPV vaccination and the risk of invasive cervical cancer. *N Engl J Med.* 2020;383(14):1340–1348. doi:10.1056/NEJMoa1917338
6. Centers for Disease Control and Prevention. Pre-exposure prophylaxis (PrEP). https://www.cdc.gov/hiv/risk/prep/index.html
7. Barth KR, Cook RL, Downs JS, Switzer GE, Fischhoff B. Social stigma and negative consequences: factors that influence college students' decisions to seek testing for sexually transmitted infections. *J Am Coll Health.* 2002;50(4):153–159. doi:10.1080/07448480209596021
8. Winskell K, Sabben G. Sexual stigma and symbolic violence experienced, enacted, and counteracted in young Africans' writing about same-sex attraction. *Soc Sci Med.* 2016;161:143–150. doi:10.1016/j.socscimed.2016.06.004
9. Morris JL, Lippman SA, Philip S, Bernstein K, Neilands TB, Lightfoot M. Sexually transmitted infection related stigma and shame among African American male youth: implications for testing practices, partner notification, and treatment. *AIDS Patient Care STDS.* 2014;28(9):499–506. doi:10.1089/apc.2013.0316
10. Goire N, Lahra MM, Chen M, et al. Molecular approaches to enhance surveillance of gonococcal antimicrobial resistance. *Nat Rev Microbiol.* 2014;12(3):223–229. doi:10.1038/nrmicro3217
11. Kidd S, Kirkcaldy R, Ye T, Papp J, Trees D, Shapiro SJ. *Ceftriaxone-Resistant* Neisseria Gonorrhoeae *Public Health Response Plan.* Centers for Disease Control and Prevention. August 2012. http://www.cdc.gov/std/treatment/Ceph-R-ResponsePlanJuly30-2012.pdf

12. World Health Organization Department of Reproductive Health and Research. *Global Action Plan to Control the Spread and Impact of Antimicrobial Resistance in* Neisseria Gonorrhoeae. 2012. http://whqlibdoc.who.int/publications/2012/9789241503501_eng.pdf

13. Krupp K, Madhivanan P. Antibiotic resistance in prevalent bacterial and protozoan sexually transmitted infections. *Indian J Sex Transm Dis AIDS.* 2015;36(1):3–8. doi:10.4103/0253-7184 .156680

14. de Vries H. Current challenges in the clinical management of sexually transmitted infections. *J Int AIDS Soc.* 2019; 22(S6):e25347. doi:10.1002/jia2.25347

15. Laga M, Manoka A, Kivuvu M, et al. Non-ulcerative sexually transmitted diseases as risk factors for HIV-1 transmission in women: results from a cohort study. *AIDS (London, England).* 1993;7(1):95–102. doi:10.1097/00002030-199301000-00015

16. Lert F. Advances in HIV treatment and prevention: should treatment optimism lead to prevention pessimism? *AIDS Care.* 2000;12(6):745–755. doi:10.1080/09540120020014291

17. Wang L, Yang B, Tso LS, et al. Prevalence of co-infections with other sexually transmitted infections in patients newly diagnosed with anogenital warts in Guangzhou, China. *Int J STD AIDS.* 2020;31(11):1073–1081. doi:10.1177/0956462419890496

18. Pagaoa M, Grey J, Torrone E, Kreisel K, Stenger M, Weinstock H. Trends in nationally notifiable sexually transmitted disease case reports during the US COVID-19 pandemic, January to December 2020. *Sex Transm Dis.*2021;48(10):798–804. doi:10.1097/OLQ.0000000000001506

19. Speaker SL. "*Fit to fight*": home front Army doctors and VD during WWI. National Library of Medicine. https://circulatingnow.nlm.nih.gov/2018/10/18/fit-to-fight-home-front-army -doctors-and-vd-during-ww-i/#:~:text=From%20April%201917%20(when%20the,in%20 6%2C804%2C818%20duty%20days%20lost

20. Deiss R, Bower RJ, Co E, et al. The association between sexually transmitted infections, length of service and other demographic factors in the U.S. military. *PLoS ONE.* 2016;11(12):e0167892. doi:10.1371/journal.pone.0167892

21. Aral SO, Hawkes S, Biddlecom A, Padian N. Disproportionate impact of sexually transmitted diseases on women. *Emerg Infect Dis.* 2004;10(11):2029–2030. doi:10.3201/eid1011.040623_02

22. Samkange-Zeeb FN, Spallek L, Zeeb H. Awareness and knowledge of sexually transmitted diseases (STDs) among school-going adolescents in Europe: a systematic review of published literature. *BMC Public Health.* 2011;11:727. doi:10.1186/1471-2458-11-727

23. Leichliter JS, Copen C, Dittus PJ. Confidentiality issues and use of sexually transmitted disease services among sexually experienced persons aged 15–25 years—United States, 2013–2015. *MMWR Morb Mortal Wkly Rep.* 2017;66:237–241. doi:10.15585/mmwr.mm6609a1

24. Harris KM, Halpern CT, Whitsel EA, et al. Cohort profile: the national longitudinal study of adolescent to adult health (add health). *Int J Epidemiol.* 2019;48(5):1415–1415k. doi:10.1093/ije/ dyz115

25. Watson J, Carlile J, Dunn A, et al. Increased gonorrhea cases—Utah, 2009–2014. *MMWR Morb Mortal Wkly Rep.* 2016;65:889–893. doi:10.15585/mmwr.mm6534a1

26. Fenton KA, Johnson AM, McManus S, Erens B. Measuring sexual behaviour: methodological challenges in survey research. *Sex Transm Infections.* 2001;77:84–92. doi:10.1136/sti.77.2.84

27. Ghosh D, Krishnan A, Gibson B, Brown SE, Latkin CA, Altice FL. Social network strategies to address HIV prevention and treatment continuum of care among at-risk and HIV-infected substance users: a systematic scoping review. *AIDS Behav.* 2017;21(4):1183–1207. doi:10.1007/ s10461-016-1413-y

28. Hunter RF, de la Haye K, Murray JM, et al. Social network interventions for health behaviours and outcomes: a systematic review and meta-analysis. *PLoS Med.* 2019;16(9):e1002890. doi:10.1371/journal.pmed.1002890

29. Nagelkerke NJ, Brunham RC, Moses S, Plummer FA. Estimating the effective rate of sex partner change from individuals with sexually transmitted diseases. *Sex Transm Dis.* 1994;21(4):226– 230. doi:10.1097/00007435-199407000-00009

30. Larson RB. Controlling social desirability bias. *Int J Mark Res.* 2019;61(5):534–547. doi:10 .1177/1470785318805305

31. Brook. Our story. https://www.brook.org.uk/about-brook/our-story

32. Rusterholz C. "If we can show that we are helping adolescents to understand themselves, their feelings and their needs, then we are doing [a] valuable job": counselling young people on sexual health in the Brook Advisory Centre (1965–1985). *Med Humanit.* Published online August 23, 2021. doi:10.1136/medhum-2021-012206

33. Ortalyi N, Ringheim K, Collins L, Sladden T. Sexually transmitted infections: progress and challenges since the 1994 International Conference on Population and Development (ICPD). *Contraception.* 2014;90(6):S22–S31. doi:10.1016/j.contraception.2014.06.024

CHAPTER 7

GASTROINTESTINAL OR FOOD-BORNE DISEASE

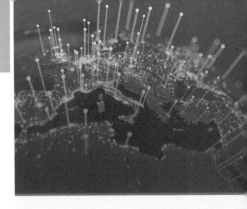

INTRODUCTION

What is healthier than water? It's refreshing and hydrating. What about those nutritious leafy greens? Will they prevent your risk of stomach cancer? Obesity? Heart disease? Leafy greens are great! With high fiber, minerals, and vitamins content, eating leafy greens seems to be the answer to everything. But when improperly handled, these healthy options are the source of stomach cramps, diarrhea, vomiting, and sometimes long-lasting disability or even death.

Take, for example, a county fair: rides, funnel cakes, lemonade, and crushed ice. New York's largest agricultural fair is held in Washington County where more than 100,000 visitors tromp through farm animal displays, rides, and concession stands in just 1 week. However, runoff contaminated a well that was subsequently used for ice and beverages; as a result, about 1,000 people were sick, 65 were hospitalized, and two died. The causal organisms: Escherichia coli 0157:H7 *and* Campylobacter.

LEARNING OBJECTIVES

By the end of this chapter, readers will be able to:

- Describe the effects of food-borne disease on health.
- List the unique epidemiologic approaches to assess a food-borne exposure.
- Discuss proven preventive measures to prevent food-borne disease.
- Explain the effect of climate change on food security.

FOOD- AND WATER-BORNE DISEASE BURDEN

In September 1999, the New York Department of Health received reports of at least 10 children with bloody diarrhea. All of those children, along with about 108,000 other people, had attended the Washington County Fair. By the end of the outbreak investigation, 921 fair attendees reported diarrhea, 65 were hospitalized, 11 children developed the potentially life-threatening hemolytic uremic syndrome (HUS), and two people died. Six defendants, including a university and its cooperative extension, were sued for $10 million in damages. Read more about this outbreak at www.cdc.gov/mmwr/preview/mmwrhtml/mm4836a4.htm.

Globally, food-borne disease is the cause of about 600 million cases (one in 10 people get ill), resulting in 420,000 deaths, approximately 30% of which occur among children under 5 years old.[1] According to the U.S. Centers for Disease Control and Prevention (CDC), about one in six Americans get sick each year because of a food-borne disease.[2] Among these cases, there are about 130,000 hospitalizations and 3,000 deaths.[3] However, these are believed to be underestimated and the pathogen is identified in only about 20% of cases.[4] To count a case of food-borne disease, it must be reported, which means it needs to be tested in a laboratory, which requires that an environmental or host sample needs to be collected, which usually requires the person to seek care, which means the symptoms were severe (Figure 7.1). Thus, the reported cases of food-borne disease are, like many other diseases, only the tip of the iceberg of the actual burden of these diseases.

Tracking and estimating the impact of these illnesses can be challenging, not just because of the underreported information, but also in the story the data can tell. There are many different ways to describe food-borne disease and its effects on human health and no one statistic can adequately capture this diversity. While there are approximately 30 pathogens that constitute the major food-borne disease pathogens, a far fewer number of pathogens are responsible for 90% of food-borne disease (Figure 7.2). When we start to think about impact, we can consider various approaches to measuring the burden of food-borne disease. While over half of food-borne illness is caused by norovirus, non-typhoidal *Salmonella spp.* is the most common cause of death, accounting for about a quarter of all food-borne disease deaths.[2,4]

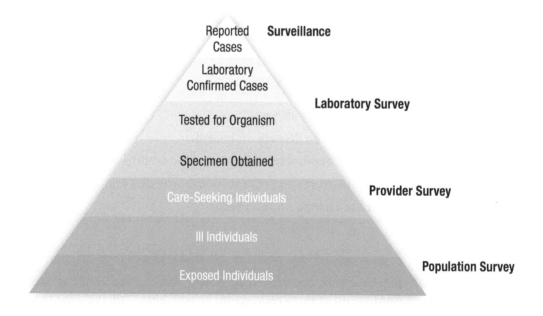

Figure 7.1 **The disease burden pyramid. For many diseases, including food-borne diseases,** where symptoms vary from mild to life-threatening and even death, the cases that are reported are only a very small percentage of the actual number of cases that occur.

Source: Centers for Disease Control and Prevention. Foodborne Diseases Active Surveillance Network (FoodNet): FoodNet surveillance. https://www.cdc.gov/foodnet/surveillance.html

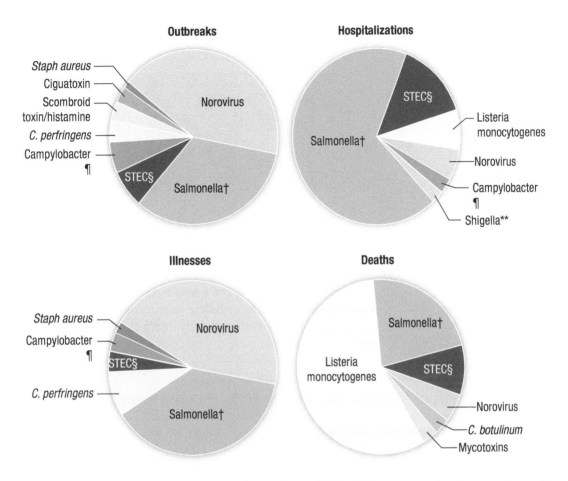

Figure 7.2 These pathogens account for at least 90% of the reported outcomes in each category (outbreaks, hospitalizations, illnesses, deaths).

† 22 Salmonella serotypes causing more than five outbreaks; § 10 STEC serogroups; ¶ multiple known and unknown Campylobacter species; ** multiple known and unknown Shigella species.

STEC, Shiga-toxin-producing *Escherichia coli*.

Source: Data from Dewey-Mattia D, Manikonda K, Hall AJ, Wise ME, Crowe SJ. Surveillance for food-borne disease outbreaks — United States, 2009–2015. *MMWR Surveill Summ*. 2018;67(No. SS-10):1–11. doi:10.15585/mmwr.ss6710a1

While counting cases (incidence) and deaths (mortality rates and case fatality rates) is helpful in comparing and characterizing the effects of food-borne diseases, they provide only a partial view of the burden of these diseases. **Disability-adjusted life years (DALY)** is an alternative measure of the burden of disease which combines years of life lost to premature mortality with the years of life lost due to living in less than full health (i.e., healthy life lost due to disability). Relatedly, the **quality adjusted life years (QALY)** is the reciprocal of the DALY, focusing on the length of time in a healthy state (Figure 7.3). These metrics are helpful for diseases that don't cause death but do cause disability. It is estimated that 14 of the major food-borne pathogens incur about 61,000 QALY per year[5] and diarrheal diseases alone, for which food- and water-borne diseases are the primary cause, are responsible for 3.6% of total DALY worldwide.[6] It is worth noting, though, that the burden of diarrheal diseases has decreased by 85.4% between 1990 and 2017 as a result of considerable improvements in hygiene and sanitation, access to better nutrition, increased

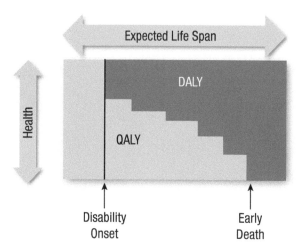

Figure 7.3 The relationship between quality-adjusted life years (QALY) and disability-adjusted life years (DALY). The expected life span is shown along the x-axis and health indicated on the y-axis. If a food-borne illness were to occur early in life with long-term increasingly debilitating sequelae, the QALY would decrease as DALY increased until early death.

breastfeeding, better supplemental feeding, increased use of oral rehydration therapy (commonly known as ORT), and certain immunizations.[7] Perhaps more than case counting, DALY captures the disproportionate effect these diseases exact.

In addition to considering the health burden, food-borne disease carries a clear economic burden. Within the United States, the economic burden from food-borne disease is estimated at $15.5 billion annually.[4] Among low- and middle-income economies, the World Bank estimates the economic burden is about $110 billion.[8] These economic costs include work or school absenteeism, with resultant lost wages and treatment costs incurred for the infected individual. If the source is also contaminated food at a food production, processing, or distribution site, there may also be the cost of recalls and destroying contaminated foods, as well as reductions in sales and potential job loss (Figure 7.4). For example, a 2015 Listeria outbreak at an ice cream production company that resulted in 10 cases across four U.S. states and three deaths also resulted in almost 1,500 workers (37% of the company's employees) losing their job due to the production shutdown.[9] Because a large proportion of the costs could be avoided through improvement in food handling, companies are being held accountable when they are responsible for outbreaks. That 2015 Listeria outbreak also garnered a fine of $17.25 million in criminal penalties to the company responsible, citing conditions in violation of the Food, Drug and Cosmetic Act.[10]

disability-adjusted life years (DALY): An alternative measure of the burden of disease which combines years of life lost to premature mortality with the years of life lost due to living in less than full health (i.e., healthy life lost due to disability).

quality-adjusted life years (QALY): An alternative measure of the burden of disease which is a measure of the quality and quantity of life lived.

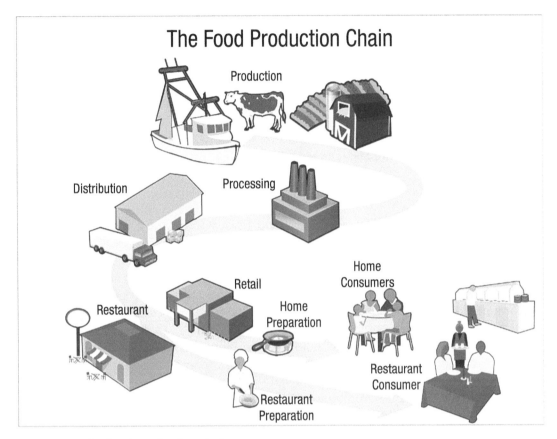

Figure 7.4 **The food production chain.**

Source: Centers for Disease Control and Prevention. Foodborne outbreaks. November 20, 2013. https://www.cdc.gov/foodsafety/outbreaks/investigating-outbreaks/figure_food_production.html

Common Food-Borne Disease Pathogens

While it is hard to rank the most important food-borne disease because of the myriad of effects they have (most cases, most hospitalizations, high case fatality rates, great economic burden), there are some common food-borne pathogens most commonly reported in the United States.

ESCHERICHIA COLI

Escherichia coli (*E. coli*) are a group of gram-negative, motile bacteria that naturally infect the intestinal tracts of humans and other animals. Most strains are nonpathogenic, but some can cause mild to severe diarrhea. *E. coli* are grouped onto **pathotypes** based on their virulence, as well as their pathogenic, mechanic, and clinical manifestations: shiga toxin-producing *E. coli* (STEC), enterotoxigenic *E. coli* (ETEC), enteropathogenic *E. coli* (EPEC), enteroaggregative *E. coli* (EAEC), enteroinvasive *E. coli* (EIEC), and diffusely adherent *E. coli* (DAEC). STEC, sometimes also called verocytotoxin-producing (VTEC) or enterohemorrhagic (EHEC), is the type most commonly associated with food-borne outbreaks.[11]

Symptoms vary by pathotype but include stomach cramps, diarrhea (often bloody), and vomiting. Most people will recover without treatment within about a week, but the dehydration due to vomiting and diarrhea can be severe. About 5% to 10% of those who are diagnosed with STEC may develop HUS, which can be life-threatening. Transmission is typically fecal-oral. Fresh produce that is contaminated pre-harvest and ground beef that is contaminated during the slaughtering process are common infection sources. *E. coli* can survive in soil for long periods of time, potentially contaminating fruits and vegetables.

pathotype: A further classification of microorganism which distinguishes within species based on differences in virulence and the pathology (i.e., disease it causes).

NOROVIRUS

Noroviruses are non-enveloped, single-stranded RNA viruses in the Caliciviridae group that are the most common cause of food-borne illness. Nearly 60% of cases occur among older adults and those in nursing care facilities. Norovirus is highly contagious. While fewer than 100 viral particles are needed to infect a person, a sick individual may shed billions, and these particles may survive on improperly cleaned surfaces for days or even weeks.

Norovirus outbreaks are those we often associate with large groups of people coming together, like cruise ships, nursing care homes, and schools. The most common transmission modes are direct contact with an infected person, contaminated food or water, or contact with contaminated surfaces and subsequently putting contaminated hands in one's mouth. Foods eaten raw or "ready to eat" foods are the most commonly implicated food sources, which may be contaminated during food handling. Norovirus primarily causes acute gastroenteritis (inflammation of the stomach and/or intestines), resulting in rapid onset vomiting and diarrhea.

SALMONELLA

Salmonella are rod-shaped, gram-negative bacteria of the family Enterobacteriaceae. The bacteria infect the intestines of people and animals. Illness due to most types of *Salmonella* is called salmonellosis, but certain strains cause typhoid fever or paratyphoid fever. While consuming contaminated food or water is the most common source of most infections, exposure to infected animals, especially chickens and reptiles, their feces, or their environment, are additional sources. Contact with pets and animals at petting zoos, farms, fairs, and schools may also result in *Salmonella* exposure.

Most people recover without treatment, although antibiotics may be necessary for severe or high-risk cases. However, resistance to essential antibiotics is increasing, which can limit treatment options for people with severe infections. With more than 2,000 serotypes of *Salmonella*, the diversity in symptoms is correspondingly large. Diarrhea—sometimes bloody—fever, and stomach cramps are common symptoms though some people may also experience nausea, vomiting, or headache.

Many of us know the story of Typhoid Mary Mallon, the household cook who ignored public health orders and spread typhoid to multiple families in the northeastern United States until finally stopped only through imprisonment. *Salmonella* serotype Typhi and *Salmonella* serotype Paratyphi are the causal agents for the life-threatening illnesses typhoid fever and paratyphoid fever, respectively. In modern times, most U.S. cases of typhoid fever or paratyphoid fever are the result of travel to countries where these diseases are common. Vaccination against typhoid fever is recommended for travelers to endemic areas.

CLOSTRIDIUM PERFRINGENS

Clostridium perfringens are gram-positive, rod-shaped, spore-forming bacteria in the same genus as the pathogens that cause botulism and tetanus. *C. perfringens* infect raw meat and poultry and are naturally occurring in animal intestines and the environment. The bacteria are able to form a spore which supports its survival by protecting them from adverse conditions.

Food maintained at unsafe temperatures after cooking supports the rapid growth of these bacteria. After ingestion, the bacteria produce a toxin (poison) that causes diarrhea. Symptoms like diarrhea and stomach cramping occur soon after consuming contaminated food, but just as there is rapid onset, it usually lasts less than a day. Most people who are infected with *C. perfringens* do not get a diagnosis. When treatment is necessary, antibiotics may be effective; however, dehydration due to diarrhea is the primary concern. Fever or vomiting are rare, and the pathogen is not passed from person to person.

CAMPYLOBACTER

Campylobacter is a genus of gram-negative bacteria which are comma- or s-shaped and motile. Raw or undercooked poultry, or something that was contaminated by raw or undercooked poultry, are the most common infection sources. Other foods, such as seafood, meat, or produce, as well as contact with animals or drinking untreated water, are also potential sources.

Symptoms of *Campylobacter* infection include diarrhea (often bloody), fever, and stomach cramps. For some people nausea and vomiting may also occur. Symptoms start within 2 to 5 days after infection and usually last about a week. On rare occasions, *Campylobacter* can spread into the bloodstream and result in life-threatening infection, particularly among immunocompromised individuals. Most infections are self-limiting, but antibiotic treatment may be necessary in severe cases.

STAPHYLOCOCCUS AUREUS (STAPH)

S. aureus is a gram-positive nonsporulating bacteria that is ubiquitous. It is naturally present in the skin, hair, and nasal passages of about a quarter of all humans and other animals. In most healthy people, it is nonpathogenic, but the bacteria can produce a toxin. Unsafe food handling is a common source of contamination; while heating food will kill the bacteria, it will not deactivate the toxin.

Symptoms, including nausea, vomiting, stomach cramping, and diarrhea, can occur as soon as 30 minutes after ingestion of food contaminated with *S. aureus*. Severe illness is uncommon, and symptoms usually dissipate within 24 hours. Because unsafe food-handling is associated with transmission, foods implicated are those that require preparation like salads. *S. aureus* is a bacterial disease, so antibiotics are a front-line treatment for very sick individuals. However, the pathogen has adapted: methicillin-resistant *Staphylococcus aureus* (MRSA) is a form of the bacteria that is exceptionally hard to treat because of its acquisition of resistance to several antibiotics. Untreated, it can be severe and cause sepsis, and it is particularly problematic if an outbreak occurs in hospitals or nursing homes because of the combination of treatment challenge and susceptible populations.

Think about the classic food-borne disease outbreaks you've heard about. Using just the food involved and the circumstances around transmission, can you classify the likely pathogen into one of these groups? For example, what was the likely contamination source for egg salad at a summer picnic? What about jalapeño peppers from the grocery store: When were they contaminated and which pathogens would you test for first?

HOW DO WE ASSESS AN EXPOSURE

Stool samples from the hospitalized children were positive for E. coli O157:H7, *while* Campylobacter jejuni *was later identified among other fair attendees. Hospitals and laboratories in the region were asked to test stool specimens for both pathogens. To determine risk factors for infection, a case-control study was initiated where controls were frequency-matched by age group. These individuals, who were also residents of Washington County and had attended the fair, were selected from the telephone directory. Through this analysis, the infection source at the fair was found to be associated with infection (OR = 23.3, 95% CI: 6.3–86.9).*[12]

When alerted to a possible food-borne disease outbreak, three types of data support identifying the source: (a) epidemiologic, (b) traceback, and (c) food and environmental testing (Figure 7.5). **Epidemiologic data** help to uncover the patterns by looking at where and when cases are occurring and comparing them to prior outbreaks. The next source of data is **traceback data**, which documents the distribution and production chain of an implicated food-borne disease source. These data are generated by careful interview and record review and are useful to (a) identify the trail from source to market of implicated food so it can be removed, and to (b) discriminate between possible sources. Finally, **food and environmental testing data** are integral to identifying the specific causal pathogen. The pathogen is defined through the collection of food items, patient samples, and environmental samples that might be sources of infection. Molecular assays can be used to explicitly identify the causative agent.

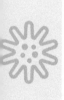

epidemiologic data: Data describing the person, place, and time of an exposure or outcome of interest.

traceback data: Data generated by tracing back from the marketplace to the source which describes the distribution chain in an effort to identify the contamination course.

food and environmental testing data: Laboratory data used to confirm the pathogen from food and environmental samples.

Case-Control Study

In trying to discover the extent of an outbreak, two primary epidemiologic tools are commonly used: first, the case-control study, and second, a cohort study. Both need a strong case definition which usually includes both clinical symptomatology as well as any available diagnostic tests. The **case definition** is a set of criteria used to classify individuals as

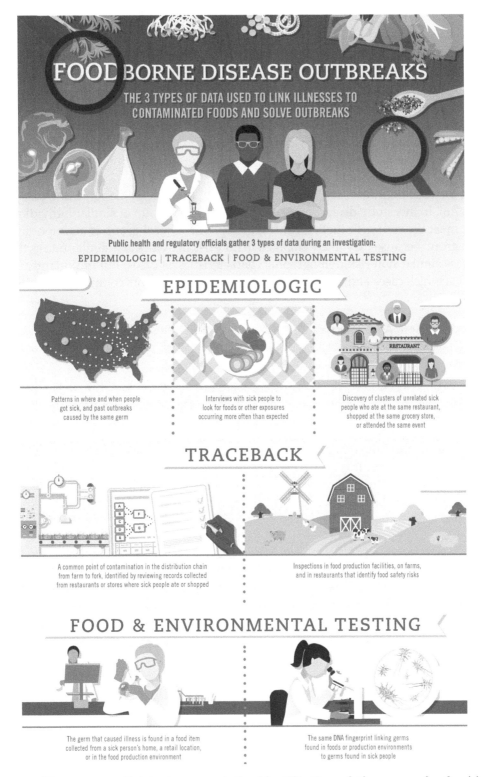

Figure 7.5 Three types of data to support the identification of the source for food-borne disease outbreaks.

Source: Centers for Disease Control and Prevention. Foodborne disease outbreaks. Accessed July 9, 2022. https://www.cdc.gov/foodsafety/outbreaks/pdfs/outbreak-infographic.pdf

having the health condition being assessed. For Nationally Notifiable Diseases Surveillance, there are accepted surveillance case definitions which are agreed upon and adopted by Council of State and Territorial Epidemiologists, the CDC, and other organizations. Occasionally, when the infection is unknown or when specific situations necessitate, outbreak-specific criteria may be set, and a broad food and exposure questionnaire is used to narrow down possible exposures. A standard case definition ensures the same criteria are applied at any location, any time, and by any member of the investigation/diagnostic team and allows for comparisons between outbreaks, locations, and times. It also ensures that observed differences are actual differences and not because of differences in how a case was classified.

With the case definition set, the most commonly used study design is the case-control (Figure 7.6). In this study design, cases are compared to a group of similar individuals who did not meet the case definition, a **control** group. The control group is an important comparison group because they likely engaged in non-risk activities at a similar rate as the cases or possess similar non-risk demographic characteristics as cases. But importantly, the key factors via which cases and controls differ may be the risk factors contributing to disease.

case definition: A set of criteria used to classify individuals as having the health condition being assessed; they may include only symptomology or may include laboratory confirmation.

odds ratio: The ratio of the odds of exposure among cases over the odds among non-exposed. It is the commonly calculated measure of effect for case-control studies.

The case-control study is an *observational study* because the researchers do not manipulate the exposures. It is also an *analytical study* design because it can be used to test hypotheses, specifically that cases and controls differ by key characteristics which might explain the higher disease rates among the former. Case-control studies are known as prevalence studies because they start with existing cases, rather than identifying new

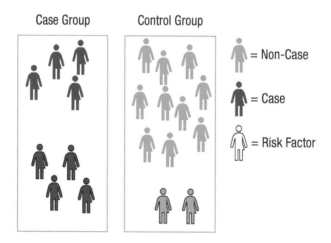

Figure 7.6 Schematic of a case-control study. Notice that we select the groups based on case or control, and then identify those individuals who were exposed or have the risk factor of interest.

cases. Because we start the case-control study with existing cases, we can calculate an **odds ratio** to compare potential exposures between cases and controls.

$$\text{Odds ratio} = \frac{\dfrac{\text{Exposed cases}}{\text{Unexposed cases}}}{\dfrac{\text{Exposed controls}}{\text{Unexposed controls}}}$$

Interpreting this comparison, we look at both the point estimate, the OR, and the confidence interval. When the point estimate is equal to 1, then there is no difference in the numerator (odds of exposure among cases) and the denominator (odds of exposure among controls) and it is unlikely that the exposure is associated with the observed outcome. When the OR is greater than 1, the exposure is more common in cases. When it is less than 1, the exposure is less common in cases and may be said to have a protective effect. These associations are significant only when the confidence interval doesn't include 1, the point estimate for no association.

THOUGHT QUESTION

If proportionally more cases were exposed than controls, will the odds ratio be greater than or less than one?

PREVENTING FOOD-BORNE DISEASE

In response to the Washington County Fair outbreak and the blatant link between a well used for beverages and the effluent from the cow barn, the state health commissioner issued a summary order to improve water supply monitoring at fairgrounds without a monitored public water supply. At about the same time the CDC was working to integrate food-borne disease data across federal, state, regional, and local health departments, including the establishment of FoodNet in 1996.

For an ongoing outbreak, the goal of prevention is to limit the outbreak and identify the gaps that led to the outbreak. While there are multiple versions of the steps to an outbreak investigation, the CDC describes seven steps to food-borne outbreak investigations (Figure 7.7)[13] The first step is to detect, or identify, that there is something going on that needs to be addressed. Typically, this is triggered through public health surveillance, medical illness reports, or informal observations. Once detected, a case needs to be defined and cases need to be found. These data help to more robustly describe the size, timing, and severity

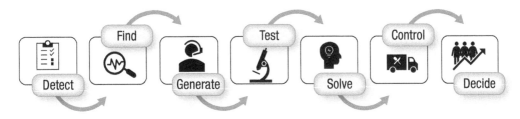

Figure 7.7 **The CDC's seven steps in a food-borne outbreak investigation.**
Source: Centers for Disease Control and Prevention. Foodborne outbreaks: steps in a foodborne outbreak investigation. https://www.cdc.gov/foodsafety/outbreaks/investigating-outbreaks/investigations/index.html

of the outbreak, as well as identifying possible sources. A good case definition and epidemic curves are critical tools at this stage. Step 3 is to generate hypotheses about the most likely sources for the exposure. This is an ongoing process, which is refined as more information is collected through home visits, interviews, and questionnaires sent to people in the area of the outbreak. With a good hypothesis about the likely source, the next step is to test whether that hypothesis is the correct source. Here the epidemiologists on the team will engage in case-control studies to compare the exposures among cases and comparable controls and the environmental or biological scientists will test food, environmental, or human samples. Step 3, generating hypotheses; Step 4, testing the hypothesis; and Step 5, solving the point source, are highly integrated and iterative. They use the three types of data that we see for food-borne disease outbreaks: epidemiologic, traceback, and food/environmental testing. The final two steps are to control the outbreak once the pathogen and source have been identified, and to decide that the outbreak has been controlled. Should the outbreak not yet be controlled, the investigations will continue.

When prevention fails, the faster an outbreak is identified and controlled the better the eventual outcome. While there are many efforts to better track and investigate food-borne disease, two concerted efforts in the United States were designed to support food-borne disease response. Since 2011, SEDRIC, the System for Enteric Disease Response, Investigation, and Coordination, has existed to support the sharing of data and information. The coordinated response pulls together the three data sources, namely epidemiologic, traceback, and laboratory data, securely and quickly.[14] FoodNet is an active surveillance network and one of the products is an online data visualization tool to help track food-borne infection trends. Currently, 15% of U.S. citizens fall within the FoodNet's 10 surveillance areas, and surveillance data are collected for nine different food-borne pathogens.[15] FoodNet is an active surveillance system, meaning that the public health officials responsible for the FoodNet data actively reach out to over 700 clinical laboratories to ensure that infections are being reported.

HEADS UP!

What's the fuss about surveillance? Active surveillance is when public health officials actively reach out and collect information from providers and laboratories. Passive surveillance still requires action, but on behalf of the provider, laboratory, or person who submits the notification to the surveillance system. Active versus passive is defined from the viewpoint of the surveillance system. If public health officials of the surveillance system actively reach out for data, it is active, whereas if the data is sent to them, the surveillance system is passive. Active is more accurate and timely, but it is labor intensive and might then have to be more limited in scope. Passive surveillance is less expensive, but takes time for the reports to come in.

Food-borne diseases are largely preventable. Contamination can happen anywhere along the production chain, from the farm where the food is grown, to processing sites, the transport, or, once it becomes available for the public, at stores or restaurants. Whether at the home or at a restaurant, once the food is being prepared, four actions can help to protect us from food-borne disease (Figure 7.8).[16] The first, and potentially the biggest public health advancement of all time, is to wash hands and food preparation surfaces frequently. These actions can limit the spread of pathogens between contact with additional surfaces. They do require access to clean water and soap. The second action is to limit cross-contamination

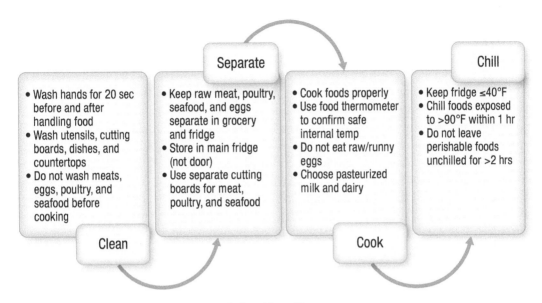

Figure 7.8 Four actions to promote safe food handling.

by keeping meats, poultry, seafood, and eggs separate from other "ready-to-eat" food. This action includes using different cutting boards and plates, different grocery bags, and storing them in different parts of the refrigerator. The next action that supports safe food handling is to ensure that foods are cooked to the right temperature. Meats, fish, ground meats, poultry, and leftovers all have their own safe internal temperature that should be measured using an internal cooking thermometer. Finally, keep foods chilled. This includes keeping your refrigerator cooled to 40°F (4.4°C) or below and throwing out food when questionable. And, when foods are set out, like at a picnic or transporting to a party, refrigerate within 2 hours (1 hour if temperatures are above 90°F [32.2°C]).

THOUGHT QUESTION

Think about the next picnic, dinner party at a friend's house, or even Thanksgiving if you celebrate it. What have you learned so far that might change your behavior?

THE FUTURE OF FOOD-BORNE DISEASE

In the traceback and environmental testing for the 1999 Washington County Fair outbreak, the source of infection was eventually determined: using untreated water that was drawn near livestock and sewage. While most of the vendors at the fair used treated water, at least one part of the fair used water from an untreated well to make beverages and ice.[12] Preceding the infections, a heavy rain even occurred, likely washing through the surrounding cattle fields, barns, and manure piles and into the wells.[17]

The interactions of human behavior, environmental stressors, and animal hosts that can lead to food-borne illness are complex. These interactions will change as our social structures change with migration and urbanization, isolation, and aging. They will change in how we engage with our environment, including changes to agriculture, deforestation, and encroachment into natural areas. Further, all of these effects will be stressed through the effects of a changing climate. As a result, predicting the future of food-borne disease, as well as many other environmentally linked diseases, is inherently wrought with uncertainty. While we may not be able to explicitly predict how many new cases of food-borne disease will occur in a given city in 2035, there are some certainties about predicting climate change effects on food safety and food security. Namely, we know that temperatures will increase, flooding risks will increase due to rising sea levels, and increased extreme weather events like heavy rains or hurricanes, will occur, and that these events will affect food supply and production. These extreme weather events may also impact the safety of our food—for example, many coastal communities are concerned with high temperature and the safety of harvested seafood during the summer months. In order to assess these effects, there is a need for improved surveillance and better communication across sectors and regions (cross-border, within states/regions, and between countries).[18]

What is also known is that health effects of climate change will disproportionately affect the most marginalized,[19] including communities of color, Indigenous peoples, children and pregnant women, older adults, certain occupational groups (e.g., outdoor workers), persons with disabilities, and persons with chronic medical conditions.[20] Regionally, fecal-oral pathogens and climate change-driven increases in diarrheal disease, many of which are food-borne, will increase in Asia and eastern Africa with an estimated 3% to 11% increased risk per 1.8°F (1°C).[21]

Food Safety and Food Security

Food safety and food security are interconnected. **Food safety** describes the access to food that is safe and free of contaminants. **Food security** is concerned with steady and reliable access to food. In the Washington County Fair example, a rain event preceded the outbreak, washing effluent from a cow barn into an unprotected and unmonitored well. Warmer temperatures support the growth of many of the pathogenic microorganisms that are responsible for food-borne disease. Food storage temperatures in our homes, at picnics and parties, and during transportation will be influenced by warmer temperatures. Warmer temperatures can also influence livestock and crop susceptibility to infection and growth of the pathogen in contaminated soil—all of these are issues of food safety.

food safety: Access to contaminant-free foods.

food security: A steady and reliable access to food.

The effects of climate on food security include reductions in crop productivity, changes in crop yield due to drought and extreme weather events, loss of crop land due to rising sea level, water demand changes, disruption of distribution, and increases in pests and disease.[21] Soil degradation due to increased fertilizer and pesticide use to counter the warming effects can result in less diverse foods, decreased yields, and reduced nutritional value.[22] Livestock and fisheries as well will be affected with stress, increased pathogens and resulting toxins, changes in ranges, and reduced yields.[23] The supply and production chains can also be disrupted by extreme weather events.

Climate change will cause food shortages which can result in humanitarian and national security crises. Combatting these inevitable outcomes includes not only a concerted effort to mitigate climate change but also the effort to take a holistic One Health approach to adapting for future risks. Priorities may include incorporating both the social and ecological factors that contribute to disease and identification of and prioritization of those populations most at risk.[24] WASH—water sanitation and hygiene interventions—can support community adaptation and prevention of food-borne disease, especially in low- and middle-income countries.[25]

THOUGHT QUESTION

As a public health specialist, how do you think you can support and engage with agricultural sectors regarding food safety and food security, particularly as it relates to the warming climate? What is the role for you and who else needs to be in the room?

CASE STUDY

While known for many other things, Louis Pasteur is known for making our food safer through pasteurization. In the late 1800s Pasteur discovered that heating beverages, like milk and wine, to a high temperature, cooling it quickly, and then storing it would help keep it from spoiling. We continue to use this heat-treating process, pasteurization, to kill the bacteria in certain foods and improve their shelf-life. And remember Typhoid Mary? Drastic reduction in typhoid in the early 1900s is attributed in part to the efforts in improving water treatment by Maryland Department of Health worker Abel Wolman. But what about since then? Modern food-borne disease heroes are working in every corner of the world to improve access to safe food and water. Take for instance Faisal Chohan, whose solution to flooding in Pakistan improved sanitation for 2 million people. Or Doc Hendley, founder of Wine To Water, which has worked in almost 1,000 communities in 48 countries to improve access to clean, safe water. Or researcher Rita Colwell, who showed that simply filtering water through layers of old, cheap sari cloth significantly reduced the risk of cholera (Figure 7.9). These amazing people show us that simple solutions can work to improve the lives of thousands and the importance of working within communities to support those changes.

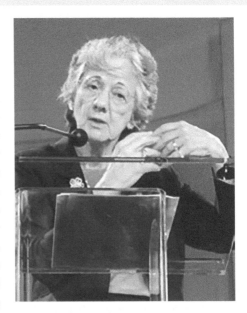

Figure 7.9 Rita R. Colwell (b. 1934), 11th director of the National Science Foundation. Dr. Colwell discovered that simple water filtration significantly reduces the risk of cholera.

Source: NIH Record. https://nihrecord.nih.gov/sites/recordNIH/files/pdf/2011/NIH-Record-2011-12-09.pdf

CONCLUSION

One source of optimism for food-borne disease is that much of it is preventable by simple actions like handwashing, improved sanitation, access to clean water, and, when available, vaccination. The challenge is that those important public health measures have been known since the 1850s, yet 3.6 billion (nearly 50%) global citizens still do not have access to basic sanitation and two billion do not have safe water in their homes.[26] Climate change will exacerbate these challenges. However, increased testing and data sharing will help to quickly and efficiently find areas for improvement to aid in controlling and preventing food-borne disease.[27] Progress is being made. Organizations like the CDC and the WHO are working to collect and share data on easy, user-friendly platforms so that outbreaks can be more quickly detected. Trans-sector interdisciplinary teams are joining together to share data, respond to outbreaks, and plan for future food-borne disease.

TEACHING CORNER

DID YOU KNOW?

While food contamination can happen anywhere along the food production chain, the classic food-borne disease outbreak is the case of a community picnic or other gathering. The outbreak investigation tools are similar regardless of source.

Shortly after attending a quinceañera celebration, 17 attendees became severely ill. Their contact information was sent to you by your state health department with a suspicion of a food-borne disease outbreak. You contact all of the guests to the celebration and identify an additional 10 cases who experienced milder symptoms. You decide a case-control study is warranted to identify the source. You interview all of the ill and at least one non-ill person of similar age/gender for every sick person interviewed. A total of 67 people were interviewed to determine what foods they ate. Of the ill persons, 12 reported eating chicken enchiladas and 18 ate tacos with fresh salsa. For those that did not get sick, 14 ate enchiladas and 26 ate tacos.

What do you think might be the culprit? Why?

TRY THIS

Organize these data into tables: one table for each exposure, two columns (cases and controls), two rows (exposed/unexposed). Use the information provided to fill in the cells.

TAKE IT A STEP FURTHER

Calculate the appropriate measure (OR or RR) for the association between each exposure and becoming ill.

Name the food you think made people sick and justify your answer.

QUESTIONS FOR FURTHER DISCUSSION

1. List some explicit examples of strategies to control food-borne disease.

2. Imagine a house party or Thanksgiving dinner. Now, walk yourself through the four actions to prevent food-borne illness in the home. List the actions and then describe a situation where that action might be violated.

3. Distinguish between the terms "food safety" and "food security." How are these both affected by a changing climate?

4. While this chapter keeps referring to food-borne disease, describe other related modes of transmission by which an individual can contract a "food-borne" pathogen.

SPRINGER PUBLISHING
CONNECT™

A robust set of instructor resources designed to supplement this text is located at http://connect.springerpub.com/Content/book/978-0-8261-5674-7. Qualifying instructors may request access by emailing textbook@springerpub.com.

REFERENCES

1. World Health Organization. Webinar: Burden of foodborne diseases - how can we estimate it, and why do we need it? June 29, 2021. https://www.who.int/news-room/events/detail/2021/06/29/default-calendar/webinar-burden-of-foodborne-diseases-how-can-we-estimate-it-and-why-do-we-need-it

2. Scallan E, Hoekstra RM, Angulo FJ, et al. Foodborne illness acquired in the United States—major pathogens. *Emerg Infect Dis.* 2011;17(1):7–15. doi:10.3201/eid1701.p11101

3. Centers for Disease Control and Prevention. Burden of foodborne illness: findings. https://www.cdc.gov/foodborneburden/2011-foodborne-estimates.html

4. Hoffmann S, Maculloch B, Batz M. Economic burden of major foodborne illnesses acquired in the United States [EIB-140]. U.S. Department of Agriculture, Economic Research Service. May 2015. https://econpapers.repec.org/paper/agsuersib/205081.htm

5. Hoffmann S, Batz MB, Morris JG Jr. Annual cost of illness and quality-adjusted life year losses in the United States due to 14 foodborne pathogens. *J Food Prot.* 2012;75(7):1292–1302. doi:10.4315/0362-028X.JFP-11-417

6. Murray CJL, Vos T, Lozano R, et al. Disability-adjusted life years (DALYs) for 291 diseases and injuries in 21 regions, 1990–2010: a systematic analysis for the global burden of disease study 2010. *Lancet.* 2012;380:2197–2223. doi:10.1016/S0140-6736(12)61689-4

7. Karambizi NU, McMahan CS, Blue CN, Temesvari LA. Global estimated disability-adjusted life-years (DALYs) of diarrheal diseases: a systematic analysis of data from 28 years of the global burden of disease study. *PLoS One.* 2021;16(10):e0259077. doi:10.1371/journal.pone.0259077

8. Jaffee S, Henson S, Unnevehr L, Grace D, Cassou E. *The Safe Food Imperative: Accelerating Progress in Low- and Middle-Income Countries. Agriculture and Food Series.* World Bank; 2019. https://openknowledge.worldbank.org/handle/10986/30568

9. Tribune Wire Reports. 1,450 Blue Bell workers losing jobs after listeria problems. *Chicago Tribune.* May 16, 2015. https://www.chicagotribune.com/business/ct-blue-bell-job-cuts-listeria-20150515-story.html

10. U.S. Department of Justice. Blue Bell Creameries ordered to pay $17.25 million in criminal penalties in connection with 2015 *Listeria* contamination. September 17, 2020. https://www.justice.gov/opa/pr/blue-bell-creameries-ordered-pay-1725-million-criminal-penalties-connection-2015-listeria

11. Centers for Disease Control and Prevention. *E. coli (Escherichia coli):* Questions and answers. https://www.cdc.gov/ecoli/general/index.html

12. Public Health Dispatch. Outbreak of *Escherichia coli* O157:H7 and *Campylobacter* among attendees of the Washington County Fair—New York, 1999. *MMWR Morb Mortal Wkly Rep.* 1999;48(36):803. https://www.cdc.gov/mmwr/preview/mmwrhtml/mm4836a4.htm

13. Centers for Disease Control and Prevention. Steps in a foodborne outbreak investigation. https://www.cdc.gov/foodsafety/outbreaks/investigating-outbreaks/investigations/index.html

14. Centers for Disease Control and Prevention. SEDRIC: System for Enteric Disease Response, Investigation, and Coordination. https://www.cdc.gov/foodsafety/outbreaks/investigating-outbreaks/sedric.html

15. Centers for Disease Control and Prevention. About FoodNet. Accessed September 23, 2021. https://www.cdc.gov/foodnet/about.html

16. Centers for Disease Control and Prevention. Four steps to food safety: clean, separate, cook, chill. Accessed October 15, 2021. https://www.cdc.gov/foodsafety/keep-food-safe.html

17. Barstow D. A deadly germ taints a tradition; *E. coli* devastates families and leaves a fair in doubt. *New York Times.* September 20, 1999. https://www.nytimes.com/1999/09/20/nyregion/deadly-germ-taints-tradition-e-coli-devastates-families-leaves-fair-doubt.html

18. Lake IR, Barker GC. Climate change, foodborne pathogens and illness in higher-income countries. *Curr Environ Health Rep.* 2018;5(1):187–196. doi:10.1007/s40572-018-0189-9

19. Sauerborn R, Kjellstrom T, Nilsson M. 2009. Invited editorial: health as a crucial driver for climate policy. *Glob Health Action.* 2009;2(1):2104. doi:10.3402/gha.v2i0.2104

20. Gamble JL, Balbus J, Berger M, et al. Populations of concern. In: Crimmins A, Balbus J, Gamble J, et al. eds. *Impacts of Climate Change on Human Health in the United States: A Scientific Assessment.* U.S. Global Change Research Program; 2016:247–286.
21. World Health Organization. *Quantitative Risk Sssessment of the Effects of Climate Change on Selected Causes of Death, 2030s and 2050s.* WHO Press; 2014. https://apps .who.int/iris/bitstream/handle/10665/134014/9789241507691_eng.pdf
22. Meehl GA, Stocker TF, Collins WD, et al. Global climate projections. In: Solomon S, Qin D, Manning M, eds. *Climate Change 2007: The Physical Science Basis. Contribution of Working Group I to the Fourth Assessment Report of the Intergovernmental Panel on Climate Change.* Cambridge University Press; 2007:747–846.
23. Ziska L, Crimmins A, Auclair A, et al. Ch. 7: food safety, nutrition, and distribution. In: Crimmins A, Balbus J, Gamble J, et al., eds. *The Impacts of Climate Change on Human Health in the United States: A Scientific Assessment.* U.S. Global Change Research Program; 2016:189–216. doi:10.7930/J0ZP4417
24. Levy K, Smith SM, Carlton EJ. Climate change impacts on waterborne diseases: moving toward designing interventions. *Curr Environ Health Rep.* 2018;5(2):272–282. doi:10.1007/s40572 -018-0199-7
25. Cissé G. Food-borne and water-borne diseases under climate change in low- and middle-income countries: further efforts needed for reducing environmental health exposure risks. *Acta Trop.* 2019;194:181–188. doi:10.1016/j.actatropica.2019.03.012
26. Centers for Disease Control and Prevention. Global WASH fast facts. Accessed December 8, 2021. https://www.cdc.gov/healthywater/global/wash_statistics.html
27. Doyle MP, Erickson MC, Alali W, et al. The food industry's current and future role in preventing microbial foodborne illness within the United States. *Clin Infect Dis.* 2015;61(2):252–259. doi:10.1093/cid/civ253

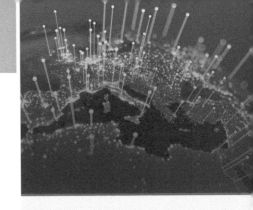

PART III

INFECTIOUS
DISEASES IN CONTEXT

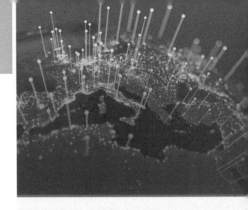

CHAPTER 8

BEHAVIORAL AND CULTURAL ASPECTS OF INFECTIOUS DISEASE

INTRODUCTION

Ebola virus disease (EVD) is a rare but deadly disease caused by infection by a group of four viruses (genus Ebolavirus) among people, as well as another virus that causes disease in nonhuman primates and pigs. Since its discovery in 1976 in the Democratic Republic of Congo in a village near the Ebola River, the virus has led to sporadic outbreaks of disease in different countries in Africa. The virus spreads to people through direct contact with body fluids or tissues of animals, spreading quickly between people through contact with someone sick with or dead from EVD. The virus is likely to spread through broken skin, mucous membranes, or sexual contact. The 2014 to 2016 Ebola outbreak in West Africa quickly spread from rural Guinea through urban areas and across borders, spreading to countries worldwide. Two and a half years after the first case was discovered, the outbreak ended with more than 28,600 cases and 11,325 deaths. Nearly 20% of all EVD cases occurred in children under 15 years of age, and an estimated 30,000 children became orphans during the epidemic. To read and listen to compelling personal stories of the outbreak, go to the story Life After Death (apps.npr.org/life -after-death/#b03g04f20b15).

LEARNING OBJECTIVES

By the end of this chapter, readers will be able to:

- Describe the influence of culture and behavior on the distribution and transmission of infectious disease.
- Examine the role of culture and behavior on disease control.
- Explain social mechanisms of disease transmission.
- Indicate how ecological study designs are used to study health outcomes.

THE INFLUENCE OF BEHAVIOR AND CULTURE ON DISEASE TRANSMISSION

The 2014 to 2016 Ebola outbreak was the deadliest in history, primarily as a result of the behavior of individuals, families, and communities. Transmission occurred in healthcare facilities, among family members when someone was sick, and during funeral practices after death. Since traditional funeral rituals in West Africa required washing, touching, and kissing the body of the dead person, the virus spread rapidly from person to person.

Useful Frameworks in Approaching Infectious Diseases

The central forces shaping disease burden are often social, rather than biological. The connections that define social relations are also those that often determine the spread of an infectious disease.

For example, as we think about human behavior and culture, it is the structure of the family or the community that defines how people interact, which in turn is shaped by broader expectations of schooling, employment, and socializing.[1] To add another layer of complexity, we can consider how behavioral patterns of humans interact with their **built environment**.[2] In other words, people pass through a variety of spaces over time, interacting with different people through their day. This **spatiotemporal** perspective can better allow us to understand the process of disease transmission (Figure 8.1). Even more

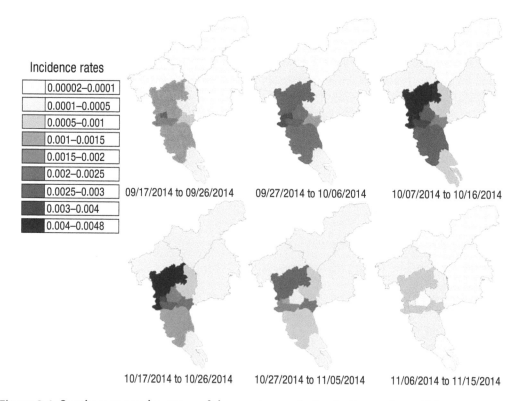

Figure 8.1 Spatio-temporal pattern of dengue transmission in Guangzhou, China.

Source: From Zhu G, Liu J, Tan Q, Shi B. Inferring the spatio-temporal patterns of dengue transmission from surveillance data in Guangzhou, China. *PLOS Negl Trop Dis*. 2016;10(4):e0004633. doi:10.1371/journal.pntd.0004633

broadly, global city networks may produce areas with higher disease potential through movement of "microbial traffic."[3] Both social activity as well as broader mobility and migration patterns that increase population density have been shown to drive outbreaks such as influenza and measles, and even vector-borne diseases (VBDs) like dengue.[4-6]

Ebola provides an example of a disease for which little has been known about how the virus first passes to humans, with subsequent waves of human-to-human transmission and high transmission and mortality. We know that the first patient in past outbreaks typically becomes infected through close contact with an infected animal, such as a fruit bat or primate, in what is known as a **spillover event**. In parts of Africa, infection has been documented through the handling and bushmeat trade of infected chimpanzees, gorillas, fruit bats, monkeys, forest antelope, and porcupines found dead or ill in the rainforest. Person-to-person transmission typically follows and can lead to large numbers of infected people. In some past Ebola outbreaks, primates were also affected by Ebola, and multiple spillover events occurred when people touched or ate infected primates while unaware that they were infected (Figure 8.2).

When we consider behavior and culture, there are substantial implications as to how social interactions and norms may fuel transmission. For Ebola, the disease is one of close social contact, with close family members bearing the highest risks of further infection.

Transmission has been well-documented in hospitals, through healthcare workers, use of insufficient precautions (e.g., unsafe injections), or close contact. Similarly, many examples exist within homes and communities, where close contacts may occur through family or friends. An additional consideration is that infectiousness (i.e., viral load) of body fluids increases as a patient becomes more ill, such that remains of individuals who died from the infection are themselves highly infectious. This means that additional contacts and subsequent transmission occur through both caring for the ill and through funeral practices.

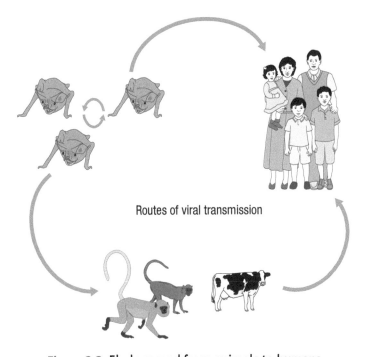

Routes of viral transmission

Figure 8.2 **Ebola spread from animals to humans.**

built environment: Areas created by humans and used by people for living, working, and recreation.

spatiotemporal: In the context of epidemiology, data collected across time (temporal) as well as space (spatio), allowing for an assessment or, when mapped, visualization of changes in disease patterns across a landscape or other surface.

spillover event: A single event during which a pathogen from one species moves into another species, potentially resulting in a new disease outbreak.

THE ROLE OF CULTURE AND BEHAVIOR ON DISEASE CONTROL

"The need for a social science perspective became clear from an early stage in the outbreak in West Africa. Some of the interventions typical of Western medicine and science clashed, at times violently, with social norms and traditional beliefs."[7para3]

Cultural diversity shapes nations between and within countries and can have a profound influence on social cohesion and communication, particularly during times of upheaval. For example, in Africa, Liberia has at least 16 major ethnic and cultural groups, each described by a specific language and associated dialects, religions, traditions, and customs.[8] Ebola, with its close person-to-person transmission, is particularly influenced by cultural and behavioral practices that occur at the household and community levels and within a hospital setting (e.g., patient care, family involvement and role, health-seeking behaviors and responses). Consequently, there is no one "community" and the cultural diversity that defines the region needs to be considered in local disease emergence prevention as well as public health response. Because the main routes of transmission of the virus are linked to everyday life, and especially influence people like health workers or caregivers, public health recommendations can appear antithetical to many, and may create opposition or resistance. For example, it was prohibited to wash or clean corpses for fear of transmission. Cremation of the deceased was also not permitted.[9] It is now clear that doing so likely prevented an additional 10,000 cases of this deadly disease. For example, leakproof bags that were puncture-resistant and sealed to prevent any leakage during handling and transport were developed, with very specific step-by-step guidelines allowing for minimal staffing and proper infection control practices, while allowing family members to see the body and escort it to the burial ground.

THOUGHT QUESTION

Which beliefs might enhance, and which might lower, health? For example, in your life as a student, what are some health-enhancing beliefs and practices? What are some health-lowering beliefs and practices? What are two to three examples in the context of Ebola?

"SOCIAL" MECHANISMS OF TRANSMISSION

Once there was realization that Ebola was a "behavioral" infectious disease, pressure increased for community engagement and social mobilization to stem the outbreak. For the first time in a global health disease emergency, a "cluster system" was created led by ministries of health to provide support around infection control, burials, protecting children, and other areas.[10] In this cluster system, coordinated efforts focused on key behaviors, for example, through developing better health messaging, and in addressing stigma and discrimination. Even small amounts of support utilized broader community supports. Behaviors indeed changed, with earlier treatment and care seeking, safer burials, better hygiene and infection control, and better reporting of infectious cases.

Ethnography is the systematic study and recording of human cultures, usually through interviews, observations, and conversations and can lend an important lens to understanding the health and health choices of a population. Inclusion of qualitative **ethnographic data** allows us to draw out detailed information about a particular social/cultural group through close study. Using qualitative approaches allows us to unpack important narratives and information that may not show up in data alone. Increasingly, qualitative approaches have been used to some effect in epidemiologic studies adding additional context to the more traditionally quantitative epidemiologic data. For example, in the Stanford Five-City Project, an integrated quantitative and qualitative approach was used to examine cardiovascular disease risks. Social networks were surveyed, and culture was stressed in interpretation, leading to a comprehensive and representative picture of that community's health.[11] Formative feedback from participants was able to guide messaging and programming for specific audiences.

Risk associated with different behaviors is also judged and understood differently among those from different cultural backgrounds and may influence people's choices about health and the social situations they engage in which might put them at potential exposure to pathogens. Risk perception often may rely on what is happening around us, and in a given culture,[12] where people may have individual motivation to seek treatment or take individual action for their risk, such as improving lifestyle practices after a disease diagnosis. Similarly, social risk explains why some groups are marginalized to unhealthy environments based on stigma or how a group is viewed. Perceptions around the harm that a disease causes or perceptions around how likely an individual is to get the disease influence their framing of risk from a given disease. For example, despite influenza having a case fatality rate around 1%, many people do not perceive it to be a bad disease and only 50% of American adults get vaccinated each year.[13,14]

Asymptomatic or mildly symptomatic individuals often do not change their behaviors during a period of infectiousness because they are either unaware of their infection or think that, with a milder infection, it is less likely to spread. However, these individuals can subsequently infect a lot of others because they maintain high contacts, inadvertently passing along disease as they do. The converse may be true, where someone with more advanced disease may have fewer social interactions because of their condition, thus reducing the chance of transmission even though they are infectious. However, there is an interplay between behavior and infection risk. In the case of Ebola, overall risks of infection peak in the final phase of the disease when vomiting, diarrhea, and bleeding occur and the person is likely to be in contact with many others engaged in trying to save their lives, or immediately after death, when family members are caring for the remains (Figure 8.3).

Sticking with the Ebola example, this disease also makes intercommunity jumps, that is, it appears in distant communities skipping over intermediate ones, and we might ask why.[15] Ethnographic data reveal that these jumps are often the result of family networking, cooperation across family units, and whether family caregivers are persuaded to collaborate in reducing risks of contact with a sick person or infected body.

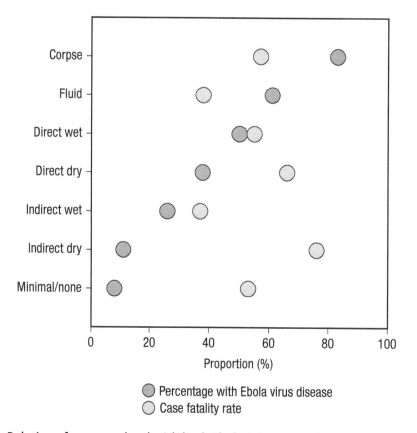

Figure 8.3 Relation of exposure level with both Ebola infection and case fatality rate.
Source: Data from Bower H, Smout E, Bangura MS, et al. Deaths, late deaths, and role of infecting dose in Ebola virus disease in Sierra Leone: retrospective cohort study. *BMJ*. 2016;353:i2403. doi:10.1136/bmj.i2403

Failure of the public health community to adhere to social customs can further and inadvertently facilitate more exposures. For example, the mass cremation policies instituted to curb the spread from highly infectious corpses in response to the outbreak had avoidable inadvertent consequences. It led to families seeking to maintain traditional burial practices continuing them in secret, without the support from public health to minimize additional exposures. Graves were left shallow and unmarked, potentially creating further exposures through grave interference. And finally, a market started for fake certificates, which listed the cause of death as something other than Ebola, undercounting the impact of the outbreak. Eventually, the recognition that this was occurring and the significance of incorporating community practices allowed for burial to be adapted to allow some contact with the dead body without putting others at risk.

Bushmeat consumption is a common practice that may have led to early Ebola transmission from animals. Bushmeat is the flesh of any wild animal. One might ask why the practice? Where meat is expensive (and potentially rare), bushmeat has always been a critical source of protein and a valuable source of income. However, increasingly it may also be handled because of its value as a commercial or black-market commodity (exotic meat) and is facilitated by logging and mining, which drives deeper into formerly protected pristine forests and jungles. Similar cultural and economic issues were seen in the H5N1 avian influenza outbreak in Vietnam, where locally produced chickens were viewed as healthy and fresh, and industrially produced chickens as not. As a result, even when local chickens were implicated in disease propagation, small-scale poultry farmers were reluctant to kill off their flocks.[16]

Another cultural way in which humans expose themselves to domestic, wild, or exotic animals, and therefore new-to-human pathogens, is through live animal markets. Markets can be wet markets, selling fresh meat, fish, and produce, or wildlife markets which sell exotic/bushmeat or live animals. These markets have important socio-cultural roles in various societies. They may act as a meeting point for people, vendors, farmers, and producers; as a source for alternative and traditional medicines that have great economic ramifications in many countries in the world; and as a means to supply fresh foods to millions of customers every day.[17] While these markets may pose a risk for disease and have been implicated in SARS, SARS-CoV-2, and avian influenza, closing them may have unintended consequences of disrupting local food supplies.[18] In China, it is estimated that this food sector alone accounts for 30% to 59% of food supplies.[19]

ethnographic data: Direct observation of users in a natural environment that allows one to gain insights into understanding how people interact. Methods are qualitative and allow for observing what is of direct significance to a community.

BEHAVIORAL FACTORS AFFECTING DISEASE SPREAD

Older people were found to be disproportionately at risk of infection and death from Ebola (Figure 8.4). This is because older family members are often heavily involved in caring for and treating the sick. As the elders often were charged with duties, and were the ones who could create safer practices, how duties were distributed in taking care of bodies mattered a lot more for infection risk than the size of the funeral.[20]

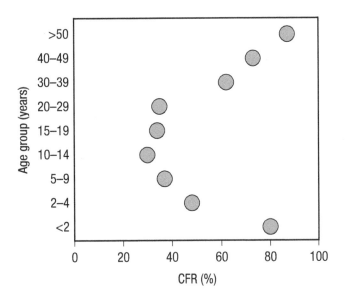

Figure 8.4 Case fatality rates by age group among individuals with Ebola virus.
Source: Data from Bower H, Smout E, Bangura MS, et al. Deaths, late deaths, and role of infecting dose in Ebola virus disease in Sierra Leone: retrospective cohort study. *BMJ*. 2016;353:i2403. doi:10.1136/bmj.i2403

More recently in the COVID-19 pandemic, the age structure of populations in different countries has played a large role in mortality patterns because of the young and old interacting and living together, along with underlying risks of severe disease by age.[21]

An epidemic may be highly heterogeneous depending on a number of socio-behavioral factors. When one hospital failed to control Ebola disease spread, there was a widespread lack of distrust in the medical system, with some sure that the disease was being deliberately spread by medical workers. Families avoided the hospital system. If access to services is poor, individuals may also take response into their own hands. People in rural areas affected by Ebola hardly visited clinics before the outbreak because there was nothing there, so the default response to Ebola was to practice home care. Several traditional and spiritual healers also falsely claimed to have the capability to cure Ebola.[22] If medical supplies were unavailable—for example, a family did not have access to a stretcher and handled the body directly—it could lead to disease spread.

Culturally inappropriate messaging may also result in disaster. For example, consumption of bushmeat, especially monkey meat, was widely warned against over the radio and on posters as a cause of infection. Villagers who never ate bushmeat, thought for religious reasons that they were safe from infection. Because they didn't take the necessary precautions to protect themselves against infection from infected individuals, they put themselves at risk. It was only late in the epidemic that this message was replaced by an emphasis on limiting body contact with persons of unknown Ebola status.

Human behavior can also play a critical role in controlling infections. Sexual behavior change has been critical to turning the tide of HIV/AIDS in Uganda.[23] In fact, disease avoidance allows the individual to avoid a metabolically costly process of then reacting to an infection. This concept of a **behavioral immune system** notes that susceptible individuals will try to avoid infection through specific behaviors.[24]

THE ROLE OF MOBILITY PATTERNS

Individual and collective patterns of human movement have been recognized as important to epidemic and pandemic emergence since at least the time of the Black Death in the 1300s. The Black Death, caused by *Yersinia pestis,* also known as plague, is a vector-borne (flea) disease transmitted both by human-to-human and human-to-animal (primarily rodents) contact. Using an **ecological study** design, researchers showed that trade routes were one of the determining factors in shaping the pattern of plague outbreak in historical Europe. During that time, the Silk Road brought not only a wealth of goods and spice from China and Asia to Europe, but likely also disease. Major trade routes were identified as the critical factor influencing areas which were plague outbreak hotspots, while navigable rivers determined the geographic patterning of more sporadic plague cases (Figure 8.5).[25]

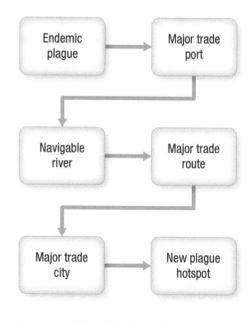

Figure 8.5 **The role of trade routes in disease transmission.**

How people move through the landscape has been linked to many introductions of infectious diseases into new regions. The introduction of smallpox into the Americas occurred due to new human movements introducing the disease from Europe where it was endemic to completely susceptible populations with devastating effects. Similarly, the speed and spread of the 1918 "Spanish Flu" is attributed to the large-scale movements of soldiers during World War I, with troops grouping together in holding and training barracks, and then being transported in tight ships to the various fronts. One can imagine how this situation could allow for person-to-person transmission through congregation in tight quarters, followed by spread into new areas. The role of travel and migration in disease spread has become even more important in recent times, with increasing numbers of international tourists and business travelers, refugees and immigrants, and greater capacity for shipping goods by sea moving in greater numbers and at higher frequency than ever before. There are now a growing number of examples of infections introduced to a new region that either temporarily wreak havoc or ultimately become endemic and more widespread. For example, chikungunya and Zika viruses appeared for the very first time in the western hemisphere in the mid-2010s with devastating impacts on communities and, especially with Zika, on future generations due to the congenital effects. While those examples seem to have wreaked havoc, they did not establish and become endemic. West Nile virus, on the other hand, was first introduced to the United States in 1999, but within just a few years it became endemic in most states of the continental United States. The 2002 SARS epidemic originated in southern China and quickly spread via air travel to 29 countries, lasting for 8 months, with 8,096 probable cases and 774 deaths.[26] In just 1 or 2 days, a traveler can move from one part to any other point on the planet, potentially spreading disease as they travel.

THOUGHT QUESTION

How can we more accurately predict where infections will spread through air or sea travel, and can this determine when the next epidemic of global health significance will occur?

ECOLOGICAL STUDIES

At the beginning of an investigation into a possible association between an infectious disease and potential risk factors, an ecological study design is often employed. Ecological studies use aggregated data to examine the association between an exposure and the occurrence of disease in the broader population or community. The actual measurement of exposure and outcome occurs at the group level, allowing for correlations across different geographies, time periods, or groups (e.g., occupational or socioeconomic class; Figure 8.6). For example, an ecologic analysis between smoking and COVID-19 incidence could ask whether countries with higher per capita cigarette consumption also have higher rates of COVID-19. Or, for example, a question was asked recently whether political proclivity (measured as voting for populist, left- or right-wing) parties was correlated with vaccine hesitancy in countries of Western Europe.[27] The data are slightly modified in Figure 8.7. Each of the 13 points represents the percent of the country voting with the populist party (x-axis) and percent of respondents who agree with a question about vaccinations (y-axis). Imagining a line that passes most closely by each of the points,

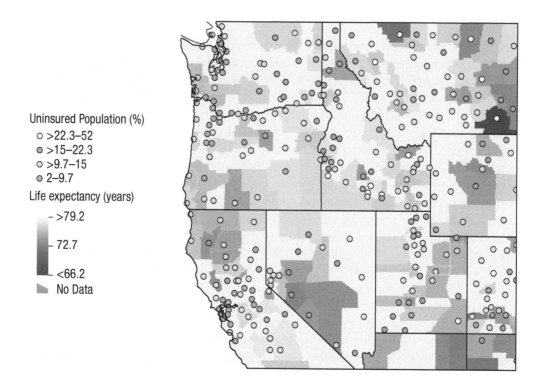

Figure 8.6 Schematic of an ecological study. Notice that participants are not recruited into the study; rather, aggregated data are used for both health outcome and exposure or risk factor status. Ecological studies often rely on secondary data and are particularly useful for generating hypotheses when little is known about an exposure–outcome association.

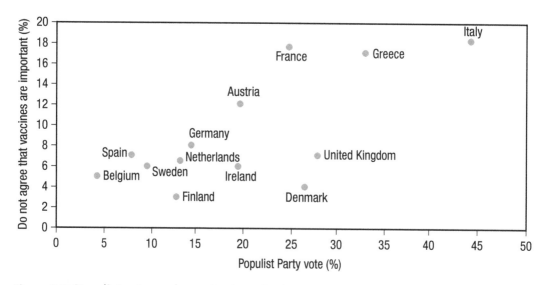

Figure 8.7 Populist votes and perceived vaccine importance.

the figure shows a highly significant positive correlation between the proportion of the electorate voting for populist parties and the percentage of people who disagree with the statement "vaccines are important for children to have." The correlation coefficient is calculated as the sum of the distances of each point to the mean in both the x and y direction over the square root of the sum of the distances squared, and here the measure of effect is a correlation coefficient of 0.79. Given that the correlation coefficient ranges from –1 (perfect negative correlation) to 1 (perfect positive correlation), the higher the level of populist votes in a country, the greater the proportion of the population that believe vaccines are not important.

Ecological studies are cheap and quick and can provide information about statistical correlations. They often use secondary data that has already been collected. They are a great and efficient first step in investigating a hypothesized association. However, they do not provide very strong study designs. This is primarily because we are using aggregated data. So, while we know how the group acts, we don't know what each individual is doing. While we might expect to find groups with greater average exposure levels to have higher rates of disease, or here more populous voting means less vaccine approval, this does not mean that the individuals with greater exposures are also the individuals with higher disease risks. The **ecological fallacy** is a type of confounding that occurs in ecological studies, occurring when relationships seen between groups are assumed to be true for individuals. For example, we saw that a smaller proportion of the population believed that vaccination was important in Italy compared to Belgium (see Figure 8.7) and that more people voted for populist parties in Italy. It would be problematic to conclude that populist party voting rates decrease vaccinations. It is possible that individuals who are not vaccinated move to Italy for some other reason (e.g., the great pizza, a perceived higher quality of life) or that another factor related to lack of vaccination is more common in Italy.

Ecological studies may also ignore confounding. In ecological studies that compare COVID-19 rates in rich versus poorer countries, confounding may occur by the population age structure. Since severity of COVID-19 is strongly linked to (older) age, younger populations will have epidemic growth that is less discernible. One approach to examining situations where both individual and population level data are available is **multilevel modeling**. This approach takes into account the clustering (and thus non-independence) of individuals within groups, for example students inside a classroom inside a school, or family members living in a household within a neighborhood.

In recent years, there has been a renewed focus on modeling behavioral changes in response to infection dynamics in order to better understand infection trajectories. The examination of broader social network dynamics allow for a broader understanding of underlying social interactions and their effects on epidemics.[28] Another approach has been to take novel data sources, such as airline flight databases, to understand how human behaviors and travel choices combine to influence which pathogen genomes circulate and continue to transmit.[29] More recently, new technologies, such as real-time global positioning systems (GPS) and use of cell phones, can allow us to track detailed human movements and to know exactly how behaviors change, and then result in spread of disease.[30] Though these technologies are restricted due to privacy, as they grow and become a larger part of our communities, they will likely lead to exciting new discoveries about the socio-behavioral aspects of disease transmission.

HEADS UP!

Know thy data. While new sources of data can provide new and exciting scientific perspectives, it is important to understand the limitations as well. For example, cell phone data sets often do not cover all populations (e.g., prisoners, children, those without smartphones), may have limited geographic coverage (e.g., less information inside a school), and can be restricted due to privacy (e.g., many of us turn on privacy settings to our devices). Imagine as well how things get complicated if someone carries multiple cell phones!

behavioral immune system: Psychological processes that facilitate immune responses that enter the body through responses to specific disease-avoidance behaviors.

ecological fallacy: An error made in thinking that relationships that are observed for groups also hold for the individuals within those groups.

ecological studies: Studies conducted at the population or group level, rather than at the individual level.

multilevel modeling: Statistical modeling techniques that recognize a clustered inter-dependent data structure. For example, individuals may be nested within a geographical area or students within a school.

THOUGHT QUESTION

To what extent would you expect human behavior and cultural practices to contribute to the likelihood of acquiring and spreading other infectious diseases? Can you think of some examples?

CASE STUDY

Often unheralded, many Ebola survivors went back to the frontlines to help others. One advantage to surviving EVD is the immunity that has allowed them to help without fear of infection. Antibodies produced by the immune system that have helped people survive are then primed when re-encountering the virus. Two female survivors are Decontee Davies and Amie Subah. Organizations such as UNICEF (The United Nations agency responsible for providing humanitarian aid to children) trained survivors on providing care and support for newly orphaned, and often stigmatized, children. Davies volunteered at an interim care center for children, playing and taking care of them. Since the children had been exposed to individuals with EVD, at times the survivors were the only ones who could touch the children. Subah was experienced as a midwife, and contracted Ebola while attending a pregnant woman. However, after recuperating, she was able to stay longer in Ebola units without need for personal protective equipment (PPE) due to her prior infection. She was able to provide psychosocial support for those with the virus, feed Ebola patients, give them medicine, and change children's diapers. She also knew firsthand how to help with the inevitable stigma these individuals would face once they had recovered. These volunteers are able to help in a way no others can, selflessly providing support based on their own lived experiences.

CONCLUSION

A biocultural approach to infectious disease work provides for a perspective on how culture and behavior shape disease dynamics. This approach emphasizes the importance of health outcomes in relation to societal and individual factors. Approaches to conducting health research in this area vary from qualitative to heavily quantitative big data methods that utilize new technologies to assess individual behavior patterns. A socio-behavioral/cultural lens to understanding disease transmission is critical to developing sustainable and implementable interventions to prevent disease spread. While human behaviors and traditions can result in greater disease transmission, they may also play a positive role in controlling infections.

TEACHING CORNER

DID YOU KNOW?

Because COVID-19 is so easily transmissible from person to person, adherence to particular individual behaviors plays a large role in disease control. During the pandemic, individuals have been asked to adhere to different behaviors that reduce contact probabilities and transmission, such as staying at home, physical distancing, masking, and avoiding interactions with individuals who are more vulnerable. The effect of these behavioral interventions is to flatten the infection curve, lowering its peaks and lowering R_e.

TRY THIS

Imagine that county A has more people who do not wear masks and indeed reported COVID-19 case rates are higher. Is it reasonable to assume that higher mask use in county B is related to fewer COVID-19 cases? Be sure to explain your reasoning why or why not.

TAKE IT A STEP FURTHER

Now consider some alternative explanations for the phenomenon presented. Which of these are plausible explanations for the observed trends in COVID-19 incidence? Be sure to explain how these alternate explanations might influence transmission.

- County A and B have different COVID-19 strains.
- County A has more people who are vaccinated.
- The two counties have different proportions of individuals with underlying exposures (e.g., frontline healthcare workers).
- The two counties have differences in their testing rates for COVID-19.
- County A has a warm climate. County B is cold.

QUESTIONS FOR FURTHER DISCUSSION

1. Would you consider behavioral and cultural factors related to infectious disease transmission and control to be most prevalent at the individual, community, or societal level? Please explain your answer.

2. For one of the behavioral practices identified in the chapter, provide a strategy to reduce the likelihood of engaging in this practice in a culturally competent manner (with the thought of reducing acquisition/transmission of disease).

3. Define an ecological study. List strengths and limitations. What strategy can you use to strengthen an ecological study design?

4. What factors influence the spread of infectious disease? How can we create safer means of travel and trade? Is it possible to have safe wildlife or live animal markets?

5. What information would you need from Figure 8.3 if we wanted to provide incidence rates?

 A robust set of instructor resources designed to supplement this text is located at http://connect.springerpub.com/Content/book/978-0-8261-5674-7. Qualifying instructors may request access by emailing **textbook@springerpub.com.**

REFERENCES

1. Prem K, Cook AR, Jit M. Projecting social contact matrices in 152 countries using contact surveys and demographic data. *PLOS Comput Biol.* 2017;13:e1005697. doi:10.1371/journal.pcbi.1005697
2. Keeler C, Emch M. Infectious-disease geography: disease outbreaks and outcomes through the lens of space and place. In: Crooks VA, Andrews GJ, Pearce J, eds. *Routledge Handbook of Health Geography.* Routledge; 2018:67–73.
3. Ali SH, Keil R. Global cities and the spread of infectious disease: the case of severe acute respiratory syndrome (SARS) in Toronto, Canada. *Urban Stud.* 2006;43:491–509. doi:10.1080/00420980500452458
4. Bharti N, Tatem AJ, Ferrari MJ, Grais RF, Djibo A, Grenfell BT. Explaining seasonal fluctuations of measles in Niger using nighttime lights imagery. *Science.* 2011;334:1424–1427. doi:10.1126/science.1210554
5. Poletti P, Visintainer R, Lepri B, Merler S. The interplay between individual social behavior and clinical symptoms in small clustered groups. *BMC Infect Dis.* 2017;17:521. doi:10.1186/s12879-017-2623-2
6. Lana RM, Gomes MFDC, Lima TFM, Honório NA, Codeço CT. The introduction of dengue follows transportation infrastructure changes in the state of Acre, Brazil: a network-based analysis. *PLoS Negl Trop Dis.* 2017;11(11):e0006070. doi:10.1371/journal.pntd.0006070
7. Makri A. Lessons from the social response to Ebola. February 10, 2015. https://www.scidev.net/global/scidev-net-at-large/lessons-social-response-ebola
8. U.S. Citizenship and Immigration Services. Resource Information Center: Liberia. https://www.uscis.gov/archive/resource-information-center-liberia-6
9. Cenetrs for Disease Control and Prevention. Guidance for safe handling of human remains of Ebola patients in U.S. hospitals and mortuaries. https://www.cdc.gov/vhf/ebola/clinicians/evd/handling-human-remains.html
10. Gillespie AM, Obregon R, El Asawi R, et al. Social mobilization and community engagement central to the Ebola response in West Africa: lessons for future public health emergencies. *Glob Health Sci Pract.* 2016;4(4):626–646. doi:10.9745/GHSP-D-16-00226
11. Fortmann SP, Varady AN. Effects of a community-wide health education program on cardiovascular disease morbidity and mortality: the Stanford Five-City Project. *Am J Epidemiol.* 2000;152(4):316–323. doi:10.1093/aje/152.4.316
12. Trostle J. *Epidemiology and Culture.* Cambridge University Press; 2005.
13. Ahmed F, Lindley M, Allred N, et al. Effect of influenza vaccination of healthcare personnel on morbidity and mortality among patients: systematic review and grading of evidence. *Clin Infect Dis.* 2014;58:50–57. doi:10.1093/cid/cit580
14. Centers for Disease Control and Prevention. Flu vaccination coverage, United States, 2020–21 influenza season. https://www.cdc.gov/flu/fluvaxview/coverage-2021estimates.htm
15. Richards P, Amara J, Ferme MC, et al. Social pathways for Ebola virus disease in rural Sierra Leone, and some implications for containment. *PLoS Negl Trop Dis.* 2015;9(4):e0003567. doi:10.1371/journal.pntd.0003567
16. Porter N. Bird flu biopower: strategies for multispecies coexistence in Viêt Nam. *Am Ethnol.* 2013;40:132–148. doi:10.1111/amet.12010

17. Si Z, Scott S, McCordic C. Wet markets, supermarkets and alternative food sources: consumers' food access in Nanjing, China. *Can J Dev Stud.* 2019;40:78–96. doi:10.1080/02255189.2018.1442 322

18. Lin B, Dietrich ML, Senior RA, Wilcove DS. A better classification of wet markets is key to safeguarding human health and biodiversity. *Lancet Planet Health.* 2021;5(6):e386–e394. doi:10.1016/S2542-5196(21)00112-1

19. Maruyama M, Wu L, Huang L. The modernization of fresh food retailing in China: the role of consumers. *J Retail Consum Serv.* 2016;30:33–39. doi:10.1016/j.jretconser.2015.12.006

20. Richards P. *Ebola: How a People's Science Helped End an Epidemic.* Zed Books; 2016.

21. Dowd JB, Rotondi V, Adriano L, Mills MC. Demographic science aids in understanding the spread and fatality rates of COVID-19. *PNAS.* 2020;117(18):9696 –9698. doi:10.1073/pnas.2004911117

22. Umeora O, Emma-Echiegu N, Umeora MC, Ajayi N. Ebola viral disease in Nigeria: the panic and cultural threat. *Af J Med Health Sci.* 2014;13(1):1–5.

23. Parkhurst JO. The Ugandan success story? Evidence and claims of HIV-1 prevention. *Lancet.* 2002;360(9326):78–80. doi:10.1016/S0140-6736(02)09340-6

24. Schaller M. The behavioural immune system and the psychology of human sociality. *Philos Trans R Soc Lond B Biol Sci.* 2011;366(1583):3418–3426. doi:10.1098/rstb.2011.0029

25. Yue RPH, Lee HF, Wu CYH. Trade routes and plague transmission in pre-industrial Europe. *Sci Rep.* 2017;7:12973. doi:10.1038/s41598-017-13481-2

26. Christian MD, Poutanen SM, Loutfy MR, Muller MP, Low DE. Severe acute respiratory syndrome. *Clin Infect Dis.* 2004;38:1420–1427. doi:10.1086/420743

27. Kennedy J. Populist politics and vaccine hesitancy in Western Europe: an analysis of national-level data. *Eur J Public Health.* 2019;29:512–516. doi:10.1093/eurpub/ckz004

28. Funk S, Salathe M, Jansen VAA. Modelling the influence of human behaviour on the spread of infectious diseases: a review. *J R Soc Interface.* 2010;7:1247. doi:10.1098/rsif.2010.0142

29. Tian H, Sun Z, Faria NR, et al. Increasing airline travel may facilitate co-circulation of multiple dengue virus serotypes in Asia. *PLoS Negl Trop Dis.* 2017;11(8):e0005694. doi:10.1371/journal.pntd.0005694

30. Levin R, Chao DL, Wenger EA, et al. Insights into population behavior during the COVID-19 pandemic from cell phone mobility data and manifold learning. *Nat Comput Sci.* 2021;1:588–597. doi:10.1038/s43588-021-00125-9

CHAPTER 9

SOCIAL DIMENSIONS AND HEALTH EQUITY

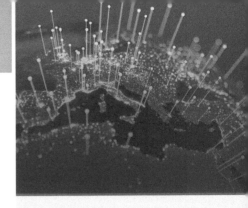

INTRODUCTION

A case series of a rare opportunistic infection among men who have sex with men (MSM) led to identification of a new infectious disease in 1983. However, even as HIV was identified as the cause of AIDS, scientists focused on laboratory studies and microbial cures for the virus, rather than on broader social factors and prevention.[1] The disease initially stigmatized the gay male community and "gay-related immunodeficiency disease" characterized the virus as one affecting only one sub-segment of the population, despite evidence to the contrary implicating cases among blood transfusion recipients, hemophiliacs, and injection drug users. In many cases, the public health measures proposed, such as condoms and clean needles, were quickly perceived as encouragement for nonmarital sex and drug use. The general biomedical response also ignored broader social constraints among those diagnosed as HIV positive. Someone diagnosed with HIV faced discrimination in housing, jobs, health insurance, and, given the lack of treatment, testing itself opened that individual up to stigma with no immediate medical benefit, and in general they faced obstacles well beyond just the delivery of healthcare services.

LEARNING OBJECTIVES

By the end of this chapter, readers will be able to:

- Assess the different factors responsible for infectious disease health disparities and inequities.
- Define key social determinants of infectious diseases.
- Debate whether social or biomedical determinants are more important in infection and transmission of disease.
- Defend the role of causality in infectious diseases.

THE IMPORTANCE OF SOCIAL FACTORS IN INFECTIOUS DISEASE

The HIV/AIDS epidemic has primarily affected socially marginalized populations. Early in the epidemic, it became clear that certain social factors made people more vulnerable to either increased individual risk of exposure to HIV or made it more difficult for individuals to protect themselves from infection. Someone who fears discrimination may not seek testing or HIV counseling and testing. They may also not disclose their HIV status to their sexual partners. Women who experience gender violence may not have control of their partner's or own use of condoms for safe sex. A number of pathways link poverty and HIV infection. Poverty decreases healthcare access, which can increase the duration of treatable sexually transmittable diseases, which, in turn, facilitates HIV transmission. People without material resources may seek to sell and buy drugs or exchange sex for drugs or money, increasing the likelihood of contracting HIV through unsafe sexual or drug practices. These social factors underlie important determinants of health.

From a purely medical perspective, people contract infectious diseases by being susceptible and subsequently becoming sufficiently exposed to a pathogen to contract disease. Traditional infectious disease epidemiology looks to characterize the patterns of those infections by person, place, and time. However, beyond individual behavior and collective culture, social factors are critical to understanding the distribution and transmission of infectious diseases. The broader conditions in which people live are critical in determining health and longevity, sometimes due to the actual quality and availability of healthcare received, but often also through direct relationships to health. Over time, the medical perspective that many infectious diseases are considered easily treatable (antibiotics) or prevented (vaccines) has limited this approach of examining what are known as upstream drivers of infection that may operate at various levels beyond the individual such as the family, community, or region (Figure 9.1). **Social determinants of health** are the conditions in which people are born, grow, live, work, and age, including the healthcare system, which influence their achieving health and well-being.[2]

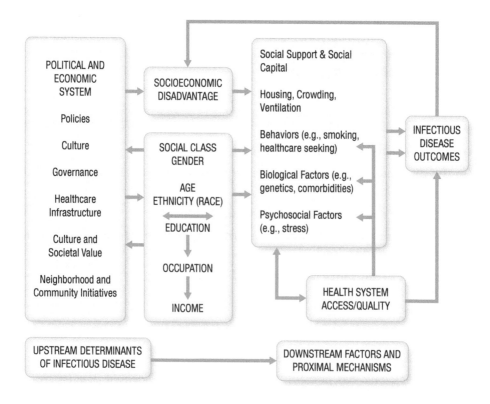

Figure 9.1 Social determinants of infectious diseases.

WHAT DO WE MEAN BY HEALTH DISPARITIES AND INEQUITIES?

An important distinction is to be made when considering terminology as it relates to differences in health outcomes. A formal definition of **health disparities** is "a particular type of health difference that is closely linked with social, economic, and/or environmental disadvantage."[3] These differences are often closely related to populations adversely affected because of their race, sex, gender, age, disability status, sexual orientation, and so on.

One can consider the broader differences in health people have as they relate to life opportunities, various exposures, stressors, and events. These might be referred to as the social determinants of health disparities. In contrast, if we examine the differences in health insurance coverage and access to and quality of care within a healthcare system, we might refer to healthcare or health services disparities. **Health equity** usually refers to individuals both achieving their full health potential, as well as those factors (or social determinants) that drive health outcomes.[4] In other words, a health inequity is not just the difference in a health state but also a commitment to reduce and get rid of health disparities by addressing the underlying determinants. Equality does not necessarily accomplish the elimination of health disparities (Figure 9.2).

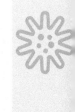

social epidemiology: The discipline within epidemiology that emphasizes the study of mechanisms and processes that produce social inequalities as they are related to health.

health disparities: Health differences closely linked with social, economic, and/or environmental disadvantage.

health equity: Individuals achieve their full health potential, through reduction of barriers that drive different health outcomes.

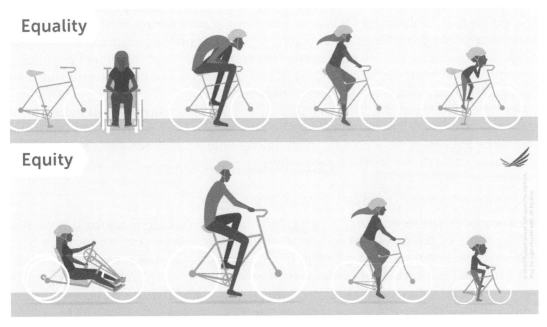

Figure 9.2 **The difference between equality and equity.**
Source: Robert Wood Johnson Foundation. Visualizing health equity: one size does not fit all infographic. 2017. https://www.rwjf.org/en/library/infographics/visualizing-health-equity.html#/download/

THOUGHT QUESTION

How might disease burden relate to disparity? That is, what if few people would benefit from your intervention even if a disparity is observed, or else not many people were affected in the first place, yet a disparity was still present?

WHAT ARE KEY SOCIAL DETERMINANTS FOR INFECTIOUS DISEASES, AND HOW DO THEY ARISE?

Social determinants of health occur due to inequities such as socioeconomic position, social structure, social class, education, occupation, income, race, and sex. Many social factors may result in a higher risk of developing and transmitting an infectious disease. Inadequate healthcare, especially for low-wage workers without paid sick days or health insurance, may directly increase exposure and vulnerability to infection when individuals are forced to decide between income and staying home to recover or must decline preventive care. Poor housing, food insecurity and malnutrition, alcohol consumption, smoking, and comorbidities are just a few other possible factors that increase susceptibility.

These social determinants may unfold in complex ways. People with HIV who have stable housing are more likely to complete treatment regimens; that is, have better treatment adherence.[5] Someone with better adherence can reduce their viral load, which is critical for both maintaining their own health and for preventing HIV transmission to others. Other important social determinants of disease transmission are population density, or differences in living in urban or rural settings.[6,7] For example, urban density may occur due to poor communities aggregating where land is cheaper or unavailable elsewhere. The transmissibility of a pathogen, measured as R_0, often increases with population density as it can spread more easily with the higher probability of contact with a susceptible host. With almost 1 billion people living in urban slums, it is easy to imagine how overcrowding, combined with poor ventilation, can provide the tinder for an infectious disease outbreak.[8] However, rural communities with typically lower population density face different disparities, where access to high-quality medical care and even transportation to medical appointments can be limited.

As we saw in Figure 9.1, these determinants may be more upstream or more downstream. That is, resulting health disparities may be due to broader societal influences and social policies, or those that are more downstream, such as behaviors and the more immediate environment in which people live.

Economic and Political Systems

Socioeconomic factors may play a particularly important role in changing disease risk during times of rapid political upheaval. For example, strong correlations have been shown across central and eastern European countries between rates of tick-borne encephalitis (a virus that attacks the nervous system once bitten by a tick) and the percentage of household expenditure on food shortly following the dissolution of the (former) Soviet Union. At least one hypothesis is that as unemployment soared, individuals picked mushrooms for additional income, with increases in encephalitis specifically observed after forest cutting activities, through additional exposures to ticks.[9] Another recent example is the opioid epidemic in the United States, where increased prescription of opioid medications led to widespread misuse and addiction. The confluence of infected needles, unprotected sex, homelessness, and lack of access to medical care resulted in increased rates of infectious disease transmission among drug users, including hepatitis C and HIV.[10] There are also times when policies may directly influence health outcomes; for example, where a mismanagement of production or redistribution of food in an inequitable manner results in famines and resultant food deserts.

Location and Neighborhood Environments

Where we live is likely to influence health as much as individual factors such as those previously described. Conditions in the neighborhoods surrounding our homes also have major health effects. These may occur through a variety of mechanisms such as the availability or accessibility of health services, and the physical and social environments of neighborhoods. If an area is polluted or has more crime, there may be direct health impacts. When the drinking water source was switched for individuals living in the city of Flint, Michigan, to the Flint River in 2014, piping was not properly treated, resulting in corrosion and lead exposure.[11] Lead exposure can result in damage to the brain and nervous system in children, and to increases in heart and kidney disease, as well as reduced fertility in adults. An individual's ability and motivation to exercise or eat a healthy diet may be reduced if there aren't reasonable exercise or healthy eating options. The neighborhood social environment is also very important—consider the role of social relationships, trust, and connectedness among residents and neighbors.

There are numerous interesting examples linking infectious diseases to neighborhood-level influence. At the neighborhood level, socioeconomic disadvantage is positively associated with both incidence of tuberculosis (TB) and increased incidence of recently transmitted TB.[12,13] For example, people living in Detroit had an average TB incidence nearly twice that of those in the rest of the state of Michigan. To add complexity, racial inequalities differed across locations in Michigan: Detroit has both higher socioeconomic disadvantage as well as a higher proportion of Blacks.[14] Black individuals also have higher prevalence of comorbidities such as coronary heart disease, asthma, and diabetes compared to Whites.

In England, a series of studies showed that human listeriosis (a serious bacterial infection usually caused by eating contaminated food) was associated with neighborhood deprivation.[15,16] Geographic areas in England were ranked according to an index of multiple deprivation by taking into account numerous socioeconomic factors such as income; employment; health deprivation and disability; barriers to housing and services; living environment; crime and disorder; and education, skills, and training. *Listeria* incidence increased with a rising deprivation index.

Social Inequality

Social inequality (or disadvantage) shapes the distribution of numerous health outcomes and is frequently captured using indicators of socioeconomic position such as income, education, and occupation.[17] Individuals who experience increased levels of social disadvantage may be more likely to live and work in environments where they are more exposed to infections and have fewer resources available to respond to these infections. There are examples of these associations in the infectious disease literature, including HIV, TB, and pandemic influenza, as well as for chronic infections such as *Helicobacter pylori* and *Chlamydia pneumonia*.[18,19] All of these infections are exacerbated by an individual's social access. The field of **social epidemiology** emphasizes the study of mechanisms and processes that produce social inequalities, placing populations at higher risk for worse health outcomes.[20] However, while diseases such as TB and cholera have long been linked to poverty and population density, there are not many examples of studies looking at the direct impacts of the social environment on infectious diseases.

Transmissible diseases can be influenced by population patterns of exposure as well as an individual's own exposure status. At the individual level, a person's prior exposure to disease, comorbidities, and general health influence their body's capacity to fight infection. At the population level, unequal distributions of housing, food, proximity to healthcare, and environmental or social conditions influence the likelihood of disease. Inequalities can also be subjective. For example, individuals who rate themselves as having lower social status compared to others have been shown to be more likely to develop symptomatic colds, independently of their actual education and income.[21] Subjective social status in fact at times predicts health and wellness better than does objective measurement, as is seen when examining health among a recent immigrant Latinx population to the United States, where individuals may better relate their stressful immigration experiences to perceived status.[22] Both objective and subjective disadvantage need to be addressed to ensure better health outcomes.

Race

Racial inequalities in health outcomes have persisted in the United States. Individuals of minority background have higher infectious disease burdens than those who identify as non-Hispanic Whites.[23] In 2019, Black people accounted for 13% of the U.S. population but 42% of new HIV/AIDS diagnoses (Figure 9.3).[24] From 1906 to 1920, African Americans

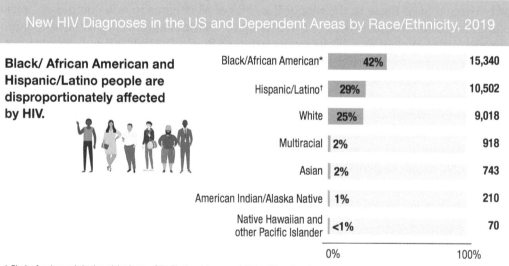

New HIV Diagnoses in the US and Dependent Areas by Race/Ethnicity, 2019

Black/ African American and Hispanic/Latino people are disproportionately affected by HIV.

Black/African American*	42%	15,340
Hispanic/Latino†	29%	10,502
White	25%	9,018
Multiracial	2%	918
Asian	2%	743
American Indian/Alaska Native	1%	210
Native Hawaiian and other Pacific Islander	<1%	70

0%   100%

* *Black* refers to people having origins in any of the Black racial groups of *Africa. African American* is a term often used for people of African descent with ancestry in North America.
† Hispanic/Latino people can be of any race.
Source: CDC. Diagnoses of HIV infection in the United States and dependent areas, 2019. *HIV Surveillance Report* 2021;32.

Figure 9.3 Proportion of AIDS cases among adults by race/ethnicity.

Source: Centers for Disease Control and Prevention. HIV in the United States and dependent areas. https://www.cdc.gov/hiv/statistics/overview/ataglance.html

in cities experienced a rate of death from infectious disease that was greater than what urban Whites experienced during the whole 1918 flu pandemic.[25] During the COVID-19 pandemic, Hispanic or Latinx persons have had hospitalization rates 2.5 times as high as White, Non-Hispanic persons.[26] These disparities are due both to historical processes of discrimination and trauma (the result of exposure to stressful events), as well as current practices that may include worse housing, healthcare access, or resources.[27] For example, numerous interviews have documented the stress from historical racism increasing substance abuse among American Indian people.[28] Similarly, prior to being forced to march on the Long Walk in 1868, Navajo diets consisted of plant-based foods with an emphasis on corn and occasional game meat or mutton. Yet at the time of this writing, there are just 13 grocery stores on the Navajo Nation, a land area roughly the size of Vermont, New Hampshire, and Massachusetts combined.[29]

Class

Social class refers to groups in different positions within a social hierarchy, often based on occupation or income. Individuals in lower social classes generally have both poorer health and shorter life expectancy.[30] For example, in a combined cross-country analysis, compared with wealthier people, those in a lower class were approximately 1.5 times more likely to die before the age of 85.

There are numerous examples pertinent to infectious disease. Human papillomavirus (HPV) infection types associated with cervical cancer are particularly common among poor women in the United States. This may be because low-income women do not have sufficient access to HPV vaccines as well as education and other preventive services.[31] Findings from the famous Whitehall study in the United Kingdom showed that employment grade was related to burden of infection as measured by detectable antibodies for three pathogens.[32] The HIV epidemic has greatly affected the economically disadvantaged in many urban areas in the United States. HIV prevalence rates in urban poverty areas are inversely related to all major socioeconomic status (SES) indicators, including education, annual household income, poverty level, employment, and homeless status, where the lower the SES, the greater the HIV prevalence rate.[33]

Social Support

Social support refers to the network of family, friends, neighbors, and community members that are available in times of need to give help and can be thought of in terms of functional and structural support.[34] Structural support refers to the level of integration of individuals into their social network, often measured by marital status or the number of relationships or cohabiting individuals in a household. Functional support refers to the different support functions fulfilled by available family/friends. Social support has shown to be clearly linked to health outcomes and has been linked directly to a decrease in risk of mortality.[35] For example, married people live longer, especially men.[36] An interesting study contrasted whether social support was associated with knowledge of, worry about, and attitudes towards AIDS and severe acute respiratory syndrome (SARS).[37] The study had differing findings for the two outcomes: Greater social support, measured using a scale, was associated with greater knowledge of AIDS, potentially because, relative to SARS, AIDS is a more common condition, with more built-in supports as a result, providing people with greater access to information.

Social network theory has shown us that individuals tend to connect with others who are more similar. This may also occur through shared behaviors and preferences, such that social networks have been shown to have positive effects through information gathering and support for prevention of influenza and pneumococcal infections through vaccination.[38] Others have shown that friends may play an important role in the adoption of infection-prevention behaviors such as handwashing and physical distancing.[39] One can consider both the number and pattern of social ties, as well as their quality (e.g., is someone socially integrated or isolated). Either way, the stronger the network, the more positive influence on health.

Social Capital

Social capital can be thought of as social networks and relationships that through coordinated efforts benefit the broader community.[40] In the case of infectious diseases, one example might be leveraging communities to spread information about the importance of distancing and encouraging community members to distance. Social capital has been linked with effective preparations during outbreaks of Ebola and Zika.[41] However, social capital may be more effective where there is also a clear governmental approach, such as in the early response to COVID-19 in Taiwan, whereas in the United States, much more variability was observed as communities made decisions about distancing that had more to do with fluctuating local government policies.[42,43]

THOUGHT QUESTION

Which social factors do you think are most important in consideration of infectious diseases? Would it be possible to prioritize one over another? How might you go about measuring these to decide?

So Which Are More Important, Social or Biomedical Measures?

In the early 20th century, large declines in TB were observed in Europe and in North America. These were likely due to better housing, less overcrowding, improved nutrition and living conditions, and milk pasteurization (Figure 9.4).[44] This dramatic reduction occurred prior to biomedical interventions against TB, with streptomycin, the first effective antibiotic drug, introduced in 1947 and childhood bacille Calmette–Guérin (BCG) vaccination in 1954.

A lively debate followed over decades whether medical or social factors were more important in driving down rates of infectious disease mortality.[45] But this has falsely provided a "either/or" proposition over the more appropriate "it's complicated." All public health measures including social, such as better housing, a clean water supply, sewage, and sanitation, and medical, such as vaccination and medication, are critical in controlling disease. While the introduction of antibiotics was instrumental in reducing disease severity and transmission and accelerated reductions in mortality, clearly social factors and an improved standard of living have played a tremendous role in the decline of mortality from infectious diseases worldwide. The complexity of disease systems is evidenced by how the greatest infectious disease killers such as TB and HIV have still not been eliminated. This is due to a complex combination of social determinants of health, coinfection (e.g., contracting TB among people living with HIV), the challenges to medication adherence, historical discrimination as it ties in to issues of trust and belief in

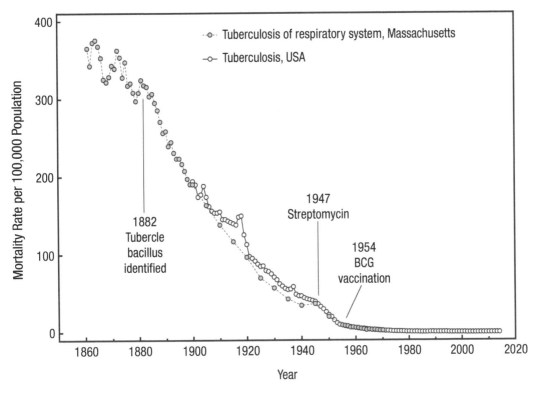

Figure 9.4 **Tuberculosis mortality rate trends over time.**
BCG, bacille Calmette–Guérin.
Source: Courtesy of Ljstalpers.

public health, and the emergence of multi-drug resistant strains of pathogens that are difficult to treat and often emerge because of inadequate access to care in the first place. Failure to consider both the medical and the social led to low adherence and low uptake with further downstream implications that undermined medical advances.

Mechanisms Relating Social Factors to Infectious Disease

Why might we see these increasing rates of disease with greater social disadvantage? We can consider the more proximal mechanisms linking a social exposure with an infectious disease outcome. One hypothesis is that as one becomes more disadvantaged, so occurs the higher likelihood of exposure to infectious diseases. This may be due to occupation, poor housing and overcrowding, or lack of material resources.[46] Someone poorer is more likely to come into contact with someone with an infectious disease, and more likely to be exposed due to overcrowding. The second major hypothesis is that of increased "wear and tear" through disadvantage, with greater chronic stress and poorer health leading to greater vulnerability to infection. For example, chronic stress related to lower income has been shown to be related to increased inflammation or decreased immune function.[47] Studies have examined the effect of social support on immune function and found associations with changes in immunity.[48] As has been noted, there could be other pathways, such as lower likelihood of accessing care or lower standard of care received. The mechanisms, or pathways, through which socioeconomic factors may influence an infectious disease outcome may operate independently or simultaneously (Figure 9.5). In order to enact effective policies and interventions to reduce the burden of disease, it is important to understand the mechanisms.

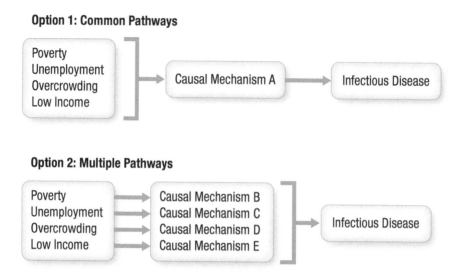

Figure 9.5 Pathways through which socioeconomic factors increase risk of infectious disease.

THOUGHT QUESTION

Is the mechanism through which social factors are associated with infectious disease less problematic than that for a chronic disease such as diabetes?

Interventions, or What Can We Do About It?

The World Health Organization's Commission on Social Determinants of Health has outlined three clear approaches to address social factors, which are highly applicable to infectious diseases.[2] The first of these is to improve daily living conditions. This can manifest both through improved living and working conditions, as well as improved education and what are known as **social protection policies**. These are initiatives designed to reduce vulnerability to poverty, mitigate the impact of economic shocks such as illness or loss of employment, and support people who suffer from disability or discrimination to secure basic livelihoods.[49] Social protection often includes providing direct transfers of food or money to poor households, with the receipt of these transfers sometimes conditional on other actions, and increasing access to microfinance opportunities to support business development. "Care" programs—particularly those focusing on strengthening families and supporting caregivers—have positive impacts on HIV infection.[50] The Sonagachi project in Calcutta, India, was a community-oriented project focused on responding to community needs, mobilizing and empowering sex worker groups, reducing HIV prevalence to 10% (from a likely baseline of 50%–90%), and increasing condom use from 3% to 90%.[51] Mathematical modeling work shows that reducing extreme poverty and expanding social protection has reduced TB incidence by up to 84.3%.[52]

The second is to tackle inequitable distribution of power, money, and resources more broadly. Racial dimensions of the HIV epidemic in the United States are very much correlated with wealth and resource gaps, which are often due to both historical and contemporary processes of segregation in housing, education, employment, incarceration, and healthcare. This approach requires a public sector that is committed to addressing such inequities, inclusive governance, accountability, and strong public health infrastructure. In Australia a combination of policy, funding, and dedicated research centers decreased the number of HIV cases in the epicenter (New South Wales) from 1993 through 2006.[53]

Finally, it is important to measure and understand health disparities and inequities. Many governments either do not acknowledge these in the first place or else have no way of tracking them. The COVID-19 pandemic has illustrated the importance of both setting up health equity surveillance systems to understand who is disproportionately affected, as well as to subsequently evaluate the health equity impact of policies and actions (Figure 9.6).

social protection policies: Initiatives designed to reduce vulnerability to poverty through education, investments, job placement, and protecting the aging population.

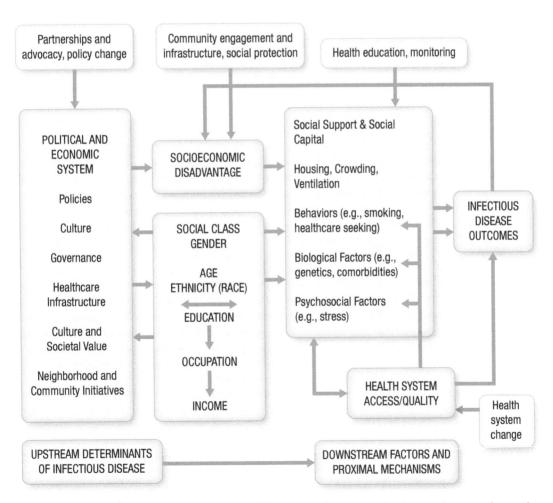

Figure 9.6 Potential interventions for different socioeconomic determinants along the continuum.

THOUGHT QUESTION

What are appropriate social interventions for infectious diseases? What social approaches could we take in reducing elements of R_0? Remember that R_0 refers to the average number of secondary cases infected and consists of frequency of contact between individuals, the probability that an interaction will lead to transmission, and how long an infected individual is contagious.

CAUSAL THINKING IN INFECTIOUS DISEASES

Epidemiologic data following HIV/AIDS patient cohorts has been key to understanding how to provide potentially toxic medications, often over a lifetime. Clinic-based cohorts have been created to follow individuals and their response to treatment. However, one can imagine how individuals become lost over time and that selection bias is probable as those remaining in studies are no longer representative of broader target populations. Various analytic approaches can be used to best understand the causal determinants of mortality among individuals beginning therapy, while understanding possible biases of the data. For example, in parts of Africa, male sex may influence loss to follow-up given that men may be engaged in migrant labor, truck driving, and trade, making them harder to track over the full period of a longitudinal study. Men may also be more likely to have deaths reported given their social status in certain countries.[54]

We have discussed causative agents and the epidemiologic triad, but the concept of causality is particularly pertinent as we think of the mechanisms and pathways through which different social factors may influence disease. There are a number of other factors that need to be considered when evaluating infectious diseases. For example, when considering infectious diseases, it is important to understand that there may be both individual-level effects (often called direct effects) as well as broader transmission effects (also called indirect effects). Some risk factors may result in an increased risk of infection for an individual (a direct effect), whereas others may increase the incidence of infection in the whole population. Complicating things further, a risk factor can have both individual and transmission effects if those exposed have an increased risk of infection, and then these individuals in turn become infectious, transmitting disease to others. While beyond the scope of this text, it is possible to examine the separate individual and transmission effects of a risk factor by looking at who else gets sick after an index case is infected in a household.[55] This can inform our understanding of infectivity based on both whether the index case has been exposed (the individual effect) as well as on whether exposed household members are susceptible to infection (the transmission effect).

THOUGHT QUESTION

Can you think of some examples of social risk factors that may have direct and indirect effects on infectious diseases?

What Makes a Cause?

So, what "counts" as a cause in infectious diseases? Causality, that a risk factor is causally associated with the outcome, is a central tenet of epidemiology. There are a number of approaches to assess the relationship between cause (an exposure or risk factor) and effect (the outcome or disease of interest). In the late 1800s, Robert Koch described four postulates that provided a starting point for standard criteria that could be used to identify whether an agent was indeed the cause of an infectious disease. However, some bacteria might be harmless under certain conditions, yet can cause disease under others (e.g., *Helicobacter pylori*, which is a naturally occurring gut bacteria, has been causally associated with certain gastric cancers). In another example, sometimes individuals are exposed to an agent, but either are not infected or do not progress to clinical disease (e.g., *Mycobacterium tuberculosis*). When epidemiologists discuss **causal inference**, we are discerning whether a causal relationship does or does not exist between a particular exposure and an outcome.

Using a case-control design, Richard Doll and Bradford Hill conducted key studies in the 1940s and 1950s establishing a strong association between smoking and lung cancer. Prior to this work, there was a lack of understanding of the risks of smoking. Almost half the population smoked. Not every smoker gets lung cancer, and the latency for lung cancer is long. But most importantly, there were no defined criteria that could be used to establish causality for a non-infectious agent. A prolonged debate followed regarding the causal nature of the association, and as a result the 1964 Surgeon General's report linked smoking cigarettes with lung cancer, and in 1965 Hill's criteria came about to weigh scientific evidence. In the text that follows we list each criterion, what question it answers, and provide an example from evidence on the causal effect of antiviral therapy on transmission of HIV.[56]

- **Strength of the association:** How large is the effect between exposure and outcome? Antiretroviral therapy is highly protective (over 90%) against HIV transmission.

- **Consistency:** Has the same association been observed by other researchers, in different populations, or using different approaches? Across 11 cohorts, the overall rate of transmission of patients treated with antiretroviral therapy decreased by 92% among couples where one partner was HIV positive.

- **Specificity:** What happens to the outcome when only the exposure is changed and nothing else? The use of antiretroviral therapy predictably prevents HIV transmission, and the therapy is independently responsible for preventing HIV transmission.

- **Temporality:** Did the exposure (the putative cause) come before the outcome? HIV antiretroviral therapy stops viral replication, so that viral load is low in bodily fluids, reducing the likelihood of HIV transmission. This can be observed in longitudinal cohort studies.

- **Biological gradient:** Is there a dose response effect where a higher exposure translates into a stronger outcome? Even small reductions in viral load result in reductions in HIV transmission. This is true for mortality as well, with less than 1% of men with low baseline HIV viral load levels dying of AIDS compared to over 18% among patients with moderate levels and almost 70% of those with high levels in a 10-year follow-up study.[57]

- **Plausibility/Coherence:** Does the observed association make sense and does the evidence fit with what is already known? The association between reduced viral load in different bodily fluids and long-term, sustained, and effective treatment is strong. When viral load is undetectable, the likelihood of HIV transmission is much lower.

- **Experiment:** Are there well-designed studies that support the association? Antiviral HIV therapy has been shown to reduce transmission from mother to child (vertical transmission) below 5%.

- **Analogy:** Are there similar associations that help support the observed one? One analogy that has been used is that treatment of genital herpes decreases viral burden and potential for herpes transmission.[58]

THOUGHT QUESTION

How do you think Hill's criteria apply for infectious diseases? Is it possible to definitively prove that something causes a case of an infectious disease? For example, COVID-19?

The Sufficient-Component Cause Model

The causal pie model was developed in 1976 by Kenneth Rothman and takes the concept of a causal pie (shaped like the one we all like to eat!), imagining the various individual causes that create that "pie" leading to a particular outcome.[59] In particular, he imagined **sufficient causes** made up of different **component causes.** For an outcome to occur, all the component causes making up the pie of a sufficient cause have to be present. If one of these components is absent, the cause is not complete, and the other components would have no effect on the outcome (Figure 9.7). The sufficient cause itself was thus not a single factor in itself but "a complete causal mechanism ... inevitably produce[ing] disease."[59] There is often more than one sufficient cause for each outcome, meaning that there are different mechanisms by which a person can get the same disease. A component cause that must be present in every sufficient cause of a given outcome is referred to as a **necessary cause**. Considering Koch's postulates, an organism is a necessary cause for the disease outcome (due to that organism). For example, in the case of HIV/AIDS, a sufficient cause could include component causes such as exposure to someone with HIV, engaging in risky sexual behavior or needle sharing with that person, and lack of appropriate treatment, and a necessary cause is that the pathogen itself, HIV, is present.

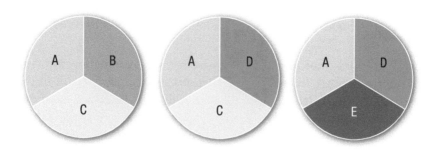

Figure 9.7 Rothman's causal pies. In each of these three sufficient cause scenarios, different sufficient causes (A to E) must be present in order for the outcome to occur.

Of course, as we know the randomized experiment provides the strongest evidence possible for causality since the exposure is manipulated by the researcher, allowing us to understand whether the outcome is attributable to the exposure or not. If we were to repeat the same experiment over and over again, and it produces the same outcome, then we would expect a given exposure to cause an outcome. However, a randomized design may not work well with social factors as exposures. This design would not be able to determine whether someone's race or sex is a "cause" of an outcome, as one cannot easily manipulate these. In contrast, while not simple, it is possible to imagine a scenario where governmental policy supplements income or provides housing assistance, allowing for a potential trial examining the effects of these social exposures.

HEADS UP!

The Blame Game. Epidemiology is very particular in considering the concept of a causal relationship. Association should not be confused with causality. If exposure X appears to lead to outcome Y, we might say the two variables are associated. However, associations can occur in both the presence and absence of a true causal relationship. For example, a third variable may be confounding the observed association (as a common cause of both the exposure and outcome). In this case a causal relationship cannot be inferred. Only if we can rule out biases such as confounding can we consider that an association also implies causation.

causal inference: Whether a causal relationship exists or does not exist between a particular exposure and an outcome.

sufficient cause: A complete causal mechanism that will inevitably produce disease.

component cause: Each participating factor in a sufficient cause that in itself does not cause disease.

necessary cause: A component cause that must be present in every sufficient cause of a given outcome.

THOUGHT QUESTION

Models of causality are shown above for infectious diseases, as with the example of HIV. Can you think of some examples of social risk factors that may have direct and indirect causal effects on infectious disease outcomes?

CASE STUDY

Mathilde Krim was an HIV/AIDS scientist, advocate, and philanthropist extraordinaire (Figure 9.8). Krim received her PhD from the University of Geneva, Switzerland, in 1953. She then moved to Israel, working in cytogenetics and cancer-causing viruses at the Weizmann Institute of Science in Israel, before moving to New York City and working at Memorial Sloan-Kettering Cancer Center, where she became involved in HIV/AIDS work when seeing patients with Kaposi's sarcoma. After dedicating her laboratory research to understanding the role of interferons—a natural substance now used in the treatment of viral and neoplastic diseases—in treating HIV/AIDS, with work spanning both basic science and epidemiology, she went on to found the AIDS Medical Foundation (AMF), the first private organization concerned with fostering and supporting AIDS research, later to become the American Foundation for AIDS Research (amfAR). President Reagan only acknowledged the existence of AIDS 2 years later, in 1985. While she was board chair, amfAR funded more than 2,200 biomedical, social/behavioral, policy, and

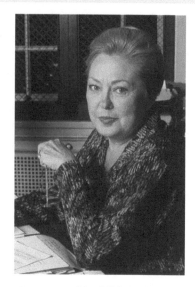

Figure 9.8 Mathilde Krim (1926–2018).

Source: Bernard Gotfryd, https://lccn.loc.gov/2020731582

education projects. Krim was an astounding advocate and fundraiser. In the 2013 documentary *The Battle of amfAR*, Krim said: "Physicians are very hesitant to announce a catastrophe and I said, it has to be said, otherwise the federal government will not pay attention. So I called as many people as I could in Washington to ask for financial support, but I got the usual stupid answer—nobody can fund it." Krim helped to get both the HOPE Act and the Ryan White CARE Act passed through Congress, which allowed for an unprecedented level of funding for AIDS prevention, education, and treatment. And who says science is boring? Krim was friends with presidents and Hollywood stars, and when she hosted a 45th birthday after-party for President John F. Kennedy, Marilyn Monroe sang him the now famous "Happy Birthday, Mr. President."

CONCLUSION

A more thorough consideration of social factors is key in thinking about how infectious diseases arise and how to reduce future morbidity and mortality. Studies need to consider the "causes of causes" and the underlying social factors that are responsible for infectious diseases. Working in conjunction with more traditional biomedical approaches such as vaccination and therapy, as well as more explicit targeting of interventions to social causes, through reducing poverty, improving living standards and nutrition, and lowering stress, can lead to an era of both greater health equity and infectious disease elimination.

TEACHING CORNER

DID YOU KNOW?

TB is a severe respiratory disease usually treated over the course of 6 months or longer, which is further complicated by multi-drug resistance and challenges with treatment adherence. High levels of overcrowding, individual-level risk factors, and lack of access to healthcare contribute to high rates of TB among individuals who are incarcerated. Incidence in prisons varies across the globe, with ranges from 30 to over 2,000 cases per 100,000 person-years. This translates into a ratio of over 27 cases to one in comparing incarcerated populations and the general population in South America.[60]

TRY THIS

Using each of Hill's criteria, build an argument that supports incarceration as a causative factor in TB incidence. Once you have worked through Hill's criteria, use Rothman's causal pies to depict two different iterations ("pies") of components and sufficient causes associated with incarceration as a cause of TB. Consider possibilities such as HIV coinfection, crowding, and other social factors.

TAKE IT A STEP FURTHER

What interventions might you recommend for targeting the social determinants of incarceration in order to reduce TB incidence? What elements of social support, social capital, and social inequity can impact a released prisoner's capacity to adhere to TB treatment?

QUESTIONS FOR FURTHER DISCUSSION

1. Define social epidemiology and describe how it is similar to the more traditional concepts of epidemiology and how it is different.

2. Choose an infectious disease and compare how disease rates and burden vary across race, class, and geographic location. What data sources were you able to find to facilitate these comparisons?

3. What are the three approaches outlined by the WHO's Commission on Social Determinants of Health to intervening to address social factors? How do they interact to promote health and what is the epidemiologist's role?

4. In the Tecumseh Study of Respiratory Illness, respiratory infection rates decreased but self-reported illness rates increased with the level of education of the head of the household.[61] Under what circumstances is that possible?

A robust set of instructor resources designed to supplement this text is located at http://connect.springerpub.com/Content/book/978-0-8261-5674-7. Qualifying instructors may request access by emailing textbook@springerpub.com.

REFERENCES

1. Fee E, Krieger N. Understanding AIDS: historical interpretations and the limits of biomedical individualism. *Am J Public Health*. 1993;83:1477–1486. doi:10.2105/ajph.83.10.1477
2. World Health Organization. Closing the gap in a generation: health equity through action on the social determinants of health—final report of the Commission on Social Determinants of Health. August 27, 2008. https://www.who.int/publications/i/item/WHO-IER-CSDH-08.1
3. Office of Disease Prevention and Health Promotion. Disparities. https://www.healthypeople.gov/2020/about/foundation-health-measures/Disparities
4. Centers for Disease Control and Prevention. Health equity. https://www.cdc.gov/chronicdisease/healthequity/index.htm
5. Rourke SB, Bacon J, McGee F, Gilbert M. Tackling the social and structural drivers of HIV in Canada. *Can Commun Dis Rep*. 2015;41(12):322–326. doi:10.14745/ccdr.v41i12a03
6. Jones KE, Patel NG, Levy MA, et al. Global trends in emerging infectious diseases. *Nature*. 2008;451:990–993. doi:10.1038/nature06536
7. Klepac P, Metcalf CJ, McLean AR, Hampson K. Towards theendgame and beyond: complexities and challenges for the elimination of infectious diseases. *Philos Trans R Soc Lond B Biol Sci*. 2013;368:20120137. doi:10.1098/rstb.2012.0137
8. United Nations. Make cities and human settlements inclusive, safe, resilient and sustainable. https://unstats.un.org/sdgs/report/2019/goal-11
9. Sumilo D, Asokliene L, Bormane A, et al. Climate change cannot explain the upsurge of tick-borne encephalitis in the baltics. *PLoS One*. 2007;2(6):e500. doi:10.1371/journal.pone.0000500
10. Association of Health Care Journalists. Connecting the dots between social determinants and infectious diseases. https://healthjournalism.org/blog/2018/09/connecting-the-dots-between-social-determinants-and-infectious-diseases/
11. Ruckart PZ, Ettinger AS, Hanna-Attisha M, et al. The Flint Water crisis: a coordinated public health emergency response and recovery initiative. *J Public Health Manag Pract*. 2019;25(suppl 1, Lead Poisoning Prevention):S84–S90. doi:10.1097/PHH.0000000000000871
12. Oren E, Koepsell T, Leroux B, Mayer J. Area-based socio-economic disadvantage and tuberculosis incidence. *Int J Tuberculosis Lung Disease*. 2012;16(7):880–885. doi:10.5588/ijtld.11.0700
13. Oren E, Narita M, Nolan C, Mayer J. Neighborhood socioeconomic position and tuberculosis transmission: a retrospective cohort study. *BMC Infect Dis*. 2014;14(1):227. doi:10.1186/1471-2334-14-227
14. Noppert GA, Clarke P, Hicken MT, Wilson ML. Understanding the intersection of race and place: the case of tuberculosis in Michigan. *BMC Public Health*. 2019;19:1669. https://gracenoppert.isr.umich.edu/wp-content/uploads/2019/12/Noppert_BMCPH.pdf
15. Gillespie IA, Mook P, Little CL, Grant KA, McLauchlin J. Human listeriosis in England, 2001–2007: association with neighbourhood deprivation. *Euro Surveill*. 2010;15(27):pii=19609. doi:10.2807/ese.15.27.19609-en
16. Semenza JC. Strategies to intervene on social determinants of infectious diseases. *Euro Surveill*. 2010;15(27):pii=19611. doi:10.2807/ese.15.27.19611-en
17. Galobardes B, Shaw M, Lawlor D, et al. Indicators of socioeconomic position. In: Oakes JM, Kaufman JS, eds. *Methods in Social Epidemiology*. Jossey-Bass; 2006:47–85.
18. Malaty HM, Graham DY. Importance of childhood socioeconomic status on the current prevalence of *Helicobacter pylori* infection. *Gut*. 1994;35(6):742–745. doi:10.1136/gut.35.6.742
19. Mamelund SE, Shelley-Egan C, Rogeberg O. The association between socioeconomic status and pandemic influenza: systematic review and meta-analysis. *PLoS One*. 2021;16(9):e0244346. doi:10.1371/journal.pone.0244346
20. Krieger N. Theories for social epidemiology in the 21st century: an ecosocial perspective. *Int J Epidemiol*. 2001;30:668–677. doi:10.1093/ije/30.4.668
21. Cohen S, Alper CM, Doyle WJ, et al. Objective and subjective socioeconomic status and susceptibility to the common cold. *Health Psychol*. 2008;27:268. doi:10.1037/0278-6133.27.2.268
22. Garza JR, Glenn BA, Mistry RS, Ponce NA, Zimmerman FJ. Subjective social status and self-reported health among US-born and immigrant Latinos. *J Immigr Minor Health*. 2017;19(1):108–119. doi:10.1007/s10903-016-0346-x

23. Zajacova A, Dowd JB, Aiello AE. Socioeconomic and race/ethnic patterns in persistent infection burden among U.S. adults. *J Gerontol A Biol Sci Med Sci*. 2009;64(2):272–279. doi:10.1093/gerona/gln012

24. Centers for Disease Control and Prevention. Diagnoses of HIV infection in the United States and dependent areas, 2018 (preliminary). November 2019. https://www.cdc.gov/hiv/pdf/library/reports/surveillance/cdc-hiv-surveillance-report-2018-preliminary-vol-30.pdf

25. Feigenbaum JJ, Muller C, Wrigley-Field E. Regional and racial inequality in infectious disease mortality in U.S. cities, 1900–1948. *Demography*. 2019;56(4):1371–1388. doi:10.1007/s13524-019-00789-z

26. Centers for Disease Control and Prevention. Risk for COVID-19 infection, hospitalization, and death by race/ethnicity. June 24, 2022. https://www.cdc.gov/coronavirus/2019-ncov/covid-data/investigations-discovery/hospitalization-death-by-race-ethnicity.html

27. Link BG, Phelan JC. Understanding sociodemographic differences in health-- the role of fundamental social causes. *Am J Public Health*. 1996;86(4):471–473. doi:10.2105/ajph.86.4.471

28. Skewes MC, Blume AW. Understanding the link between racial trauma and substance use among American Indians. *Am Psychol*. 2019;74(1):88–100. doi:10.1037/amp0000331

29. Partners in Health. Eating well: grocery program takes off in the Navajo nation. June 26, 2018. https://www.pih.org/article/eating-well-grocery-program-takes-navajo-nation

30. Stringhini S, Carmeli C, Jokela M, et al. Socioeconomic status and the 25 × 25 risk factors as determinants of premature mortality: a multicohort study and meta-analysis of 1·7 million men and women. *Lancet*. 2017;389(10075):1229–1237. doi:10.1016/S0140-6736(16)32380-7

31. Kahn JA, Lan D, Kahn RS. Sociodemographic factors associated with high-risk human papillomavirus infection. *Obstet Gynecol*. 2007;110(1):87–95. doi:10.1097/01.AOG.0000266984.23445.9c

32. Steptoe A, Shamaei-Tousi A, Gylfe A, et al. Socioeconomic status, pathogen burden, and cardiovascular disease risk. *Heart*. 2007;93:1567–1570. doi:10.1136/hrt.2006.113993

33. Centers for Disease Control and Prevention. *HIV infection, risk, prevention, and testing behaviors among heterosexually active adults at increased risk for HIV infection. National HIV Behavioral Surveillance 23 U.S. Cities, 2019*. https://www.cdc.gov/hiv/pdf/library/reports/surveillance/cdc-hiv-surveillance-special-report-number-26.pdf

34. Uchino BN. Social support and health: a review of physiological processes potentially underlying links to disease outcomes. *J Behav Med*. 2006;29(4):377–387. doi:10.1007/s10865-006-9056-5

35. Holt-Lunstad J, Smith TB, Layton JB. Social relationships and mortality risk: a meta-analytic review. *PLoS Med*. 2010;7(7):e1000316. doi:10.1371/journal.pmed.1000316

36. WebMD. Marriage tied to longer life span, new data shows. October 10, 2019. https://www.webmd.com/a-to-z-guides/news/20191010/marriage-tied-to-longer-life-span-new-data-shows

37. Nandi A, Tracy M, Aiello A, Des Jarlais DC, Galea S. Social support and response to AIDS and severe acute respiratory syndrome. *Emerg Infect Dis*. 2008;14(5):825–827. https://www.ncbi.nlm.nih.gov/pmc/articles/PMC2600224/pdf/07-1070_finalD.pdf

38. Zimmerman RK, Santibanez TA, Fine MJ, et al. Barriers and facilitators of pneumococcal vaccination among the elderly. *Vaccine*. 2003;21:1510–1517. doi:10.1016/s0264-410x(02)00698-9

39. Steijvers LCJ, Brinkhues S, Hoebe CJPA. Social networks and infectious diseases prevention behavior: a cross-sectional study in people aged 40 years and older. *PLoS One*. 2021;16(5):e0251862. https://www.ncbi.nlm.nih.gov/pmc/articles/PMC8133464/#pone.0251862.ref009

40. Putnam, Robert D. *Bowling Alone: The Collapse and Revival of American Community*. Simon & Schuster; 2000.

41. Kruk ME, MyersM, Tornorlah Varpilah S, Dahn BT. What is a resilient health system? Lessons from Ebola. *The Lancet*. 2015;385(9980):1910–1912. doi:10.1016/S0140-6736(15)60755-3

42. Shapiro D. Taiwan shows its mettle in coronavirus crisis, while the WHO is MIA. Brookings (blog). 2020. https://www.brookings.edu/blog/order-from-chaos/2020/03/19/taiwan-shows-its-mettle-in-coronavirus-crisis-while-the-who-is-mia/

43. Gibbons J, Yang T-C, Oren E. Community boosts immunity? Exploring the relationship between social capital and COVID-19 social distancing. *Spatial Demogr*. 2022;10:75–105. https://link.springer.com/article/10.1007/s40980-021-00096-5

44. Hargreaves JR, Boccia D, Evans CA, Adato M, Petticrew M, Porter JD. The social determinants of tuberculosis: from evidence to action. *Am J Public Health.* 2011;101(4):654–662. doi:10.2105/AJPH.2010.199505

45. McKeown T. *The Role of Medicine: Dream, Mirage or Nemesis?* (The Rock Carlington Fellow, 1976). Nuffield Provincial Hospital Trust; 1976.

46. Acevedo-Garcia D. Residential segregation and the epidemiology of infectious diseases. *Soc Sci Med.* 2000;51(8):1143–1161. doi:10.1016/s0277-9536(00)00016-2

47. Friedman E, Herd P. Income, education, and inflammation: differential associations in a national probability sample (the MIDUS study). *Psychosom Med.* 2010;72:290–300. doi:10.1097/PSY.0b013e3181cfe4c2

48. Roy V, Ruel S, Ivers H, et al. Stress-buffering effect of social support on immunity and infectious risk during chemotherapy for breast cancer. *Brain Behav Immun Health.* 2021;10:100186. doi:10.1016/j.bbih.2020.100186

49. Adato M, Bassett L. *What Is the Potential of Cash Transfers to Strengthen Families Affected by HIV and AIDS? A Review of the Evidence on Impacts and Key Policy Debates.* Joint Learning Initiative on Children and AIDS; 2008.

50. Visser M, Zungu N, Ndala-Magoro N. ISIBINDI, creating circles of care for orphans and vulnerable children in South Africa: post-programme outcomes. *AIDS Care.* 2015;27(8):1014–1019. doi:10.1080/09540121.2015.1018861

51. Cohen J. Sonagachi sex workers stymie HIV. *Science.* 2004;304:506. doi:10.1126/science.304.5670.506

52. Carter DJ, Glaziou P, Lönnroth K, et al. The impact of social protection and poverty elimination on global tuberculosis incidence: a statistical modelling analysis of Sustainable Development Goal 1. *Lancet Glob Health.* 2018;6:e514–e522. doi:10.1016/S2214-109X(18)30195-5

53. Zablotska IB, Prestage G, Grulich AE, Imrie J. Differing trends in sexual risk behaviours in three Australian states: New South Wales, Victoria and Queensland, 1998–2006. *Sex Health.* 2008;5:125–130. doi:10.1071/sh07076

54. Geng EH, Glidden DV, Bangsberg DR, et al. A causal framework for understanding the effect of losses to follow-up on epidemiologic analyses in clinic-based cohorts: the case of HIV-infected patients on antiretroviral therapy in Africa. *Am J Epidemiol.* 2012;175(10):1080–1087. doi:10.1093/aje/kwr444

55. Halloran ME, Struchiner CJ. Causal inference in infectious diseases. *Epidemiology.* 1995;6(2):142–151. doi:10.1097/00001648-199503000-00010

56. Nosyk B, Audoin B, Beyrer C, et al. Examining the evidence on the causal effect of HAART on transmission of HIV using the Bradford Hill criteria. *AIDS.* 2013;27(7):1159–1165. doi:10.1097/QAD.0b013e32835f1d68

57. Mellors JW, Muñoz A, Giorgi JV, et al. Plasma viral load and CD4+ lymphocytes as prognostic markers of HIV-1 infection. *Ann Intern Med.* 1997;126(12):946–954. doi:10.7326/0003-4819-126-12-199706150-00003

58. Centers for Disease Control and Prevention; Workowski KA, Berman SM. Sexually transmitted diseases treatment guidelines, 2006. *MMWR Recomm Rep.* 2006;55(RR-11):1–94. https://www.cdc.gov/mmwr/preview/mmwrhtmL/rr5511a1.htm

59. Rothman KJ. Causes. *Am J Epidemiol.* 1976;104:587–592. doi:10.1093/oxfordjournals.aje.a112335

60. Cords O, Martinez L, Warren JL, et al. Incidence and prevalence of tuberculosis in incarcerated populations: a systematic review and meta-analysis. *Lancet Public Health.* 2021;6(5):e300–e308. doi:10.1016/S2468-2667(21)00025-6

61. Monto AS, Ullman BM. Acute respiratory illness in an American community: the Tecumseh study. *JAMA.* 1974;227:164–169. doi:10.1001/jama.1974.03230150016004

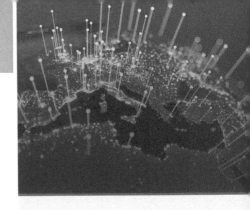

CHAPTER 10

INFECTIOUS DISEASES AND THE ENVIRONMENT

INTRODUCTION

In 2006, the livestock disease bluetongue, caused by the midge-borne bluetongue virus (BTV), first arrived in temperate Northern Europe. Prior to then, it had only been observed in the warmer climates of Africa and around the Mediterranean Sea. While a mild disease in cattle (only about 5% show symptoms and the case fatality rate [CFR] is about 1%), it is a devastating disease to sheep (70%–90% CFR) and deer (80%–90% CFR). Particularly among sheep, the tongue may swell, and the lack of oxygen causes a blueish color, giving the disease its name. The 2006 invasion into Northern Europe consisted of BTV-8, primarily being transmitted by midges in the Culicoides obsoletus *and* Culicoides pulicaris *complex; that is, a novel strain being transmitted by midges not previously known to be vectors. Read more about the distribution of BTV in Europe by Kundlacz et al. at www.mdpi.com/1999-4915/11/7/672/htm.*

ENVIRONMENTAL PREDICTORS OF INFECTIOUS DISEASE

It used to be that bluetongue virus (BTV) was restricted to the tropics and subtropics, and was only found between 40° to 50° N and 20° to 30° S latitude. Within that band, the 27 strains of BTV are somewhat selective to their Culicoides *vector and the vectors are highly selective to the environments. Across Africa, where BTV was first described, the primary vector is* Culicoides imicola *and is where most strains circulate. In central and Southeast Asia, on the other hand, BTV is primarily spread by* Culicoides brevitarsis. *Yet another pattern occurs in the more temperate United States, where the primary strain is BTV-10 and the primary vector is* Culicoides sonorensis. *The Caribbean and Central America has* Culicoides insignis *and only shares two of the same BTV strains with the United States, BTV-10 and BTV-17.*

When, *where*, and *how much* transmission of infectious disease occurs is often driven by the environment in which the disease is occurring. We intuitively know this based on nomenclature such as *winter* flu, *hay* fever, *tropical* diseases, or *Eastern* equine encephalitis, but what factors drive these patterns? How can understanding this association help us to better understand and reduce infectious disease burden?

To understand what it takes for an infectious disease to occur in a given area, we can turn back to the epidemiologic triad as a framework. *Agent:* the pathogen, be it viral, bacterial, fungal, parasitic, or prion, has to be there. *Environment:* the right habitat is necessary to support any vectors or reservoirs; the right climate must also exist to promote the pathogen's growth (Figure 10.1). *Host:* people or animals, as well as any vectors or living reservoirs, must be living there and engaging in those activities that expose them to the pathogen. Each of those connections allow for understanding of disease risk as well as for possible interventions to break the transmission cycle.

**Habitat Types
Typically Associated With Disease**

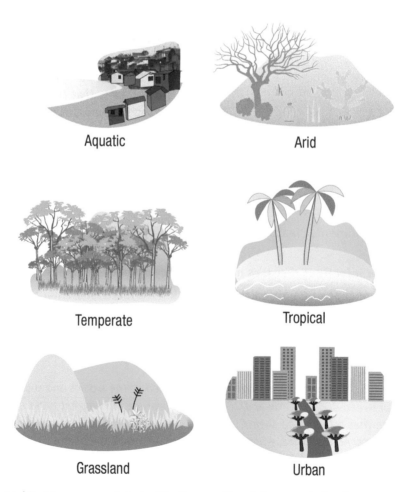

Aquatic

Arid

Temperate

Tropical

Grassland

Urban

Figure 10.1 Habitat types associated with disease. The tight association between diseases and environment does mean that knowing the habitat can give hints to the likely diseases one might encounter.

GETTING THERE

What, then, does it take for the pathogen to be in a given location? Arrival of a pathogen can occur via mutations of existing pathogens resulting in the development of new strains. Evolutionary changes in host–pathogen interactions may change the capacity for pathogens to infect new hosts. Wind, blowing vectors, or pathogenic spores have been implicated in the transmission of various diseases—sometimes locally, but sometimes at greater distances (see, for example, the role of wind and flight in BTV spread[1]).

But currently, there is also the opportunity for pathogens, vectors, and reservoirs to hitch a ride with travelers or commercial trade between endemic and susceptible areas (see, for example, travel implicated in the re-establishment of dengue in the western hemisphere[2]). Magellan took 3 years to circumnavigate the globe. Most modern ships will make it in about a year and a half, if you want to enjoy the journey, or about 2 months if you are in a rush. If you are really in a hurry, the Air France Concorde did it in about a day and a half in 1992. Layer onto that the estimated six million people in the air every day and the 100,000 flights in the sky, and we are more connected to other cities and to remote areas of the world than we ever have been. This connectivity allows us to more easily experience new cultures, collaborate and engage, and move goods quickly, but it also provides an opportunity to move pathogens around the world much more quickly.[3]

ESTABLISHING

Let us assume that our pathogen or vector has arrived to a new area. What does it take for the vector or pathogen to establish? Soil- and water-borne pathogens need a specific substrate or temperature to grow. Vector-borne and zoonotic diseases need the right vectors and reservoirs to infect. The vectors and reservoirs themselves also have habitat requirements for them to live and thrive. Suitable habitat can mean the right soil type for animals to burrow in and *Coccidioides* fungi to grow in, which will eventually aerosolize and cause Valley fever.[4] The right combination of forest-abutting peri-domestic yards allows for white-footed mice, deer ,and *Ixodes scapularis* to mix and spread Lyme disease.[5] In metapopulation models of ecology, the establishment of species is dependent upon the immigration rate (how quickly they arrive) and the extinction rate (how quickly they die out), as well as introduction of species into an area,[6] which in turn is dependent upon the degree of isolation (especially with islands, how far does the species need to travel to get to the new area) and the availability of a suitable habitat once it arrives.[6,7]

Relatedly, and by some definitions, part of a suitable habitat for organisms is a permissible climate. Most microorganisms and many animal hosts have narrow temperature tolerance ranges for optimal growth and survival. *Aedes aegypti*, the primary dengue vector, starts to exhibit increased mortality at temperatures above 104°F (40°C) or near 50°F (10°C) with low humidity.[8] But, with optimal temperature and humidity, the population grows quickly and reaches high vector densities. Temperature-driven survival thresholds are also true for the pathogen and hosts, as optimal temperatures support proliferation.

Without suitable habitat, even if a disease is introduced, it cannot establish. However, the reciprocal argument is still true, as just because there is a suitable habitat does not guarantee that disease transmission will occur. Other factors including socioeconomics, behavior, and the health and nutritional status of hosts place constraints on disease establishment.[9] If humans are not interacting with the habitat in which the pathogens, vectors, or nonhuman hosts exist, disease cannot occur. And, even when they are interacting, humans can protect themselves to minimize exposure risk.

FINDING HOSTS

Infected and susceptible hosts need to be available and exposed for a disease to occur. There are times of year when activity puts hosts (humans and other animals) at a greater risk of exposure. Examples include kids gathering for school in the fall, increasing the risk for vaccine-preventable diseases when vaccination goals aren't met, or community gatherings like summer picnics and potlucks and the resulting risk of food-borne illness when proper food safety isn't maintained; other options include families traveling for summer vacations and exposing themselves to diseases for which they have no naturally or vaccine-acquired immunity. These activities can increase one's risk by crowding and increasing the chance of contact with an infected person, exposing us to novel pathogens our immune system has yet to experience and develop an immune response to, or placing us in situations where we encounter contaminated foods or water.

Even economics can influence our risk of exposure to disease. Maintenance of window screens and bed nets keep mosquitoes at bay but have an associated cost. Proper sanitation keeps rodents and pests away, but again, it has a cost. In a study to understand the upswing in tick-borne encephalitis in the Baltics, adults in the highest and lowest income groups reported mushroom hunting in the forests: optimal mushroom growing conditions happened to coincide with tick activity as well.[10] Hantavirus is another example,

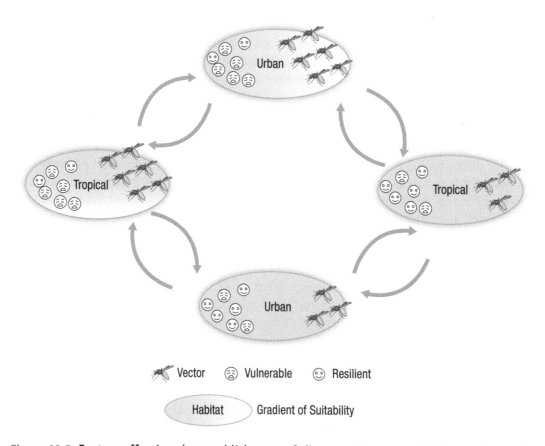

Figure 10.2 **Factors affecting the establishment of disease. Disease establishment is contingent upon a suitable habitat (denoted by the shading), the presence of necessary vectors or nonhuman hosts, and the vulnerability of hosts.**

where spring precipitation increases food resources and subsequent mild winters reduce die-off, thus increasing rodent populations and, when the rodents inundate substandard housing, put people at risk for developing hantavirus pulmonary syndrome.[11] These are just a few examples of where social factors influence exposure to disease.

This interaction is depicted in Figure 10.2. Pathogens and their vectors, and reservoirs to a lesser extent, are constantly moving around the landscape, sometimes into new habitats. If the habitat is suitable, they may establish. However, for disease to occur, hosts must be exposed and susceptible to infection. Human behavior, driven by economics or culture or other factors influences the likelihood of exposure. That risk of exposure, combined with the person's own health and capacity to respond to the infection, further dictates the likelihood that an introduced disease will establish.

THOUGHT QUESTION

If you were going to predict where the next pandemic would start or the next virus to emerge in cattle, what information would you need to know to pinpoint the starting location? How confident would you be in that prediction?

A CHANGING CLIMATE

With expansion into 12 countries within just 7 years and a concomitant movement 800 km further north; an effectively simultaneous invasion of six BTV strains; persistent transmission (overwintering); an extension of the range for the primary vector, C. imicola; and the inclusion of new vectors, the warming climate was the best explanation for the incursion of BTV into northern Europe. Read more about this incursion in Purse et al.[12]

Climate change, primarily due to greenhouse gas emissions, is expected to result in increased average annual temperatures, rising sea levels, and greater climate extremes. The latter includes hotter, longer heat waves; heavier precipitation events; longer drought events; and stronger storm surges (Figure 10.3). From a health standpoint, there are the direct effects, where hotter, more humid days mean more heat-related illness and death and exacerbation of preexisting conditions like asthma and cardiovascular disease.[13] These changes in climate also result in mental health issues due to loss of property, income, and livelihoods because of fires, floods, and agricultural losses.[14] As the changing climate affects our agriculture and food systems, so also come concerns over food security and undernutrition.[15]

But what does a changing climate mean for infectious disease? Direct effects of climate on infectious disease may include changes in the incidence and prevalence of established diseases, extension, or changes in the seasons when the diseases may be transmitted, or exposure to novel pathogens that are able to establish in previously unsuitable habitat. Vector-borne diseases are among the most cited examples of the impacts of climate change on infectious disease. This is in part because the tight association between vectors and the environment is well established. Further, even in the absence of climate change, vectors moving into and establishing in areas where they had been eliminated or into new areas are similarly well documented.

In response to the changing climate, vectors, reservoirs, and humans are migrating. **Climate refugees** are people forced to cross-borders and migrate due to weather-related disasters. Depending on resources, where they end up may put themselves at risk for disease

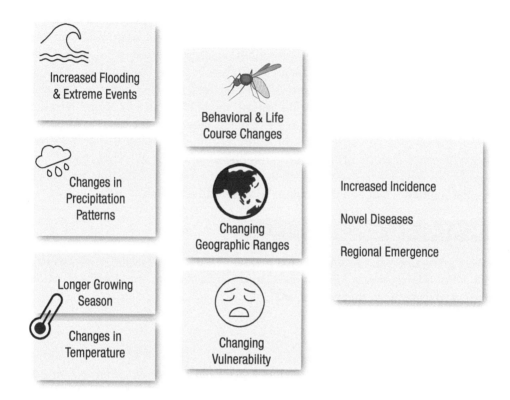

Figure 10.3 The impact of climate change on health. The climate components (extreme events, changing precipitation patterns, and increasing temperature) influence the behaviors and life cycle of vectors and reservoirs; will change the geographies of vectors, hosts, and reservoirs; and influence host vulnerability through anxiety, nutrition, and access. As a result, there will be increased disease incidence, and both novel and known diseases emerging in new areas.

or may expose others to novel disease. Relatedly, behaviors are changing in response to climate change—for example, when vectors emerge, the timing of animal breeding, or foraging behaviors may change. These indirect or downstream effects and the complex interactions of changes to human systems in response to climate change coupled with the direct effects on pathogens are slightly harder to quantitatively assess. However, the logical argument and the evidence exists, and the catalogue of definitive examples continues to grow.

 climate refugee: A person who is displaced because of climate change effects.

INCIDENCE

The very immediate impact of climate change on infectious disease is in changes in the number of new cases. In most disease systems, warming speeds the growth process. For vector-borne disease, this can mean a more rapid build-up of vector abundance which may mean an increased risk of hosts being exposed to those vectors, also known as entomologic risk. If those vectors are infected, there is a greater risk of disease transmission both from the greater number of potentially infectious vectors (increased abundance) but also because the warming can speed pathogen replication, increasing infectious dose and shortening the time to infectivity (shortened extrinsic incubation period). Increasing humidity affects vector survival by reducing an insect's or arthropod's likelihood of desiccating and influences vector activity like flight range and host-seeking activity. The same can hold for food-borne and water-borne pathogens, where the warmer climate supports the growth and development of the pathogens, increasing the pathogen levels more quickly.

While the larger body size, bigger brains, and physical capacity to move across the landscape can make zoonotic hosts and reservoirs more resilient and adaptable, they are still affected by the climate. As with vectors and pathogens, the climate influences the global distribution of hosts. Climate-related changes in food availability, as well as heat and extreme precipitation events, will affect population size through its effects on survival and reproduction, and in foraging, fighting, and mating behavior. While large animals will adapt and we are already documenting morphological changes, the adaptive response may not be sufficient for survival of some species.[16] This research focuses on the survival and extinction of species, but the subsequent human health implications of the ecological impacts of losing species in predator–prey interactions are unknown. However, one can easily imagine the downstream implications on health as the pathogens adapt or vectors switch hosts due to the loss of primary hosts, or hosts adapt to living closer to humans.

The reciprocal argument is also true: Areas formerly suitable may become inhospitable for the pathogen, its reservoirs or vectors, or even the hosts. Hosts may seek refuge in sealed, air-conditioned homes, or migrate out of the area, breaking the transmission cycle.[17] However, on average, the effects of climate change are predicted to be increasing rates of disease.

SEASONALITY

Many infectious diseases exhibit **seasonality**; that is, a trend across the year—they emerge, then populations grow, peak, and then decline at predictable times during the year. We see this seasonality in infectious diseases: Influenza in the northern hemisphere is a winter disease; most West Nile virus cases occur in mid to late summer. These trends in infectious diseases are tightly linked to seasonal trends driving host behavior (e.g., crowding for warmth, staying indoors, host-seeking) or effects on the organism's physiology (e.g., mating, emerging). With the warming climate the frost-free days will increase, and the length of the growing season will increase. This can mean that vectors emerge earlier in the year, are active longer into the fall, and, as a result, have more generations. If conditions remain permissive, populations build up to greater densities and vectors may live longer, taking more blood meals and surviving through the extrinsic incubation period. Having more, older mosquitoes active for longer means there is an increased chance of a susceptible host becoming exposed to an infectious vector. Like vectors, reservoirs such as rodents may stay active longer and increase the number of litters they have when the winters are less harsh.[18]

Changes in seasonality can also mean a shift in patterns where hosts or vector life stages that did not previously coincide now do. For example, rather than the more common vectors being infected by an infectious blood meal, co-feeding of various ticks and tick life stages has been associated with transmission of pathogens. That is, before or even without infection of the host, when infected ticks co-feed they can infect the susceptible ticks feeding near them.[19] Climate change may alter the timing of the emergence of reservoirs, hosts, and vectors, influencing the feeding habits and thus affecting disease transmission.

seasonality: Regular and predictable annual changes not just in weather but also in host behavior and disease trends.

DISTRIBUTION

Increasing temperatures and more intense and more frequent extreme precipitation events will influence the geographic distribution of infectious diseases as vectors and reservoirs move into new areas. We saw this with this chapter's case study of BTV invasion into northern Europe, but others too have shown temporal changes in the distribution of infectious diseases, especially vector-borne and zoonotic.[20] Flooding events, lead to displaced reservoirs and hosts; water- and soil-borne pathogens may also be transported into new areas and establish.

Perhaps the greatest impact will be newly susceptible populations. New hosts, that is, those with no prior immunity, will be exposed as pathogens are moved into new areas. In addition to the vulnerability due to no immune history, there may be delays in diagnosis and treatment. These delays can be due to patients not seeking treatment or providers not identifying the disease; regardless of the reason, treatment delay is associated with more severe disease.[21,22] With non-endemic diseases, the provider may not recognize the symptoms or may mistake them for more commonly occurring diseases. Further, the tests may be optimized for different strains or not be available for the pathogen, resulting in missed or misleading diagnoses. When West Nile virus first appeared in the United States it was misidentified as another flavivirus, St. Louis encephalitis, which is endemic.[23]

ADAPTATION AND MITIGATION

There is very high confidence that climate change is already impacting health and high confidence that climate change will continue to increase if we do not engage in additional **adaptation** and **mitigation** activities.[24] Across the United States and globally, cities and states are developing Climate Adaptation Plans. The United States Centers for Disease Control and Prevention (CDC) developed a 5-Step framework to aid health officials in their development of strategies to prepare for the health effects of climate change, the Building Resilience Against Climate Effects (BRACE, Figure 10.4) framework.[25]

BRACE Step 1 is to anticipate and assess; that is, to identify what climate impacts and associated health outcomes are anticipated in the region and to identify those populations most vulnerable to the identified impacts. Step 2 is to estimate or quantify the associated excess health burden that results from the identified climate impacts. Step 3 moves toward recognizing capacity by identifying health interventions that can successfully address those climate health burdens in populations likely to be most affected. With the regionally important climate effects, populations most vulnerable to the impacts, and specific interventions identified, the purpose of Step 4 is to develop and implement an adaptation plan. The plans are locally developed with **stakeholder** input and are, through the process, regionally specific. The last step of BRACE, Step 5, looks back

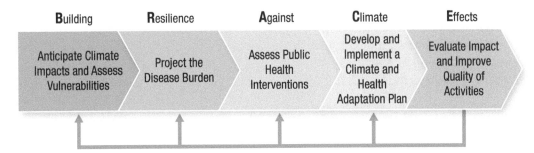

Figure 10.4 The 5-Step BRACE process to support community resilience against climate change.
Source: Adapted from Centers for Disease Control and Prevention. CDC's Building Resilience Against Climate Effects (BRACE) framework. https://www.cdc.gov/climateandhealth/BRACE.htm

to evaluate and improve any of the activities undertaken. This step ensures the work in practice matches the goals set forth by the process and, if not, allows the opportunity to reflect and redirect. This framework aims at an iterative process, using evidence and building on prior success to prepare for health impacts of climate change.

HEADS UP!

Like a Horse and Carriage. Adaptation and mitigation in the climate change world, they go together like, well, a horse and carriage, but what are they? Why do we need two words? Adaptation focuses on the actions that we must do to adapt to the existing or expected climate effects. Mitigation, on the other hand, refers to actions to reduce emissions and stabilize greenhouse gas levels in the atmosphere.

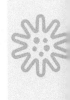

adaptation: The actions we must engage in in response to expected climate effects on health.

mitigation: The actions that can be taken to limit the effects of climate change by reducing or preventing greenhouse gas emissions into the atmosphere.

stakeholders: Those individuals with a personal stake in the project or outcome.

Climate change disproportionately affects communities of color, Indigenous peoples, children and pregnant women, older adults, certain occupational groups (e.g., outdoor workers), persons with disabilities, and persons with chronic medical conditions.[26] Through the BRACE initiative, climate preparedness and response have been strengthened at local public health agencies across the nation and health has been more broadly integrated into climate planning.[27,28] Of note is the success the program had in leveraging partnerships, refining assessment methodologies, and enhancing communication.[27]

While most deaths attributed to environmental risk are noncommunicable diseases, about one-third are infectious. It is estimated that about 25% of deaths worldwide could be prevented if certain actions could be implemented.[29] Effective actions are available at national, regional, local, and individual levels. Sauerborn et al. suggest three reasons to consider health impacts in climate policy.[30] First, the impacts are large, growing, and not equitably distributed. Second, health can motivate behavior and policy changes as we previously discussed. And third, when quantified, the health co-benefits of mitigation activities will be significant. Integrating health into climate change adaptation and mitigation planning is essential to the transformative and sustainable climate policies necessary to address the health impacts of climate change.

THOUGHT QUESTION

Not all infectious diseases will be affected by climate change. Rank the modes of transmission from most likely to least likely to be affected. Within those categories, what factors do you think will mitigate or exacerbate the effect of climate change?

IS THIS ONE HEALTH?

BTV had probably been circulating in wild ruminate for centuries but was not formally described until European sheep imported to South Africa began dying at high rates.[31] Humans do not contract BTV, although they experience the economic and emotional losses associated with lost livestock.

To understand these complex health interactions, the field of **One Health** provides a transdisciplinary approach that brings together multiple sectors to collaboratively deepen the understanding of how animal, human, and plant health are linked within a shared environment (Figure 10.5). While One Health makes theoretical sense and there is considerable support for using the approach to understand disease, implementing it for public health application has been challenging, curiously, in that the very nature of its transdisciplinary nature does not allow it to fit into traditional academic or bureaucratic silos. At its essence, One Health builds on the strengths of the various disciplines and sectors that are responsible or might be involved in responding to infectious disease problems and creates more innovative and sustainable solutions.[32]

One Health: A transdisciplinary approach that considers the linkages between animal and human health in their shared environment.

Boots to the ground, where One Health really shines is in the rapid detection, response, and containment of outbreaks facilitated by cross-sector communication. When veterinarians and human public health are in communication and working together, the detection of true zoonoses (i.e., diseases of animals in animals) can be shared with human medicine more quickly. When ecologists and entomologists work with public health, records of changes in insect patterns can be an early warning of potential shifts in the diseases vectored by disease. Antimicrobial resistance is yet another field for which a One Health approach is essential. A One Health approach will allow us to incorporate climate and anthropogenic effects on the spread of antimicrobial resistance across sectors (e.g., hospitals, communities, agriculture, and ecosystems).[33] Effective responses to the changing landscape of infectious disease require coordinated, synergistic strategies which are locally adapted to community needs.[34] The transdisciplinary nature of One Health will aid in faster detection of potential threats through faster data sharing across sectors and improved logistical support to aid in the diagnosis and treatment of ongoing outbreaks.

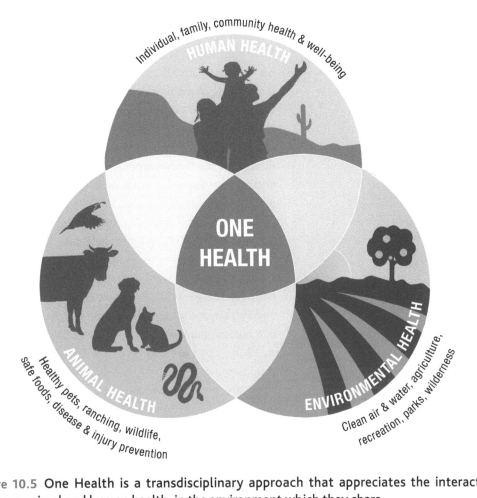

Figure 10.5 One Health is a transdisciplinary approach that appreciates the interaction between animal and human health, in the environment which they share.

Source: Courtesy of Paul Akmajian.

THOUGHT QUESTION

Are there any diseases that you believe would benefit from the One Health approach? What about those that would not? What key characteristics can you identify that distinguish between them?

CASE STUDY

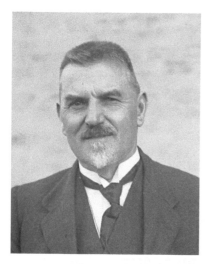

Figure 10.6 Sir Arnold Theiler (1867–1936).

Source: Library of Congress Prints and Photographs Division Washington, D.C. 20540 USA. http://hdl.loc.gov/loc.pnp/pp.print

Sir Arnold Theiler was born in Switzerland in 1867, but his work in South Africa is what gives him the claim to fame as one of the fathers of veterinary science (Figure 10.6). In his mid-twenties, he traveled to South Africa, practicing veterinary medicine, and eventually worked as the state veterinarian. He was the founder and first director of the Onderstepoort Veterinary Research Institute near Pretoria, which was the only veterinary program in South Africa until 1980.[35]

Theiler himself is credited with showing that the etiologic agent of bluetongue could pass through a filter, thereby providing evidence the disease was very small and viral in nature. Moreover, the strain that he had been using was later shown to be a relatively avirulent strain, and as a result became a somewhat effective bluetongue vaccine.[36] It was not until much later, 1944, that transmission by *Culicoides* midges was established. Interestingly, this discovery was made by an entomologist at the Onderstepoort Veterinary Research Institute established by Theiler.

Beyond BTV, Theiler, and the research teams he worked with, are credited with developing a vaccine that effectively curbed the rinderpest epidemic. Rinderpest, a devastating disease of livestock, is one of only two diseases that have been eradicated due to effective and intense use of vaccination. It was finally declared eradicated on May 25, 2011. Of note, one of his sons, Max Theiler, received the Nobel Prize in Physiology or Medicine in 1951 for his work developing the yellow fever vaccine.

CONCLUSION

Environmental factors influence the incidence, seasonality, and distribution of infectious diseases. While human actions can influence what is observed, the overpowering drive is the environmental situation in which hosts and pathogens interact. While the association may be stronger for some diseases compared with others, because of this environmental influence infectious diseases are particularly vulnerable to the effects of a changing climate. Frameworks like the CDC's BRACE framework guide the development of adaptation strategies which will hopefully help to ameliorate the health effects of climate change. One Health's transdisciplinary approach supports the understanding of the complex interactions between the environment, humans, and animals, and facilitates innovative and sustainable solutions to improving health.

END-OF-CHAPTER RESOURCES

TEACHING CORNER

DID YOU KNOW

According to a 2020 United Nations Environment Programme (UNEP) statement, 60% of infectious diseases, and 75% of emerging infectious diseases, are zoonotic and climate change contributes to these changes.[37] But how do we quantify the impact of climate change? How can we attribute changes to climate change? Enter attributable risk, which is the risk (incidence) of disease that can be *attributed* to the exposure. It assumes a causal relationship between exposure and outcome and is a measure of the disease that could be prevented if the exposure were removed. The attributable risk (AR) is calculated as the incidence in the exposed (I_e) minus the incidence in the unexposed. It is often written as a percent, by dividing the I_e.

$$AR = \left(\frac{\text{Incidence in exposed} - \text{Incidence in unexposed}}{\text{Incidence in exposed}} \right) \times 100$$

TRY THIS

Listed in Table 10.1 are Lyme disease incidence data for Canadian provinces for 2009 and 2012. If we assume that climate change is the exposure, we can calculate what proportion of Lyme disease cases can be attributed to climate change. Since incidence is already calculated, we subtract and then divide to calculate AR. Calculate the ARs, order them highest to lowest, and put the results into a sentence. Manitoba is calculated for you.

TAKE IT A STEP FURTHER

How do we interpret the AR? It is the incidence of disease that can be attributed to the exposure in a causally related association. Here, when subtracting the incidence at one time, we'll call them unexposed in 2009 (incidence was 0.3 per 100,000) from the incidence at another time (let's call 2012 "exposed" with an incidence of 1.0 per 100,000)

Table 10.1 Incidence of Reported Lyme Disease for Cases Acquired in Canada for Certain Provinces for 2009 and 2012

PROVINCE	2009	2012	AR
Manitoba	0.3	1.0	((1.0−0.3)/1.0) × 100 = 70%
Ontario	0.5	0.8	
New Brunswick	0.0	0.7	
Nova Scotia	1.5	5.3	
Prince Edward Island	0.0	0.7	

Source: Adapted from Ogden NH, Koffi JK, Lindsay LR, et al. Surveillance for Lyme disease in Canada, 2009 to 2012. *Can Commun Dis Rep.* 2015;41:132. doi:10.14745/ccdr.v41i06a03

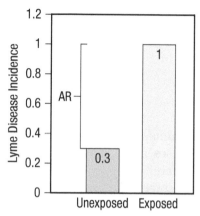

Figure 10.7 **Bar graph showing attributable risk as the difference between the incidence in the exposed and in the unexposed.**

we calculated an AR of 0.7 cases per 100,000 population, or 70% of the incidence in 2012 can be attributed to climate change between 2009 and 2012 (Figure 10.7). Critical to the AR calculation is that there is a causal relationship between the exposure and the outcome, but for climate change this can be difficult to definitively show. Using what you have learned in this chapter, compile a list of alternative exposures which may contribute to the increased incidence of Lyme disease in Canada. Know that the researchers who calculated these values were careful epidemiologists and would have adjusted for changes in population structure or reporting/surveillance changes. In their commentary in Environmental Health Perspectives (EHP), Ebi and colleagues go into depth in the challenges of definitively attributing changes in disease incidence to climate change.[38]

QUESTIONS FOR FURTHER DISCUSSION

1. Pick a favorite disease and design an intervention that is purely medical, purely public health, or purely One Health. How do the interventions differ? Which is more sustainable?

2. Which environmental factors might be relevant for food-borne or water-borne diseases? What specific environmental reservoirs might be impacted?

3. List and define the five steps to the BRACE framework.

4. Distinguish between direct and indirect effects of climate change and provide examples for each.

A robust set of instructor resources designed to supplement this text is located at http://connect.springerpub.com/Content/book/978-0-8261-5674-7. Qualifying instructors may request access by emailing textbook@springerpub.com.

REFERENCES

1. Sedda L, Brown HE, Purse BV, Burgin L, Gloster J, Rogers DJ. A new algorithm quantifies the roles of wind and midge flight activity in the bluetongue epizootic in northwest Europe. *Proc Biol Sci.* 2012;279(1737):2354–2362. doi:10.1098/rspb.2011.2555
2. Gubler DJ, Clark GG. Dengue/dengue hemorrhagic fever: the emergence of a global health problem. *Emerg Infect Dis.* 1995;1,2:55–57. doi:10.3201/eid0102.952004
3. Tatem AJ, Rogers DJ, Hay SI. Global transport networks and infectious disease spread. *Adv Parasitol.* 2006;62:293–343. doi:10.1016/S0065-308X(05)62009-X
4. Kollath DR, Miller KJ, Barker BM. The mysterious desert dwellers: *Coccidioides immitis* and *Coccidioides posadasii*, causative fungal agents of coccidioidomycosis. *Virulence.* 2019;10(1):222–233. doi:10.1080/21505594.2019.1589363
5. Li S, Hartemink N, Speybroeck N, Vanwambeke SO. Consequences of landscape fragmentation on Lyme disease risk: a cellular automata approach. *PLoS One.* 2012;7(6):e39612. doi:10.1371/journal.pone.0039612

6. Gotelli NJ. Metapopulation models: the rescue effect, the propagule rain, and the core-satellite hypothesis. *Am Nat*. 1991;138(3):768–776. http://www.jstor.org/stable/2462468

7. MacArthur RH, Wilson EO. An equilibrium theory of insular zoogeography. *Evolution*. 1963;17(4):373–387. https://www.jstor.org/stable/2407089

8. Brown HE, Barrera R, Comrie AC, Lega J. Effect of temperature thresholds on modeled *Aedes aegypti* (Diptera: Culicidae) population dynamics. *J Med Entomol*. 2017;54(4):869–877. doi:10.1093/jme/tjx041

9. Randolph SE, Rogers DJ. The arrival, establishment and spread of exotic diseases: patterns and predictions. *Nat Rev Microbiol*. 2010;8(5):361–371. doi:10.1038/nrmicro2336

10. Sumilo D, Asokliene L, Bormane A, Vasilenko V, Golovljova I, Randolph SE. Climate change cannot explain the upsurge of tick-borne encephalitis in the Baltics. *PLOS ONE*. 2007;2(6): e500. doi:10.1371/journal.pone.0000500

11. Yates TL, Mills JN, Parmenter CA, et al. The ecology and evolutionary history of an emergent disease: hantavirus pulmonary syndrome: evidence from two El Niño episodes in the American Southwest suggests that El Niño–driven precipitation, the initial catalyst of a trophic cascade that results in a delayed density-dependent rodent response, is sufficient to predict heightened risk for human contraction of hantavirus pulmonary syndrome. *BioScience*. 2002;52(11):989–998. doi:10.1641/0006-3568(2002)052[0989:TEAEHO]2.0.CO;2

12. Purse BV, Mellor PS, Rogers DJ, Samuel AR, Mertens PP, Baylis M. Climate change and the recent emergence of bluetongue in Europe [Erratum in: *Nat Rev Microbiol*. 2006;4(2):160. doi:10.1038/nrmicro1366]. *Nat Rev Microbiol*. 2005;3(2):171–181. doi:10.1038/nrmicro1090

13. Ebi KL, Hess JJ. Health risks due to climate change: inequity in causes and consequences. *Health Affairs*. 2002;39(12). doi:10.1377/hlthaff.2020.01125

14. Smith KR, Woodward A, Campbell-Lendrum D, et al. Human health: impacts, adaptation, and co-benefits. In: Field CB, Barros VR, Dokken DJ, eds. *Climate Change 2014: Impacts, Adaptation, and Vulnerability. Part A: Global and Sectoral Aspects. Contribution of Working Group II to the Fifth Assessment Report of the Intergovernmental Panel on Climate Change*. Cambridge University Press; 2014:709–754.

15. Mbow C, Rosenzweig C, Barioni LG, et al. Food security. In: Shukla PR, Skea J, Calvo Buendia E, et al., eds. *Climate Change and Land: an IPCC special report on climate change, desertification, land degradation, sustainable land management, food security, and greenhouse gas fluxes in terrestrial ecosystems*. International Panel on Climate Change; 2019.

16. Radchuk V, Reed T, Teplitsky C, et al. Adaptive responses of animals to climate change are most likely insufficient. *Nat Commun*. 2019;10:3109. doi:10.1038/s41467-019-10924-4

17. Reiter P, Lathrop S, Bunning M, et al. Texas lifestyle limits transmission of dengue virus. *Emerg Infect Dis*. 2003;9(1):86–89. doi:10.3201/eid0901.020220

18. Andreassen HP, Sundell J, Ecke F, et al. Population cycles and outbreaks of small rodents: ten essential questions we still need to solve. *Oecologia*. 2021;195:601–622. doi:10.1007/s00442-020-04810-w

19. Randolph SE. Transmission of tick-borne pathogens between co-feeding ticks: Milan Labuda's enduring paradigm. *Ticks Tick Borne Dis*. 2011;2(4):179–182. doi:10.1016/j.ttbdis.2011.07.004

20. Jones K, Patel N, Levy M, et al. Global trends in emerging infectious diseases. *Nature*. 2008;451:990–993. doi:10.1038/nature06536

21. Bastaki H, Carter J, Marston L, Cassell J, Rait G. Time delays in the diagnosis and treatment of malaria in non-endemic countries: a systematic review. *Travel Med Infect Dis*. 2018;21:21–27. doi:10.1016/j.tmaid.2017.12.002

22. Thomas C, Nambudiri VE. Delayed diagnosis of nonendemic dermatologic diseases: a retrospective review. *J Am Acad Dermatol*. 2021;84(5):1451–1453. doi:10.1016/j.jaad.2020.06.1007

23. Centers for Disease Control and Prevention. Outbreak of West Nile-like viral encephalitis--New York, 1999. *MMWR Morb Mortal Wkly Rep*. 1999;48(38):845–849. https://www.cdc.gov/mmwr/preview/mmwrhtml/mm4838a1.htm

24. Balbus JM, Luber G, Ebi KL, et al. Ch 14: Health. In Reidmiller DR, Avery CW, Easterling DR, et al., eds. *USGCRP, 2018: Impacts, Risks, and Adaptation in the United States: Fourth National Climate Assessment, Volume II*. U.S. Global Change Research Program; 2018:1515. doi:10.7930/NCA4.2018

25. Marinucci GD, Luber G, Uejio CK, Saha S, Hess JJ. Building resilience against climate effects—a novel framework to facilitate climate readiness in public health agencies. *Int J Environ Res Public Health*. 2014;11(6):6433–6458. doi:10.3390/ijerph110606433

26. Gamble JL, Balbus J, Berger M, et al. Populations of concern. In: U.S. Global Change Research Program, ed. *The Impacts of Climate Change on Human Health in the United States: A Scientific Assessment*. U.S. Global Change Research Program; 2016:247–286.

27. Sheehan MC, Fox MA, Kaye C, Resnick B. Integrating health into local climate response: lessons from the U.S. CDC climate-ready states and cities initiative. *Environ Health Perspect*. 2017;125(9):094501. doi:10.1289/EHP1838

28. Schramm PJ, Ahmed M, Siegel H, et al. Climate change and health: local solutions to local challenges. *Curr Envir Health Rep*. 2020;7:363–370. doi:10.1007/s40572-020-00294-1

29. World Health Organization. *Compendium of WHO and Other UN Guidance on Health and Environment*. World Health Organization; 2021. https://www.who.int/publications/i/item/WHO-HEP-ECH-EHD-21.02

30. Sauerborn R, Kjellstrom T, Nilsson M. Invited editorial: health as a crucial driver for climate policy. *Glob Health Action*. 2009;2. doi:10.3402/gha.v2i0.2104

31. Coetzee P, Stokstad M, Venter EH, et al. Bluetongue: a historical and epidemiological perspective with the emphasis on South Africa. *Virol J*. 2012;9:198. doi:10.1186/1743-422X-9-198

32. Kelly TR, Machalaba C, Karesh WB, et al. Implementing One Health approaches to confront emerging and re-emerging zoonotic disease threats: lessons from PREDICT. *One Health Outlook*. 2020;2:1. doi:10.1186/s42522-019-0007-9

33. Walsh TR. A One-Health approach to antimicrobial resistance. *Nat Microbiol*. 2018;3:854–855. doi:10.1038/s41564-018-0208-5

34. Osterhaus ADME, Vanlangendonck C, Barbeschi M, et al. Make science evolve into a One Health approach to improve health and security: a white paper. *One Health Outlook*. 2020;2:6. doi:10.1186/s42522-019-0009-7

35. Swan GE, Kriek NP. Veterinary education in Africa: current and future perspectives. *Onderstepoort J Vet Res*. 2009;76(1):105–114. doi:10.4102/ojvr.v76i1.73

36. Verwoerd DW. History of bluetongue research at Onderstepoort. *Onderstepoort J Vet Res*. 2009;76:99–102. https://pdfs.semanticscholar.org/4417/f34750de59e8ea95ab600c9cd35b36de5e2e.pdf

37. United Nations Environment Programme. Preventing the next pandemic: zoonotic diseases and how to break the chain of transmission. https://www.unep.org/news-and-stories/statements/preventing-next-pandemic-zoonotic-diseases-and-how-break-chain

38. Ebi KL, Ogden NH, Semenza JC, Woodward A. Detecting and attributing health burdens to climate change. *Env H Perspectives*. 2017;125(8). doi:10.1289/EHP1509

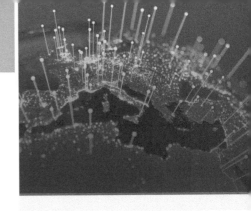

PART IV

DISEASE CONTROL, ERADICATION, AND EMERGENCE

CHAPTER 11

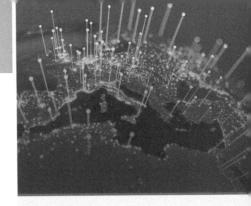

INFECTIOUS DISEASE OUTBREAK DETECTION, INVESTIGATION, AND SURVEILLANCE

INTRODUCTION

Active Bacteria Core (ABC) Surveillance was a system established by the Centers for Disease Control and Prevention (CDC) as part of its Emerging Infections Program network to monitor invasive bacterial infections of public health importance. The program expanded to 10 states by 2003, representing up to 12% of the U.S. population, depending on the pathogen. This system has led to the quick identification of a virulent pathogen on numerous occasions. Neisseria meningitidis is an important cause of meningitis, with sporadic outbreaks in the United States. Using the ABC system, data were collected on meningococcal isolates across the United States and classified, allowing for quick classification of possible spread of virulent meningococcal clones and patterns of transmission. About 10% of cases were assigned to a particular nonrandom spatial and temporal cluster, a proportion of cases higher than those identified in outbreaks using traditional epidemiologic methods. Using age-specific data from ABC, the increased risk of meningococcal disease among young adults was highlighted. Results directly contributed to the Advisory Committee on Immunization Practices policy recommendation for routine use of meningococcal conjugate vaccines in all persons 11 to 18 years of age and subsequent recommendations for a booster dose during late adolescence.[1]

LEARNING OBJECTIVES

By the end of this chapter, readers will be able to:

- Relate the steps responsible for an outbreak, practices that have contributed to the outbreak, and how we monitor and track disease outbreaks over time.
- Explain how we conduct disease surveillance and reporting.
- Describe the mechanisms to monitor and evaluate public health surveillance systems.
- Relate the differences between sensitivity, specificity, and positive predictive value (PPV).

WHAT IS AN OUTBREAK INVESTIGATION?

In the 1980s, invasive group A streptococcus (GAS) was responsible for a number of public health emergencies, including necrotizing fasciitis and toxic shock syndrome. ABC data was used to estimate that approximately 9,400 cases and 1,200 deaths were due to invasive GAS by 1999. Case clusters were reported in various community and household units, and the ABC system was used to estimate attack rates for confirmed GAS disease as well as severe GAS-compatible disease among household contacts. Of 680 eligible index–patient households, 525 (77.2%) were enrolled in surveillance. Households were investigated for GAS cases. Among these households, only one confirmed GAS case in a household contact was reported and one additional household contact had severe GAS-compatible illness without confirmation. The confirmed case still represented an estimated risk of 66.1 per 100,000 household contacts, a much higher attack rate as compared to incidence in the general population (3.5 per 100,000).[2]

In the 18th and 19th centuries, yellow fever (caused by a virus and transmitted by the *Aedes aegypti* mosquito) was seemingly everywhere. Ten percent of Philadelphia's population was dead in a matter of months in 1793, prompting the federal government to flee the city. Brooklyn had an epidemic in 1856 that may have been concentrated near the dockside due to contaminated cargo.[3] An outbreak in Philadelphia began in 1870 when a "filthy" ship arrived at the Lazaretto quarantine station—the captain died en route and an additional 18 people who were in some way associated with or near the quarantine station passed away. Outbreaks followed in New Orleans and in the Caribbean. When the United States invaded Cuba at the end of the 19th century, 13 people died of yellow fever for every soldier who died in battle.[4] At the time, there was no clear approach to investigating and controlling these outbreaks. Germ Theory was still in its infancy, and anti-contagionists, as they were known at the time, came up with alternative theories for disease transmission, including attributing disease to heat, humidity, filth, and poor ventilation. Many years later, in the late 19th century, once yellow fever was verified as a mosquito-borne infection, better disease control and sanitation efforts helped to eliminate the disease from these cities. But how does an epidemiologist know when an outbreak exists? And what are the steps needed to investigate an outbreak?

While the classic definition of an outbreak is the occurrence of more cases of disease than expected in a given area or population, there are additional considerations that need to be taken into account. These include the following:

- Is there clustering of cases in the same time and place, or among individuals with similar demographics and risk factors? A cluster of disease may have a common cause or may be due to unrelated reasons.

- Related to the previous note, are there clear **epidemiologic links** tying individuals together? These are characteristics, often across person, place, and time, that might connect two cases.

- Are viruses or bacteria related to each other, and thus due to the same chain of transmission? **Whole genome sequencing (WGS)** is one high-resolution approach to examine a large fraction of a pathogen's genome for its overall patterns and diversity.[5] WGS may help confirm epidemiologic links or vice versa.

- Does transmission continue despite disease control efforts? If transmission continues in a steady (or exponential) manner, personnel and infrastructure might be stretched thin, necessitating increased urgency or additional resources.

- What is the public health importance of the outbreak? In other words, beyond a lot of new cases, is the disease severe? Are a lot of people dying? Are people unable to go to work or school?

It is also important to consider whether a larger number of cases is due to some other reason. Was there recently a change in how cases were reported? In the definition of a case? Did the procedures used to diagnose a case improve or change?

epidemiologic links: Characteristic that links two cases, such as close contact between two people or a common exposure, such as spending time in the same place together.

whole genome sequencing: A laboratory process used to determine a complete DNA or RNA sequence, which can be useful in tracking disease outbreaks.

In the early stages of an outbreak in particular, epidemiologists play key roles in collecting, managing, and analyzing data to ascertain whether a signal is truly indicative of an outbreak, and a true increase in disease is occurring. One such model is illustrated in Figure 11.1.

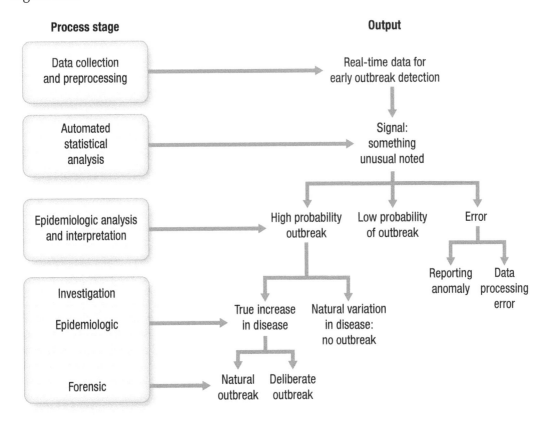

Figure 11.1 Process model for early outbreak detection. Note that the model shows the role of the epidemiologist in the left column and the decisions made based on the investigation in the outputs on the right.

Source: Adapted from Buehler JW, Hopkins RS, Overhage JM, Sosin DM, Tong V. Framework for evaluating public health surveillance systems for early detection of outbreaks: recommendations from the CDC Working Group. *MMWR Recomm Rep.* 2004;53(RR-5):1–11. https://www.cdc.gov/mmwr/preview/mmwrhtml/rr5305a1.htm

WHY IS INVESTIGATING OUTBREAKS IMPORTANT?

While it might seem obvious that outbreak investigation can prevent individuals and larger groups from getting sick, there are broader motivations to keeping a disease from spreading. The main reason is to identify the source so that the current outbreak can be controlled and also to initiate strategies that will prevent future episodes of disease (or outbreaks). At times, such as in the case of the Ebola virus, investigations may discover a completely new pathogen.[6] Outbreak investigations may shed light on behaviors or practices that need to be changed to reduce the risk of disease. They are also useful training grounds for public health professionals in epidemiologic methods and in learning more about public health response and mechanisms for transmission.

Steps of an Outbreak Investigation

Outbreak investigation follows a systematic step-by-step process, with steps occurring sequentially or sometimes concurrently depending on urgency and resource coordination. An outbreak team may consist of epidemiologists, clinicians, microbiologists or laboratorians, veterinarians, environmental health specialists and others. The team might seek to answer the following questions:

1. What is the etiological agent responsible for an outbreak or epidemic?

2. What is/are the predominant modes of transmission?

3. What specific source(s) of disease can be identified?

4. What specific practices or environmental deficiencies have contributed to an outbreak?

5. What is the chain of events that led to an outbreak?

6. How rapid is the progress toward specified goals in reducing disease incidence/ transmission?

7. What are future public health priorities, policies, and strategies based on the data?

The following are steps in a typical outbreak investigation:[7]

STEP 1: CONFIRM THE EXISTENCE OF AN OUTBREAK

Beyond the criteria outlined earlier establishing when an outbreak exists, it is important to consider other factors relevant to the situation, such as the agent (if known), since the background rate of a disease will determine whether to consider a small or large number of cases of an outbreak. In addition, the size of a community and community factors, that either place the population at higher risk for disease (such as age) or that might influence disease rates (such as population density), are important to keep in mind. Data may be collected through surveys, registries, hospital discharge records, or other sources.

STEP 2: VERIFY THE DIAGNOSIS

The next step is to confirm the diagnosis to ensure the disease has been properly identified as well as to rule out any clinical or laboratory errors. A clinical diagnosis may thus be confirmed by a laboratory, and additional work may take place to get a better understanding of those affected. Identifying the agent through methods such as genetic sequencing can help to assess whether patients have similar disease strains. Speaking directly with patients as well as with providers can give valuable information regarding exposures, epidemiologic links, and potential clusters. The distribution of clinical features such as symptoms is summarized and can provide important information in understanding the scope and validity of the diagnosis.

STEP 3: DEFINE AND IDENTIFY CASES

Case definitions provide a set of uniform criteria used to categorize a disease. If an individual fits the case definition, they are classified as having the condition of interest and included in the "set" of individuals meeting the outbreak diagnosis. A case definition typically includes both clinical criteria as well as clear criteria regarding person, place, and time. For the former, the criteria are ideally simple and objective. For example, for acute watery diarrhea, one might consider "three or more abnormally loose or fluid stools in the past 24 hours with or without dehydration." Restrictions by person (e.g., age, risk factors, certain groups), place (e.g., a building, a bar), or time (e.g., disease onset within the past week) help to further refine the definition so that those who are included are in fact linked to the outbreak. In examining acute lower respiratory tract infection in children less than 5 years of age, a definition might be provided that includes: "Cough or difficult breathing; and breathing 50 or more times per minute for infants aged 2 months to 1 year; or breathing 40 or more times per minute for children aged 1 to 5 years."[8] If the suspected source of the outbreak is included in the case definition, all included cases will have exposure to that source and the hypothesis will be nontestable because by definition all included cases will have the exposure.

Cases are often grouped as confirmed, probable, or possible depending on the certainty of the diagnosis. While a confirmed case has the typical clinical features of the agent and usually laboratory confirmation of the pathogen, a probable case is suspected and may not have needed verification of diagnosis or epidemiologic links to other cases. A possible case may either have pending laboratory results, or fewer clinical features matching the agent. There are numerous approaches to case finding in an outbreak. While some cases may be reported proactively, they are likely to represent just a small fraction of the total number. **Active surveillance** refers to the process of case finding through initiation of data collection for cases by obtaining information directly from providers, facilities, and laboratories. This may further extend to outreach to businesses, schools, or other locations to contact those individuals who may have been exposed in order to screen as a possible case. Individuals who are cases themselves may also be interviewed to see if they know of others who are sick. In contrast, **passive surveillance** refers to a less resource-intensive approach, examining existing data to identify cases, or else sending more generic communications with requests to provide information on cases. It is clearly important to actively search for additional cases associated with each outbreak, not only to get a sense of the true magnitude of the outbreak, but also to accurately characterize the outbreak and identify a potential cause, and to be sufficiently **powered** to make statistical inference from the study findings.

case definition: A set of criteria used to classify individuals as having the health condition being assessed; they may include only symptomology or may include laboratory confirmation.

active surveillance: Systematic identification and location of cases of disease, including screening, diagnosis, and treatment.

passive surveillance: Detection of cases among those seeking medical care and who are both aware of their own symptoms and have access to healthcare facilities.

STEP 4: MANAGE AND ANALYZE THE DATA

To systematically categorize key characteristics of cases, and using descriptive epidemiology, epidemiologists summarize key variables, often by person, place, and time. The epidemic curve provides one approach to understanding the natural course of an outbreak and see both the magnitude and time trend of the disease in question. Another approach is to compile a **line listing**, information organized in a tabular format with each row representing a case and each column a particular variable of interest (Figure 11.2). The line listing can be easily reorganized or updated and allows for visualization, hypothesis generation, and analysis.

STEP 5: DEVELOP, TEST, AND (RE-)EVALUATE HYPOTHESES

As the investigation progresses, the team develops and refines hypotheses as to the outbreak source. Hypotheses should always be testable, in order to either settle on the factor responsible for the outbreak or move on. Some approaches to hypothesis development include through discussions with both case providers and health department staff, through further examination of the data, and through what might already be known about a particular agent. Specific study designs can be used to then assess or evaluate whether a particular hypothesis is plausible. Analytic epidemiologic tools such as case-control or retrospective cohort studies are commonly used to investigate outbreaks. Typically, the overall goal is to understand whether observed numbers or trends among cases or exposed individuals are higher than those that might be seen (or expected) among non-cases or non-exposed individuals.

STEP 6: IMPLEMENT CONTROL AND PREVENTION MEASURES

At this stage the outbreak team may begin to consider longer-term approaches and collaborations to control the outbreak and to prevent additional cases and chains of transmission. Sometimes, health agencies respond with measures with even small numbers of cases, or even a single case of disease, that may not exceed the expected or usual number of cases. The agent itself, severity of the illness, the potential for spread, availability of control measures, political considerations, available resources, and other factors such as community buy-in may influence the decision regarding which control and prevention measures to use. Since the idea is to stop a given chain of infection, control measures and interventions will interface with a particular part of the chain. For example, interventions aimed at stopping a mode of transmission may isolate someone sick or else quarantine those exposed in the event that they go on to become sick. Interventions such as vaccinations improve a host's defenses through antibodies that protect against infection (Figure 11.3).

STEP 7: COMMUNICATE FINDINGS

Findings from the investigation must be communicated, either at given strategic timepoints, or at the conclusion. Communications take place with other public health professionals, sometimes through the CDC's Epidemic Information Exchange (Epi-X), a secure network facilitating discussions. In addition, government and local authorities are informed regarding key points, and the broader public may be briefed through the media or else through official channels through health departments. If there is great urgency in stopping disease spread, the broader public may be notified through public service announcements, phone calls, text messages, or social media.

COVID-19 and Respiratory Outbreak Line List for Long-Term Care Facilities
For Symptomatic RESIDENTS

COUNTY OF LOS ANGELES
Public Health

Facility Name: _____   Date: _____   Contact Person/Phone No.: _____

Outbreak Number: _____   Total Number of Residents at time of outbreak: _____

Resident Information				Vaccination status		Illness Description										Diagnostics									Outcome		
Resident Name	Date of birth or Age	Sex (M/F)	Room #	Resident Location Unit/Ward	Influenza (Y/N), if yes, provide date	Pneumococcal (Y/N), if yes, provide date	Date of illness onset	Fever (Y/N) or highest temperature (°F)*	Cough (Y/N)	Myalgia/Body Aches (Y/N)	Chills (Y/N)	Sore throat (Y/N)	Shortness of breath (Y/N)	Other (Y/N)	Chest X-ray confirmed pneumonia (Y/N)	Doctor visit (Y/N)	Specimen collected (Y/N)	Specimen Type (NP, Sputum, Other)	Diagnosis/Lab Result	Antivirals (Y/N), Date started/Date ended	Antibiotics (Y/N), Date started/Date ended	Final Diagnosis (COVID-19, Influenza, other)	Hospitalized (Y/N)	Died (Y/N, if yes, date)
1.																								
2.																								
3.																								
4.																								
5.																								
6.																								
7.																								
8.																								
9.																								
10.																								

*Self-reported or highest temperature: measured oral, under armpit or rectal

Figure 11.2 Sample line listing for COVID-19 in long-term care facilities.

Source: County of Los Angeles Public Health Department. *COVID-19 and Respiratory Outbreak Line List for Long-Term Care Facilities for Symptomatic Residents.* March 18, 2020. http://publichealth.lacounty.gov/acd/Diseases/EpiForms/COVID_LTCFOBLineList_Residents.pdf

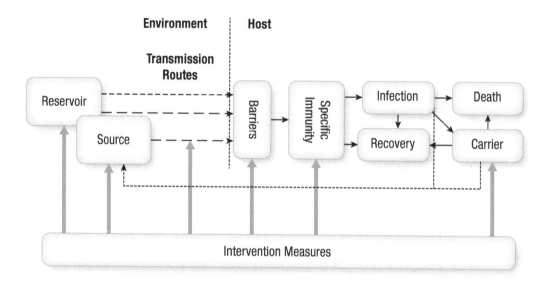

Figure 11.3 Intervention points across the chain of infection.

What factors might change a case definition beyond those listed in the preceding text?

line listing: A table containing key information about each case in an outbreak, with each row representing a case and each column representing a variable such as demographic, clinical, and epidemiologic information.

HOW DO WE STOP POTENTIAL OUTBREAKS FROM SPREADING? THE ROLE OF PUBLIC HEALTH SURVEILLANCE

In the late 1990s, ABCs detected a large reduction in invasive pneumococcal disease (IPD) among children under 5 years old due to Streptococcus pneumoniae. Vaccination with a new 7-serotype pneumococcal conjugate vaccine was partly responsible for the decrease as were the adults who were now protected due to increased herd immunity. At the same time, ABCs noted an uptake in IPD rates caused by S. pneumoniae serotypes that were absent from the vaccine—which resulted in the rapid approval of a pneumococcal vaccine protecting against 13 serotypes. ABCs in turn detected another decrease in IPD.[9]

An effective surveillance system picks up disease outbreaks rapidly and efficiently before lives are lost and the disease can spread broadly. Surveillance is in fact one of the most important tasks of an epidemiologist! Surveillance is the primary way by which we track diseases over time, allowing us to compare places and time periods, as well as assess the presence of outbreaks. The CDC defines public health surveillance as the *"ongoing, systematic* collection, analysis, interpretation, and dissemination of data regarding a *health-related event* for use *in public health action to reduce morbidity and mortality* and to improve health."[10]

This definition provides several clues to the nature of a surveillance system. Surveillance cannot be short-term and must be ongoing to be effective and informative. The approach to surveillance must be standardized and clear. Surveillance is not just about detecting a specific disease outcome, and can refer to broader healthcare, including health behaviors, access, adverse events following a drug or vaccine, or exposure to an environmental hazard. Finally, it is critical that the data collected are used for public health impact. That is, the data are interpreted and provided to decision-makers to take action.

Public health surveillance thus seeks to meet a variety of objectives. These include detection of outbreaks, but also the documenting of the distribution and spread of a disease, monitoring changes, detecting changes in public health or healthcare practice, and generating hypotheses about causes of the disease. By providing baseline or comparison data to assess the state of an outbreak or threat to public health, surveillance also provides information for evaluation of existing public health programs and allows for future planning efforts. Surveillance may also stimulate research through hypothesis generation or innovative methodologic approaches to a given problem. An effective surveillance system should be timely, secure, simple, and flexible, with high data quality—that is, accurate, acceptable to the user, stable, and representative of actual events in a population.[10] Some examples of what is monitored and the approach to monitoring in the United States are shown in Table 11.1. Several of these surveillance systems are population-based surveys that have well-defined sampling schemes allowing for broader generalizability and representativeness of a broader population.

Data Sources

Numerous data sources are available for public health surveillance. These vary by purpose and function. Typically, they may come from individuals (e.g., surveys), from healthcare providers or facilities, or from direct collection from the environment (e.g., animals, vectors, or water samples). Sometimes they may come from administrative, financial, or legal data sources as well. Vital statistics data provide critical information on births, marriages, divorces, and deaths in the United States.[19] Disease registries are population-based compilations of all individuals diagnosed with a health condition of interest. The National Cancer Institute's Surveillance, Epidemiology and End Results (SEER) program, along with CDC's National Program of Cancer Registries, together collect data on all cancer cases and deaths in the United States.[20] So how does one choose the correct data source? Several factors might be important, such as the severity of illness; whether confirmation of diagnosis is important; the quality, timeliness, and reliability of the data; and the prevalence of the condition.

Disease Reporting

As with outbreaks, after establishing the public health need for a system and developing case definitions for given diseases or health events, the next steps are to consider the format and frequency of data collection. Most surveillance systems are set up to collect data with no set end date. However, the frequency of data collection should be responsive to the public health need (e.g., influenza data collection occurring weekly during influenza season). Timely reporting is essential, but the definition of timeliness may differ. For example, reporting on a mass casualty event may require a much quicker response compared to a chronic disease. In addition, more rapid reporting is likely to miss or incorrectly diagnose cases, while a more complete report might not arrive on time.

Table 11.1 Examples of Public Health Surveillance Data Sources

SURVEILLANCE SYSTEM	WHAT IS BEING MONITORED	APPROACH
Behavioral Risk Factor Surveillance System (BRFSS)[11]	Health-risk behaviors, use of preventive health services in the United States	Telephone surveys across all 50 states and United States territories; more than 400,000 adult interviews per year
Chronic Kidney Disease Surveillance System[12]	Kidney Disease in the United States	Various data sources tracking adults in the United States
National Adult Tobacco Survey (NATS)[13]	Prevalence of tobacco use in the United States	National, landline, and cell phone survey of non-institutionalized adults aged 18 years and older residing in the 50 states or D.C.
Pregnancy Mortality Surveillance System[14]	Circumstances of pregnancy-related death	52 reporting areas send copies of death certificates for all women who died during pregnancy or within 1 year of pregnancy
9–11 World Trade Center (WTC) Health Program[15]	Medical monitoring and treatment of WTC-related health conditions for 9/11 responders and survivors	Ongoing services and monitoring of those who were present (responders and survivors) during and after attacks of September 11, 2001. Sub-cohort enrolled in WTC Screening, Monitoring, and Treatment Program
ArboNET[16]	Arthropod borne viral (mosquito and tick-borne) infections among humans and animals	Passive surveillance system used by clinicians reporting the diagnosis of an arboviral disease and obtaining the appropriate diagnostic test
Vaccine Adverse Event Reporting System (VAERS)[17]	National early warning system to detect possible safety problems in U.S.-licensed vaccines	Passive reporting system that relies on individuals to send in reports of their experiences to CDC and FDA. Healthcare providers are required by law to report certain adverse events.
System for Enteric Disease Response, Investigation, and Coordination (SEDRIC)[18]	Multistate outbreaks of food-borne disease	Integrates multiple surveillance data sources and visualizes outbreak data to improve collaborative enteric disease investigations

The burden of illness pyramid provides a model for understanding disease reporting (Figure 11.4). Part of the population is exposed to a pathogen, but only some of these individuals become ill. Some of those who are ill, perhaps those with more severe disease or better access to care, in turn seek medical care. Of those who seek care, a specimen or sample is obtained from some and passed on to a clinical laboratory. The laboratory tests some or all of the specimens for one or more pathogens. Some of the tests are positive for the pathogen(s) and are considered a confirmed case. It is only once these cases are officially reported to the local health department that they are entered into the surveillance system.

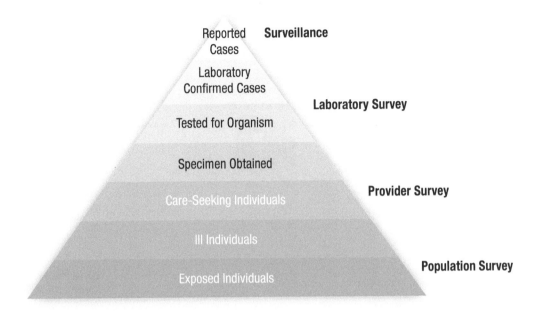

Figure 11.4 The disease burden pyramid. For many diseases, including food-borne diseases, where symptoms vary from mild to life-threatening and even death, the cases that are reported are only a very small percentage of the actual number of cases that occur.

Source: Centers for Disease Control and Prevention. Foodborne Diseases Active Surveillance Network (FoodNet). https://www.cdc.gov/foodnet/surveillance.html.

Each state in the United States has a list of reportable conditions and definitions. About 120 of these are considered national notifiable infectious diseases and conditions. CDC conducts case surveillance through the National Notifiable Diseases Surveillance System (NNDSS) through which about 3,000 health departments gather data on disease to protect their communities. These are largely passive surveillance systems, relying on the laboratory or provider to submit their case findings. Data are generally published weekly, with an annual report published in the *Morbidity and Mortality Weekly Report* (*MMWR*) to represent official case counts for the year.[21] Completeness of notifiable diseases and conditions is highly variable and related to the disease or condition being reported. Different notifiable conditions have their own unique reporting systems and forms.

Information is gathered through a standard data flow, with data reported from hospitals, healthcare providers, and laboratories to state, local, and territorial public health departments (Figure 11.5). In turn, these health departments report data to the CDC, where data is aggregated at a national level. CDC reports certain conditions on to the World Health Organization. Data are reported based on the **International Health Regulations**, which govern how country signatories detect, assess, report, and respond to public health diseases and emergencies.

More recently, electronic case reporting (eCR) allows for automated generation and transmission of case reports from an electronic health record to public health agencies. This is both faster and often more complete than manual reporting and timesaving for

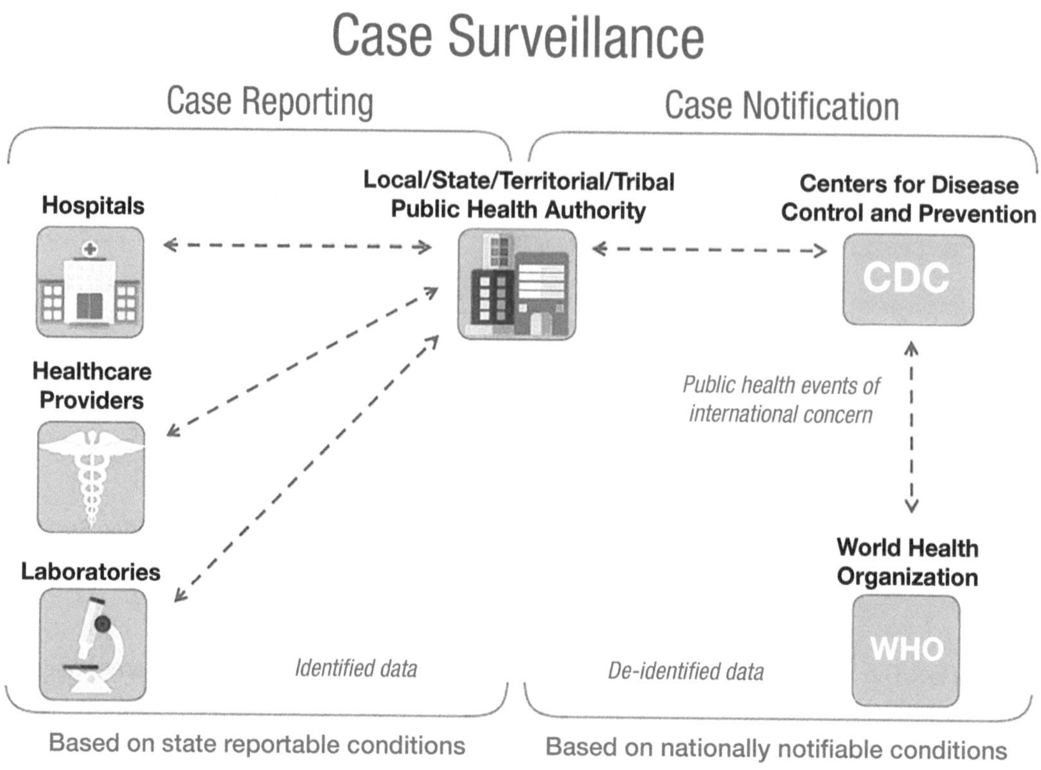

Case Surveillance

Figure 11.5 Case surveillance flow from the local to international level.

Source: Adapted from Centers for Disease Control and Prevention. FAQ: COVID-19 data and surveillance. https://www.cdc.gov/coronavirus/2019-ncov/covid-data/faq-surveillance.html.

healthcare personnel. As of January 1, 2022, it is now required for eligible hospitals and clinicians (Figure 11.6).

At times, surveillance systems cannot be based on a single diagnostic criterion, and instead use a number of signs and symptoms that are somewhat less specific. **Syndromic surveillance** may use a constellation of symptoms or "syndrome" instead of a disease as an early warning system for whether there is a sudden or unusual increase in the disease. In syndromic surveillance, rather than a specific disease, what is being monitored is the grouping of particular symptoms that are flagged. Emergency department visits are a common location for these systems, and (bio-) terrorism events may be another circumstance when these are used. An innovative project called the "Healthy Cup" app was developed to improve public health surveillance in the Brazilian Unified Health System (Sistema Único de Saúde [SUS]) during the 2014 FIFA World Cup, as part of a *participatory surveillance* system. The system relied on visitors or residents in Brazil to voluntarily participate by reporting their health status through information on 10 signs/symptoms (fever, cough, sore throat, shortness of breath, nausea and vomiting, diarrhea, joint pain, headache, bleeding, and exanthema [rash]).[22] Syndromic surveillance systems can be critical in under-resourced areas where laboratory detection may not be feasible, or areas of conflict where sample collection may be restricted.

Imagine a sentinel guard keeping watch. **Sentinel surveillance** enrolls a small number of health facilities reporting on health events generalizable to the whole population.

HOW DOES ELECTRONIC CASE REPORTING (eCR) WORK?

| Patient is diagnosed with a reportable condition, such as COVID-19 | Healthcare provider enters patient's information into the electronic health record (EHR) | Data in the EHR automatically triggers a case report that is validated and sent to the appropriate public health agency if it meets reportability criteria | The public health agency receives the case report in real time and a response about reportability is sent back to the provider | State or local health department reaches out to patient for contact tracing, services, or other public health action |

cdc.gov/eCR

CS328445-A   12/3/2021 11 AM

Figure 11.6 **Electronic case reporting (eCR).**
Source: Centers for Disease Control and Prevention. Electronic case reporting (eCR). https://www .cdc.gov/ecr/digital-resources.html

Events of interest are collected only from this sample of sentinel sites which may provide an early warning signal or red alert for a particular disease. This can be particularly useful when the goal is to gather information on disease trends, as opposed to individual cases, or if sites serve very particular populations.[23] For example, the Outpatient Influenza-like Illness Surveillance Network (ILINet) is a program conducted by the CDC and state health departments to gather influenza surveillance data from volunteer sentinel healthcare providers.[24] More recently, some states have instituted systems to monitor community transmission of SARS-CoV-2 and other respiratory pathogens at sentinel testing sites.[25]

Challenges in Surveillance Systems

Surveillance systems are critical for improving public health and help to prioritize public health actions and identify emerging infectious diseases of public health importance. However, they are only as good as the data they collect. There are numerous limitations to surveillance, with many of these highlighted during the COVID-19 pandemic. For example, we saw in 2020 how case definitions necessarily changed over time as more information became available, and how, before testing was available, individuals with milder disease were less likely to be reported such that the proportion of infections captured by surveillance likely dropped. This resulted in lower incidence estimates and a higher CFR than in reality. Local testing practices, laboratory capacity, and medical resources were also variable across different regions, again distorting the ability to make meaningful comparisons between areas. All of these factors made comparisons of rates difficult across areas, as it became important to also keep in mind the number of tests performed, the proportion of tests that were positive for SARS-CoV-2, testing policies, excess deaths, and hospital and ICU admission rates.

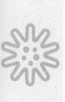

sentinel surveillance: A system of ongoing data collection and monitoring from selected sites or populations that allows for rapid identification of possible outbreaks and public health events.

syndromic surveillance: Categorizing symptoms and diagnoses into syndromes to identify illness clusters early, often before diagnoses are confirmed and reported to public health agencies, and to mobilize a rapid response.

THOUGHT QUESTION

What might be the impact of inconsistent reporting on demographic data (e.g., age, sex, race) for a COVID-19 case surveillance system?

EVALUATION OF SURVEILLANCE SYSTEMS

ABCs also conduct special studies that use the same surveillance infrastructure but require collection of additional data. For example, molecular subtyping of pathogen isolates may occur, as in the case of Haemophilus influenzae, *a bacterium that causes many infections, including pneumonia and meningitis. ABCs use core indicators to monitor system performance, including sensitivity of greater than 90% for active surveillance, which is based on the total cases detected by surveillance and a laboratory validation audit, collection of greater than 85% of isolates from cases, and enrollment of 90% of eligible participants into special studies.* [26]

Surveillance system attributes were mentioned earlier, and systems should be evaluated frequently to ensure that findings improve prevention and control efforts. Different characteristics must be balanced to meet the objectives of the different surveillance systems. A key concept related to the performance of a surveillance system is its accuracy, or its correctness. **Sensitivity** refers to the proportion of cases of a disease or event correctly detected (Table 11.2). In other words, these are the number of cases detected (A) divided by all actual cases of the disease (A+C), which might be detected by a "gold standard." A higher sensitivity would include identification of more of the actual cases in a sample or population. A more sensitive diagnostic test, for example, will capture more of the cases. **Specificity,** meanwhile, refers to correctly excluding individuals that don't meet the outbreak definition. This allows for exclusion of those individuals who truly do not have

Table 11.2 Calculating Performance of a Surveillance System

DETECTED BY SURVEILLANCE SYSTEM	CONDITION PRESENT		TOTAL
	YES	NO	
Yes	True positive (A)	False positive (B)	A+B
No	False negative (C)	True negative (D)	C+D
Total	A+C	B+D	A+B+C+D

the disease of interest. Often investigations begin with a more sensitive definition so as not to exclude true cases. To understand the sensitivity of a surveillance system requires collection of or access to data external to the system to determine the true frequency of the condition in the population under surveillance.

A positive predictive value (PPV) refers to the proportion of reported cases that actually have the disease or event under surveillance. In this scenario, the true cases detected by the surveillance system (A) are divided by the total number of cases detected, including false positives (A+B).

A surveillance system with low PPV, meaning more false-positive case reports, would lead to misdirected resources and heightened, perhaps unnecessary, concern and alarm.

Increasing sensitivity and PPV mean that a system is more representative of the broader population. There is usually a trade-off between sensitivity and PPV. eCR from laboratory test results often has high PPV for diseases that have laboratory tests that are both specific and have rare positives.[27]

Case definitions similarly must balance sensitivity and specificity. Ideally a case definition includes all cases (high sensitivity) while excluding those who do not have the disease (high specificity). There is a trade-off; a sensitive case definition will detect many cases but may also count individuals who do not have the disease. A more specific case definition is more likely to include only persons who truly have the disease under investigation but as a result also more likely to miss some cases.

Since screening tests for diseases are often imperfect, similar terminology is useful to identify the presence or absence of a condition of interest. People are assigned to cells A through D in a similar manner as previously noted, only now whether the screening test yielded a positive result (the person appears to have the condition) or a negative result (the person appears not to have the condition) is noted. One additional important concept is that of **negative predictive value (NPV)**, the proportion of individuals who are truly diagnosed as negative out of all those who have negative tests (including those who were incorrectly diagnosed as healthy). PPVs and NPVs are influenced by the prevalence of disease in the population that is being tested. If we test in a high prevalence setting, it is more likely that persons who test positive truly have disease than if the test is performed in a population with low prevalence.

sensitivity: Proportion of cases correctly detected/tested positive. A higher sensitivity implies fewer false-negative results.

specificity: Proportion of healthy individuals who are correctly detected/tested negative. A higher specificity implies fewer false-positive results.

positive predictive value (PPV): The proportion of cases who have a truly positive test result/event out of all those who have positive test results/are detected.

negative predictive value (NPV): The proportion of healthy individuals truly diagnosed as negative out of all those individuals who have a negative test result.

THOUGHT QUESTION

How else might the sensitivity of a surveillance system be improved?

HEADS UP!

Welcome to the 21st Century. The COVID-19 pandemic has illustrated the need for a rapid, modernized, and complete data surveillance system. After years of under-investment in data systems, the pandemic has created new opportunities for the CDC to share real-time data from many sources, respond more flexibly, and focus more on health equity. Public resources such as the COVID-19 data tracker have provided critical data needs, such as case and mortality data by vaccination status.

CASE STUDY

Alexander Langmuir was the CDC's chief epidemiologist and directed the vaunted Epidemic Intelligence Services (EIS) for 21 years. Beyond helping to contribute to the elimination of polio in the United States and other epidemiologic accomplishments, under his tenure a malaria surveillance system in the early 1950s revealed that malaria had disappeared from the United States. Influenza surveillance began to track the spread of the influenza virus in 1957 and led to attempts to develop tailor-made vaccines. Even with polio, he used detailed information from people with polio (an early surveillance system) to predict the expected size of an epidemic due to early administration of the polio vaccine. Langmuir was also an outbreak investigation pioneer. Toxic shock syndrome was found to be associated with certain kinds of tampons, leading to product withdrawals and new policy guidelines.[28] Similarly, the use of aspirin during illness with either chickenpox or influenza increased children's risk of a severe condition known as Reye's syndrome.[29] The legacy of the EIS is immense, assigning public health officers to various governments or universities around the country and globe, and investigating disease outbreaks and events to this day. EIS officers serve for 2 years, and many then go on to take leadership positions in public health across the country.

CONCLUSION

Persistent infectious disease public health threats mandate clear and standardized outbreak response and surveillance systems. Epidemiologic expertise is needed from the design of data systems, to using a variety of types of health information and data sources, to analyzing, interpreting, and communicating complex data. Responses also require coordinated multidisciplinary efforts with all levels of public health working together to protect the population's health. The single word "surveillance" encompasses a variety of ways in which surveillance data are collected and collated. Evaluating surveillance systems requires both qualitative and quantitative approaches. All surveillance data systems should lead to public health action and continual improvement of public health programs.

TEACHING CORNER

DID YOU KNOW?

Whooping cough (pertussis) is a highly contagious bacterial infection. Whooping cough spreads easily by coughing and sneezing and mainly affects the respiratory system. Pertussis is so contagious that 8 of 10 non-immune people will be infected when exposed to someone with the disease. Following the introduction of pertussis vaccines in the 1940s when case counts frequently exceeded 100,000 cases per year, reports declined dramatically to fewer than 10,000 by 1965. Since the 1980s, the number of reported pertussis cases in the United States as reported through ABC has been gradually increasing: 48,277 cases reported in 2012 represented the largest number of cases since 1955.

TRY THIS

Some people have whooping cough without knowing it, so they may not see a doctor and it could go undiagnosed and unreported. Assume that (a) approximately one in every 10 people with pertussis goes to the doctor, (b) based on symptoms, doctors request submission of a nasopharyngeal or blood specimen from approximately one in every five patients, and (c) approximately two in every three specimens are properly tested for pertussis and are reported through the ABC surveillance system. Given these assumptions, what is the true burden and incidence rate of pertussis? In 2019, the *reported* pertussis incidence rate was 5.7 cases per 100,000 population, or 18,617 cases.[30]

TAKE IT A STEP FURTHER

The diagnostic tools used for confirming a pertussis case are not perfect. Polymerase chain reaction (PCR) is sensitive, but not all that specific; culture confirmation is less sensitive, but close to 100% specific. For example, a recent study found that culture was 64.0% sensitive while PCR was 90.6% sensitive overall.[31] When compared to culture results, PCR was 93.0% sensitive and 99% specific. In this study 545 individuals were tested by both of these methods. Assume 14 of these tested positive by culture. How many people would need to test positive by PCR for these results to be observed? What might be a factor that could influence the results?

QUESTIONS FOR FURTHER DISCUSSION

1. Which of these scenarios would you consider to be an outbreak? Be sure to explain your reasoning.
   a. A single case of botulism is reported in Arkansas after the individual ate canned green beans.
   b. Ten cases of influenza are reported in Boston in December.
   c. One case of smallpox is reported based on the same stock used in a live laboratory at the CDC.
   d. Eight clustered cases of tuberculosis are reported in an immigrant neighborhood in Los Angeles.

2. What are some factors that might affect the sensitivity of a public health surveillance system?

3. What is one existing source of data you can think of for conducting surveillance on Legionella?

4. What are some advantages and disadvantages for conducting a phone survey of the U.S. population to obtain information about diabetes prevalence and incidence in the past year?

5. Why wouldn't we include the suspected source of an outbreak (i.e., the hypothesis you are trying to test in the investigation) in the case definition?

6. What will happen to the apparent prevalence of a disease when you make a case definition more sensitive? What will happen if it is more specific?

 A robust set of instructor resources designed to supplement this text is located at http://connect.springerpub.com/content/book/978-0-8261-5674-7. Qualifying instructors may request access by emailing textbook@springerpub.com.

REFERENCES

1. Wiringa AE, Shutt KA, Marsh JW, et al. Geotemporal analysis of *Neisseria meningitidis* clones in the United States: 2000–2005. *PLoS ONE*. 2013;8(12):e82048. doi:10.1371/journal.pone.0082048

2. Robinson KA, Rothrock G, Phan Q, et al. Risk for severe group A streptococcal disease among patients' household contacts. *Emerg Infect Dis*. 2003;9(4):443–447. doi:10.3201/eid0904.020369

3. Cavins HM. The National Quarantine and Sanitary Conventions of 1857 to 1860 and the beginnings of the American Public Health Association. *Bull Hist Med*. 1943;13(4):404–426. https://www.jstor.org/stable/44440798

4. Bryan CS, Moss SW, Kahn RJ. Yellow fever in the Americas. *Infect Dis Clin North Am*. 2004;18(2):275–292. doi:10.1016/j.idc.2004.01.007

5. Walker TM, Ip CL, Harrell RH, et al. Whole-genome sequencing to delineate *Mycobacterium tuberculosis* outbreaks: a retrospective observational study. *Lancet Infect Dis*. 2013;13(2):137–146. doi:10.1016/S1473-3099(12)70277-3

6. Emond RT, Evans B, Bowen ET, Lloyd G. A case of Ebola virus infection. *Br Med J*. 1977;2(6086):541–544. doi:10.1136/bmj.2.6086.541

7. Dicker R, Coronado F, Koo D, Parrish RG. *Principles of Epidemiology in Public Health Practice*. 3rd ed. Centers for Disease Control and Prevention; 2006

8. World Health Organization. *Acute Respiratory Infections in Children: Case Management in Small Hospitals in Developing Countries*. World Health Organization; 1994. https://apps.who.int/iris/bitstream/handle/10665/61873/WHO_ARI_90.5.pdf

9. Moore MR, Link-Gelles R, Schaffner W, et al. Effectiveness of 13-valent pneumococcal conjugate vaccine for prevention of invasive pneumococcal disease in children in the USA: a matched case-control study. *Lancet Respir Med*. 2016;4(5):399–406. doi:10.1016/S2213-2600(16)00052-7

10. Centers for Disease Control and Prevention. Updated guidelines for evaluating public health surveillance systems. https://www.cdc.gov/mmwr/preview/mmwrhtml/rr5013a1.htm

11. Centers for Disease Control and Prevention. Behavioral Risk Factor Surveillance System. https://www.cdc.gov/brfss/index.html

12. Centers for Disease Control and Prevention. Chronic Kidney Disease (CKD) Surveillance System. https://nccd.cdc.gov/ckd/default.aspx

13. Centers for Disease Control and Prevention. National Adult Tobacco Survey (NATS). https://www.cdc.gov/tobacco/data_statistics/surveys/nats/index.htm

14. Centers for Disease Control and Prevention. Pregnancy Mortality Surveillance System. https://www.cdc.gov/reproductivehealth/maternal-mortality/pregnancy-mortality -surveillance-system.htm

15. Centers for Disease Control and Prevention. 9.11 World Trade Center Health Program. https://www.cdc.gov/wtc/index.html

16. Centers for Disease Control and Prevention. ArboNET disease maps. https://wwwn.cdc.gov/arbonet/Maps/ADB_Diseases_Map/index.html

17. U.S. Department of Health and Human Services. Vaccine Adverse Event Reporting System. https://vaers.hhs.gov

18. Centers for Disease Control and Prevention. SEDRIC: System for Enteric Disease Response, Investigation, and Coordination. https://www.cdc.gov/foodsafety/outbreaks/investigating-outbreaks/sedric.html

19. Centers for Disease Control and Prevention. National VitalStatistics System. https://www.cdc.gov/nchs/nvss/index.htm

20. Centers for Disease Control and Prevention. U.S. cancer statistics public use databases. https://www.cdc.gov/cancer/uscs/public-use/index.htm

21. Centers for Disease Control and Prevention. *MMWR*: summary of notifiable infectious diseases. https://www.cdc.gov/mmwr/mmwr_nd/index.html

22. Leal Neto O, Dimech GS, Libel M, et al. Saúde na Copa: the world's first application of participatory surveillance for a mass gathering at FIFA World Cup 2014, Brazil. *JMIR Public Health Surveill*. 2017;3(2):e26. doi:10.2196/publichealth.7313

23. Thacker SB, Redmond S, Rothenberg RB, Spitz SB, Choi K, White MC. A controlled trial of disease surveillance strategies. *Am J Prev Med*. 1986;2(6):345–350. doi:10.1016/S0749-3797(18)31307-2

24. Centers for Disease Control and Prevention. U.S. influenza surveillance: purpose and methods. https://www.cdc.gov/flu/weekly/overview.htm#anchor_1539281266932

25. Cooksey GLS, Morales C, Linde L, et al. Severe acute respiratory syndrome coronavirus 2 and respiratory virus sentinel surveillance, California, USA, May 10, 2020–June 12, 2021. *Emerg Infect Dis*. 2022;28(1):9–19. doi:10.3201/eid2801.211682

26. Schuchat A, Hilger T, Zell E, et al. Active Bacterial Core Surveillance of the emerging infections program network. *Emerg Infect Dis*. 2001;7(1):92–99. doi:10.3201/eid0701.010114

27. Panackal AA, M'ikanatha NM, Tsui FC, et al. Automatic electronic laboratory-based reporting of notifiable infectious diseases at a large health system. *Emerg Infect Dis*. 2002;8(7):685–691. doi:10.3201/eid0807.010493

28. Shands KN, Dan BB, Schmid GP. Toxic shock syndrome: the emerging picture. (Editorial). *Ann Intern Med*. 1981;94: 264–266. doi:10.7326/0003-4819-94-2-264

29. Waldman RJ, Hall WN, McGee H, Van Amburg G. Aspirin as a risk factor in Reye's syndrome. *JAMA*. 1982;247:3089–3094. doi:10.1001/jama.1982.03320470035029

30. Centers for Disease Control and Prevention. *2019 Final Pertussis Surveillance Report*. https://www.cdc.gov/pertussis/downloads/pertuss-surv-report-2019-508.pdf

31. Lee AD, Cassiday PK, Pawloski LC, et al. Clinical evaluation and validation of laboratory methods for the diagnosis of *Bordetella pertussis* infection: culture, polymerase chain reaction (PCR) and anti-pertussis toxin IgG serology (IgG-PT). *PLoS ONE*. 2018;13(4):e0195979. doi:10.1371/journal.pone.0195979

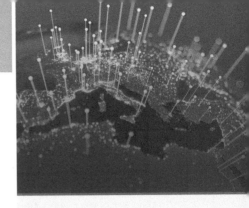

CHAPTER 12

VACCINES: IMPACT, QUESTIONS, AND CHALLENGES

INTRODUCTION

Poliomyelitis, more commonly known as polio, is a contagious viral disease transmitted through the fecal-oral route. While most people who become infected do not get sick, in about 1% of infected individuals the virus attacks the central nervous system and destroys spinal cord motor cells. In this form, flaccid paralysis occurs where muscles become limp and cannot contract. The extent of flaccid paralysis depends on where the virus attacks and the number of cells it damages.

The earliest description of the disease was made in 1789 by British physician Michael Underwood, followed by identification of the viral cause in 1908 by Karl Landsteiner and Erwin Popper. However, a priest with the withered lower leg and foot that is typical of polio is clear in a stele dating from 1570 to 1342 BCE and the mummy of Pharaoh Siptah (who ruled from 1197 to 1191 BCE) shows similar physical characteristics. While the disease has been around since antiquity, in the late 19th century polio epidemiology changed toward large epidemics with significant health outcomes. There is no cure for polio, but there are effective vaccines and, because only humans are hosts, eradication is possible. Since the launch of the Global Polio Eradication Initiative in 1988, polio cases have been reduced by 99%, it is endemic to only two countries, and five of the six World Health Organization (WHO) regions are certified wild polio virus free.[1] Read more about the public–private partnership to eradicate polio at Polioeradication.org.

LEARNING OBJECTIVES

By the end of this chapter, readers will be able to:

- Describe how vaccines work and discuss why vaccines matter.
- Relate vaccination to concepts of innate and acquired immunity.
- Evaluate factors associated with the vaccine-preventable disease burden.
- Propose methods to combat misinformation and disinformation that may contribute to vaccine hesitancy.

HOW DO VACCINES WORK? PART 1: EPIDEMIOLOGY

Transmission of the poliovirus occurs by direct contact with individuals infected with the virus, or through contaminated water or food. The fecal-oral transmission cycle can be broken with proper hygiene and sanitation. Circumstantial evidence suggests that public sanitation and improved hygiene delayed infants' exposure from 6 to 12 months, when they likely still had passive immunity through nursing, to 12 months when passive antibodies waned.[2] Since the 1930s, population density, specifically the baby boom, has been associated with increased regularity and size of U.S. pandemics.[3]

Immunization, along with sanitation, are the greatest, most efficient, and cost-effective public health achievements. It is estimated that between 4 to 5 million deaths are prevented each year because of vaccines and vaccination programs.[4] The benefits of vaccination go beyond illnesses or deaths averted to include education and economic attainment through wellness (e.g., less absenteeism). It is because of vaccination that we no longer worry over smallpox, which had a 30% case fatality rate (CFR) and left survivors visibly scarred and sometimes blind.[5]

Vaccination does not change the innate transmissibility of the disease, R_0, but reduces the effective reproductive number, R_e (Figure 12.1). The goals of vaccination are twofold: (1) to protect the individual from the disease and its devastating side effects, and (2) to reduce the spread of disease, thereby protecting the community. Vaccination is an active prevention strategy in that, at the community or population level, it is ongoing and must be maintained. Each generation brings new susceptible individuals who need to be protected; even among those fully vaccinated, immunity wanes with age, and previously protected individuals may become susceptible as the pathogen evolves or as our immune system changes.

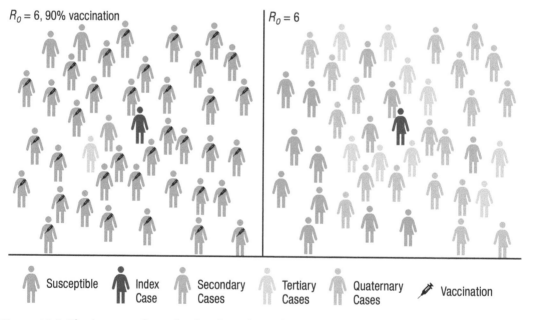

$R_0 = 6$, 90% vaccination $R_0 = 6$

| Susceptible | Index Case | Secondary Cases | Tertiary Cases | Quaternary Cases | Vaccination |

Figure 12.1 The impact of vaccination for a hypothetical disease where, in a fully susceptible population, each case would result in six new cases. The left panel shows the impact of vaccination, if 90% vaccination were achieved. Notice that the people in the upper left corner do not become infected despite not being vaccinated. The right panel is an $R_0 = 6$ in a fully susceptible population.

How Effective Is a Vaccine?

Two related words are important when considering how effective a vaccine is: efficacy and effectiveness. **Vaccine efficacy (VE)** is an innate property of the vaccine. It answers the question: Under ideal conditions, how well does the vaccine work to prevent disease? VE is calculated from clinical trials, controlled experiments where carefully selected individuals are given the vaccine or a placebo and cumulative incidence is (number of cases as a percentage of each group) compared. Typically, the outcome of disease is definitively confirmed with laboratory testing. The trade-off with clinical trials is that the tight constraints necessary for the experimental conditions may reduce **generalizability**. That is, they only let us know how well the vaccine works on people who look like the people included in the trial.

vaccine efficacy: A measure of the reduction in incidence in a vaccinated group compared to an unvaccinated group under ideal conditions.

vaccine effectiveness: A measure of the ability of a vaccine to prevent disease under "real-world" conditions.

Vaccine effectiveness is the real-world counterpart, which answers the question, how well does the vaccine prevent disease in a population or community? Effectiveness is influenced by other **comorbidities**, diversity in population characteristics such as age and sex, and prior exposures. It is also influenced by the vaccine requirements; for example, storage and transport, refrigeration requirements, and administration to individuals. Typically, vaccine effectiveness is measured through observational studies and surveillance data.

Unlike the randomized controlled trial (RCT), observational studies, which are used to assess vaccine effectiveness, are more vulnerable to **validity** threats. RCTs are favored and considered the gold standard because the random selection into the vaccine or placebo group helps to control for many biases and confounding. **Confounding** is when a third factor exerts influence on both the exposure, here the likelihood to get the vaccine, as well as the outcome, the likelihood to contract the disease. For example, people with chronic illnesses may be targeted with specific vaccine messaging to increase vaccine uptake, and they are also those more likely to have severe outcomes if they get the disease or might be less likely to elicit a full immune response from the vaccine. Another concern in observational studies is called selection bias. **Selection bias** happens in observational studies when the people who opt in to taking the vaccine are different from the people who opt out. For example, people who engage in riskier behavior may be less likely to get vaccinated and be more likely to become exposed, thereby potentially overestimating the observed association between the vaccine and the outcome and limiting the generalizability. Any of these factors can influence how much we can trust the results of an observational study; that is, the validity. Despite these threats to validity, **observational studies** are integral to estimating vaccine effectiveness.

validity: The degree to which the information collected answers the research question.

confounding: A third factor, not the exposure or outcome variable, that is a common cause of both the exposure and the outcome, that may result in a spurious association between the exposure and outcome. It is biologically important to understand its role.

selection bias: A systematic error where those who are selected to participate are different from those who are not.

A well-designed observational study considers, tests for, and controls for these threats and helps to strengthen the study's validity. While we cannot randomly assign people in an observational study, sometimes we can compare those who opt out to see if they differ in any way from those opting in. This helps to control for selection bias by identifying whether other factors might be driving any observed differences in the two groups. Stratified analysis—that is, comparing effects within groups sorted by a third variable—can be a way to identify confounding in an observational study. For example, if you know that age might influence VE, then comparing within age groups can help minimize confounding. The ability to estimate the effectiveness of a vaccine requires a strong, careful, and well documented study design.

THOUGHT QUESTION

In the polio example that starts this section, we learned that maternal antibodies and population density influenced the dynamics of polio from an infrequent disease to one causing large epidemics. Use the concept of R_0 to explain this phenomenon and be sure to consider additional factors that might influence such a change.

HOW DO VACCINES WORK, PART 2: BIOLOGY

Within about 5 years of each other, two polio vaccines were developed that changed the course of polio. The first was developed in 1955 in the laboratory of Jonas Salk. Salk trained in medicine at New York University and was, at the time, working at the University of Pittsburgh with the National Foundation for Infantile Paralysis. Having prior experience with a killed virus vaccine for influenza, he naturally turned toward those same methods in developing this first successful polio vaccine. With the vaccine showing safety and efficacy, over 1 million children (about the population of Delaware) were randomized to receive the vaccine or a placebo in 1954. Incidence was 50% lower in the vaccinated group and breakthrough infections led to less severe, nonparalytic, disease.[6] Albert Sabin looked to the route of infection for inspiration in vaccine development. Observing that the digestive system was the point of entry before the virus attacked the nervous system, Albert Sabin developed an oral, live attenuated vaccine. By 1960, Sabin's oral vaccine was licensed for use in the United States. Eventually, Sabin's live attenuated vaccine showed greater effectiveness and replaced Salk's killed vaccine. However, since 2000, the oral vaccine is no longer used in the U.S., replaced by an Inactivated poliovirus vaccine.

When a pathogen infects a host, the host's immune system responds at a cellular level with immune cells which fight the infection. Three primary immune cells which fight infection are macrophages, B-lymphocytes, and T-lymphocytes. The macrophage phagocytizes—that is, engulfs—and then destroys the pathogen. Hence the name: *macro,* meaning "large"; *phage,* meaning "to eat." Macrophages are among those immune cells, along with the physical barrier provided by skin or coughing, and chemical barriers like stomach pH or tears, that make up **innate immunity**. Innate immunity is nonspecific and seeks to protect against any pathogen.

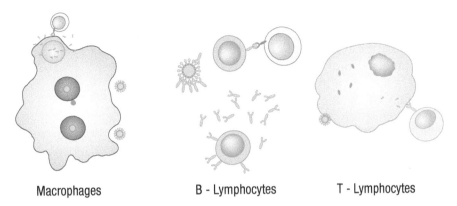

Macrophages   B - Lymphocytes   T - Lymphocytes

Figure 12.2 The primary cellular immune responses. First, macrophages engulf the pathogen. B-cells then use the antigens that are released to generate antibodies as plasma cells and B-memory cells to remember prior exposures. These cells are then primed to respond to specific antigens. Killer T-cells, a specific type of lymphocyte, also recognize the foreign antigen but in infected host cells.

In the process of phagocytosis, macrophages break down and express pieces of the pathogen called antigens. With helper cells, these antigens are recognized and can be attacked by two other immune cell types: T-lymphocytes and B-lymphocytes. While both immune cell types recognize antigens, B-lymphocytes attack the antigens of the pathogen, while T-lymphocytes attack host cells which express the antigen after being infected. In this context, B-cells and T-cells are adaptive immune responses (also known as **acquired immunity**) because they develop in specific response to prior exposure (Figure 12.2).

innate immunity: Nonspecific immune response that we are born with and includes physical, chemical, and certain immune cells.

acquired immunity: The adaptive immune response which is acquired over the lifetime by natural infection or immunization and is specific to specific antigens.

Vaccine Types

Vaccines, are an acquired immunity as they present the body with a less pathogenic or nonpathogenic version of the pathogen which stimulates the body's immune system. The primary types of vaccines are live attenuated, inactivated, toxoid, subunit/conjugate, mRNA, and viral vectors. Live attenuated vaccines are most like a natural infection because they are live but weakened versions of the pathogen. The MMR (measles, mumps, and rubella vaccine) and chickenpox vaccines are two examples. Inactivated vaccines present your body with inactive or killed vaccines. These may require multiple doses to achieve immunity. Polio and human papillomavirus (HPV) vaccines are examples of inactivated vaccines. Toxoid vaccines use toxoids as antigens to stimulate the immune response against certain bacterial infections. They are stable vaccines, but like the inactivated vaccines, often require boosters to maintain immunity. The tetanus vaccine is an example. The subunit or conjugate vaccines use only specific pieces of the pathogen to elicit the immune response. While they do generate a strong response to that component of the pathogen, they may require boosters. The pertussis component of the DTaP (diphtheria, tetanus, and pertussis) vaccine is a conjugate vaccine.

mRNA and viral vector vaccines work differently. Rather than presenting your body with a pathogen or a part of the pathogen, these vaccines enter your cells and instruct your body to make the antigen. mRNA vaccines are wrapped in a fatty barrier to stabilize the mRNA. Similarly, viral vector vaccines use either DNA or mRNA to instruct your body to make a specific antigen which then elicits the immune response, but they are encased in a nonpathogenic virus which *vectors* the material to your cells. Rather than growing the pathogen in the laboratory as is necessary with more traditional vaccines, these vaccines provide the instructions and rely on your body to do the work. The rapidly developed COVID vaccines in response to the COVID-19 pandemic were mRNA (e.g., Moderna) or viral vector (e.g., Johnson & Johnson) vaccines.

Regardless of the vaccine type, laboratories follow strict protocols to ensure the safety of the vaccine. Once candidate vaccines are developed, clinical development involves yet further rigorous tests to ensure that the vaccine works as it should and that it is safe (Figure 12.3). These tests are called **clinical trials**. In the United States, there are three phases, with each building on the representativeness of the test population and ensuring statistical power. In Phase I clinical trials, only small, carefully selected individuals are given the candidate vaccine. In the second phase, Phase II, a larger, more diverse group is recruited for the trial. Finally, Phase III involves recruiting thousands of individuals. In all stages, the participants are carefully monitored for adverse outcomes and the efficacy and safety of the vaccine is documented. Once the vaccine is determined to be safe, it must be reviewed and approved before manufacturing and distribution can start. In the United States, the Center for Biologics Evaluation and Research (CBER) of the Food and Drug Administration (FDA) regulates vaccines. A vaccine will only be approved if it is safe and effective and if the benefits outweigh the side effects. After approval, evidence-based recommendations are made on how to use the vaccine for disease control by a committee of medical and public health experts, the Advisory

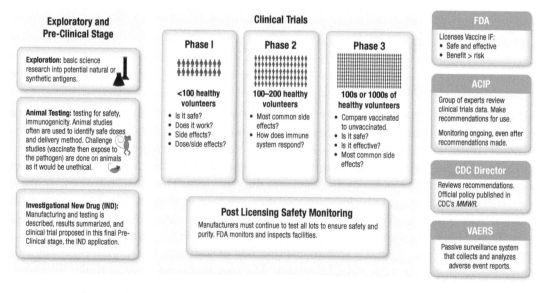

Figure 12.3 **Phases of vaccine development. Prior to the submission of an investigational new drug, manufacturing companies conduct laboratory-based exploratory and preliminary work to develop a candidate vaccine. If the candidate vaccine shows the promise of safety and efficacy, it will move to clinical trials.**

Committee on Immunization Practices (ACIP). ACIP provides their recommendations for approval by the CDC director and the U.S. Department of Health and Human Services (HHS). When approved and published in the CDC's *Morbidity and Mortality Weekly Report*, the *MMWR*, the vaccine is then considered officially recommended for use in the United States.

Safety testing continues even after approval and recommendations for use are published. The manufacturer must continually test the vaccines themselves and allow the FDA to inspect the facility for quality and safety. Monitoring continues outside the manufacturing process as well. A CDC- and FDA-sponsored surveillance program, the Vaccine Adverse Event Reporting System (VAERS), is a **passive surveillance** system to collect and analyze adverse events (side effects).[7]

passive surveillance: Systematic surveillance of health outcomes or exposures; in contrast to systems in which providers and laboratories are contacted, passive surveillance relies on submissions by the wider public.

THOUGHT QUESTION

Immunity is far more complicated than how we've explained it here, but this section gives an introduction to understanding the role an epidemiologist might have in vaccine development. Looking at the phases of vaccine development, describe how you might shorten the timeline, as was done for COVID-19. Where do you think most of the "loss" is in each stage with no vaccine ultimately being developed?

VACCINE-PREVENTABLE DISEASE BURDEN

In 1988, the WHO set 2000 as the date for global polio eradication.[8] The success of this program has led to a 99% reduction in the number of polio cases. However, vaccine hesitancy, along with lack of human resources and access to healthcare and vaccine stock, jeopardizes eradication. In 2019, despite nearly two decades of wild poliovirus-free status, the Philippines experienced an outbreak. Fifteen cases of vaccine-derived poliovirus (VDPV) were reported. VDPV is extremely rare, but the live attenuated oral polio vaccine can accumulate mutations and, in regions with low vaccination rates and poor sanitation, infection may occur when susceptible children are exposed to the vaccine virus, which can be excreted with feces.

Global Progress to Elimination

Vaccination is among the cheapest, most effective interventions that has come out of medicine, with impacts that go beyond the individual receiving the vaccine. It is estimated that for every $1 invested in immunization in low- and middle-income countries, the return is $16 in healthcare savings and improved economic productivity alone.[9] Past successes and the positive impact of vaccination has led to new initiatives to further reduce the vaccine-preventable disease burden. Ultimately, the goal of these initiatives is high vaccine coverage, that is, to get enough people immunized to limit the spread of disease. The CDC has identified five goals to support this effort, which are grouped as those that improve capacity and those which support capacity (Figure 12.4).

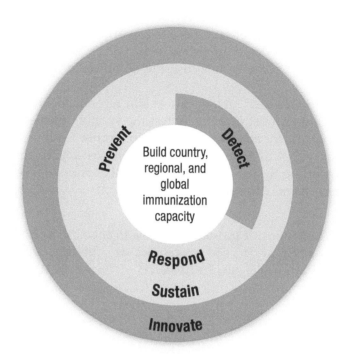

Figure 12.4 CDC Global Immunization Strategic Framework. The CDC's Global Immunization Strategic Framework set five goals to reduce vaccine-preventable disease burden.
Source: Adapted from Centers for Disease Control and Prevention. *CDC Global Immunization Strategic Framework*. 2022. https://www.cdc.gov/globalhealth/immunization/framework/index.html

Three goals support improving capacity: (1) improving immunization services to prevent, (2) improving surveillance to detect, and (3) supporting outbreak response and preparedness to limit vaccine-preventable disease outbreaks. Two additional goals span these capacity improvement goals, namely (4) sustained support to immunization programs and (5) innovation in increasing the reach of vaccination programs.[10] To achieve these goals, the CDC Global Immunization Strategic Framework uses high-quality data analytics in an integrated holistic approach to foster partnerships across organizations.

Despite the observed declines in diseases for which there are vaccines, there is no consensus on how to define the impact of vaccination. For example, VE and vaccine effectiveness are measures of the difference in risk between unvaccinated and vaccinated, standardized over (divided by) the risk among vaccinated, but one could also measure the impact as the reduction in incidence rate before and after vaccination (again standardized over the prevaccination incidence rate).[11] However, these underestimate the impact of vaccines by assuming that the unvaccinated are not impacted by the vaccinated, that is, by the indirect effects of reduced transmission. Moreover, neither measure adequately captures the broader benefits of vaccination including the economic benefits to the country as well as the individual, reductions in long-term disability due to avoided infection, or educational and occupational gains when protected individuals do not miss work or school.[12]

Herd Immunity

Vaccines do not need to reach 100% efficacy to be effective at reducing the disease burden in a community nor does **coverage**, the percent of people receiving a specific vaccine, need to be 100%. Rather, it is a balance of efficacy and coverage along with consideration of population dynamics, the proportion of recovered individuals, the lasting effects of immunity, and disease control capacity. When enough people have been immunized, the proportion of susceptible individuals in the population decreases and the effective reproductive number can drop below 1 even if coverage is not 100%. Those too young to be vaccinated, those who have had severe adverse reactions in the past, those with certain immune disorders, or those for whom the vaccine did not elicit sufficient immunity will still be protected. This is the concept of **herd immunity,** which is the protection of the group when enough of the group is immunized and protected against disease. The lack of prior exposure and thus any immunity against the communicable diseases of European settlers arriving to North America between 1616 and 1619 contributed to a 90% reduction of the Native American population.[13] Refer to Figure 12.1 showing the same hypothetical disease with an R_0 of 6 under circumstances of high vaccine coverage versus none. Critical vaccination coverage refers to the proportion of people who are vaccinated to block disease transmission.

herd immunity: Indirect protection to groups when enough of the group is immunized such that those unable to be vaccinated or those who did not develop sufficient immunity to thwart the infection are still protected.

Herd immunity is an active process that must be maintained until the disease is globally eradicated. Each year new susceptible individuals are born into a population and additional individuals age into reduced immunity (immunity wanes as people get older), pathogens may mutate, and the vaccine becomes less efficacious. In addition, there are always individuals who get vaccinated but whose bodies do not elicit a sufficient immune response. Diseases like measles clear the immune system memory T-lymphocytes, causing immunologic amnesia and rendering previously immune individuals susceptible again.[14] Vaccine-hesitant individuals additionally, for a variety of reasons, do not get vaccinated and "vaccine freeloaders" rely on herd immunity to save themselves the vaccine side effects. For these reasons, herd immunity requires constant attention and cannot be assumed to ensure that those who can be vaccinated have access to and receive the appropriate vaccine.

Determining how many people need to be immunized to reduce transmission is related to how transmissible the disease is, namely, R_0. Specifically

$$\text{Herd immunity} = 1 - (1/R_0)$$

Plotting R_0 by herd immunity, we see that the more transmissible the pathogen, the greater number of individuals who must be immunized to reduce transmission (Figure 12.5). For highly transmissible diseases like measles, which has an R_0 of around 17, it is estimated that at least 95% of the population needs to be vaccinated to reach herd immunity. For less transmissible diseases like polio ($R_0 = 4$–6), the number of immunized needed is nearer to 80%.

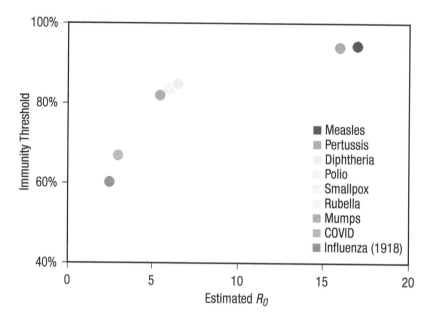

Figure 12.5 Association between immunity threshold and transmissibility. The association between the immunity threshold (y-axis) and the reproductive number (x-axis) for common vaccine-preventable diseases shows that the more transmissible the pathogen the greater the number of individuals who must be immunized in order to reduce transmission.

Source: R_0 estimates based on Fine PE. Herd immunity: history, theory, practice. *Epidemiol Rev.* 1993;15:265–302. doi:10.1093/oxfordjournals.epirev.a036121

Getting to Eradication

Two diseases—smallpox and rinderpest (an animal disease)—have been successfully eliminated globally, that is eradicated, both through successful vaccination programs. Regionally, vaccination has also led to the elimination of measles, rubella, mumps, and diphtheria in the United States. Four additional diseases—polio, yaws, dracunculiasis (Guinea worm), and malaria—are targeted for eradication. Polio has been dramatically reduced through vaccination. Yaws is treatable with antibiotics, but progress to eradication is hampered by asymptomatic infections.[15] Guinea worm, like yaws, will be eliminated through surveillance to detect cases, as well as containment and treatment to reduce secondary exposures. This has led to the reduction of cases into the 20s, but the recent discovery of increasing incidence in dogs has forced the WHO to move the eradication target back to 2030.[16] Malaria is proving to be more challenging. Between 2000 and 2015, incidence was reduced by 41% and 17 fewer countries are endemic, but millions of cases and almost half a million deaths continue to occur each year.[17] Technical, operational, and financial challenges hinder progress, though perhaps the October 2021 WHO recommendation for widespread use of a newly developed malaria vaccine will turn the course for eradication.[18] That so much has been achieved cannot be underestimated, but that so few diseases have been eradicated or eliminated shows the continued challenges in infectious disease control. As we have discussed in this text, development of a safe and effective vaccine is expensive and challenging, and, even once it is developed, active and honest engagement with those communities that are affected is necessary to support the vaccines' successful adoption.

Eliminate the negative. Both elimination and eradication refer to bringing case numbers to zero, so why two terms? *Elimination* means no cases, but it is restricted to a defined geographic region. *Eradication* is reserved for permanent worldwide reduction to zero new cases. While many diseases have been regionally eliminated, only smallpox and rinderpest have been eradicated. Hopefully, Guinea worm is soon added to that list too!

Despite the progress, vaccine-preventable diseases continue to extoll a burden globally. An additional 1.5 million deaths could be avoided if vaccine coverage were improved.[18] Since 2010, global immunization coverage has increased by only 1% and 25 countries reported a net *decrease* in immunization coverage (Figure 12.6).[19]

Among the challenges to disease control is vaccine development. On average, it takes 10 to 15 years for vaccine development and approval, and the cost of getting a candidate vaccine to the end of Phase 2 is $319 to $469 million.[20,21] The very nature of a "vaccine trial" can be intimidating and recruiting volunteers can be a challenge. Innovative vaccine trial designs, such as 1:1 allocation of vaccine and placebo or 2:1 in favor of the vaccine, may increase enrollment for trials. Additional innovation in estimating the role of vaccination to consider broader effects—models that account for the evolving pathogenicity and risk of the disease and prioritizing vulnerable populations or those most likely to transmit or to be exposed—can aid in improving the pathway to vaccination.[22]

Once a vaccine is developed, safe, and approved, there are the challenges of distribution. While the speed at which COVID-19 vaccines were made was unprecedented, the distribution of the vaccine had the same challenges as any other vaccine: logistics and maintaining the cold-chain (a temperature-controlled supply chain), community education, equitable distribution, and administration.[23] During the pandemic, vaccination rollout was layered upon an already burdened healthcare system, further straining resources.

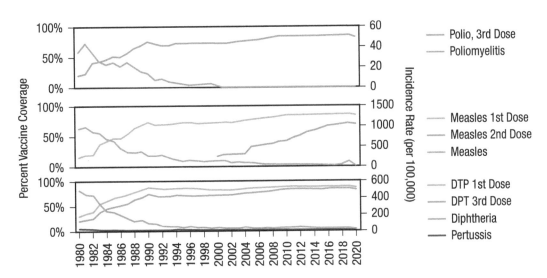

Figure 12.6 WHO global data comparing immunization coverage with incidence for poliomyelitis, measles, diphtheria, and pertussis.

Source: Data from World Health Organization. Immunization data. https://immunizationdata.who.int /listing.html?topic=incidence&location=Global

There were the logistic issues of getting vaccines, properly maintained, to providers and into people's arms before they expired. Partnering with local organizations (e.g., schools, houses of worship, local healthcare) can help to improve uptake and reduce disparities.[24] Yet issues remain on who and how to prioritize, how to get vaccines to harder-to-reach populations, and getting vaccines into low-income countries when most of the vaccine was reserved and manufactured by wealthy countries.[25,26]

THOUGHT QUESTION

Figure 12.3 in the prior section walked us through the steps from idea to vaccine approval. Continue the process: create an infographic to describe the next steps from approval to herd immunity.

REDUCING VACCINE HESITANCY

During the polio vaccine roll-out of the 1950s, vaccine hesitancy was hindering progress. In 1956, only 0.6% of American teens were vaccinated despite 60,000 children becoming infected annually.[27] A solution: teens and teen idols. In 1956, teen idol and performer Elvis Presley got his polio vaccine on the "Ed Sullivan Show." Within 6 months, vaccination in this age group rose to 80%.[27]

There is a worrying trend that the continued success of immunization programs will be thwarted by anti-vaccine sentiment.[28] Most cases of vaccine-preventable diseases that occur in the United States occur among those who chose not to be vaccinated.[29,30] But understanding vaccine hesitancy is itself a complex endeavor.

vaccine hesitancy: Reluctance or refusal to vaccinate despite the availability of services.

Many factors affect individuals' uptake of vaccines, including vaccine supply, access to health services, affordability, awareness, acceptance, and motivation; these are sometimes categorized as *The 5As of Vaccine Uptake*—Access, Affordability, Awareness, Acceptance, and Activation—as well as thoughts and feelings.[31] **Vaccine hesitancy** is the reluctance or refusal to vaccinate despite the availability of services and it has been identified by the WHO as one of the top 10 global health threats.[32,33]

Vaccine hesitancy has been around since the very first vaccine, with concerns over adverse effects, misinformation about the efficacy and side effects of the vaccine, and mistrust of the motivation for those promoting vaccination. Even the success of vaccination at reducing disease has compromised vaccine uptake, because the perceived risk from the vaccine becomes greater than the perceived risk of the disease. Vaccine mandates (i.e., requiring vaccination for school or work) can be effective, but at what cost to the community? With mandates, marginalized communities can be further marginalized and cut-off from education and employment opportunities.

In engaging with communities to promote vaccination, education can be helpful to explain the benefits of vaccination and how they work. In trying to address vaccine hesitancy, focusing on the positive messages can be helpful, while disagreeing or telling people they are wrong is not helpful. Worse, corrective information may further reduce intent to vaccinate among those with high levels of concern.[34] Acknowledging that vaccines do have side effects and there can be adverse effects is honest and maintains credibility. It can even be helpful to talk about how side effects like soreness and redness or minor swelling can be indicative of the body's immune response to the vaccine. Critical to continuing the successful use of vaccination, those promoting vaccination must recognize that vaccine hesitancy falls in a greater context of trust, history, and experience of the community.[32] Failing to engage with that greater context will further increase hesitancy around vaccination.

THOUGHT QUESTION

Imagine that you are promoting a vaccine for HPV in a rural community. Because of the impact of HPV on fertility, you are focusing on adolescent girls. What might you do to engage with the community to improve the success of your program? What alternative measures of success might you consider beyond how many girls are vaccinated? Here is a helpful commentary to get you started: https://doi.org/10.1038/d41586-018-07034-4

CASE STUDY

Salk and Sabin are by far the most commonly associated names with polio and the polio vaccine. But like most science, their work was built with and on the work of teams of scientists: one such scientist was Dorothy Horstmann (Figure 12.7). Dr. Horstmann was born in the state of Washington in 1911, just 5 years before one of the worst polio epidemics in the United States. She attended UC Berkeley for undergraduate studies and then UC San Francisco for medicine. After a residency at Vanderbilt University, she was the Commonwealth Fellow in Preventive Medicine in New Haven, Connecticut, in 1942. She was the first woman to earn tenure at Yale University's School of Medicine and was the first woman to receive an endowed chair.

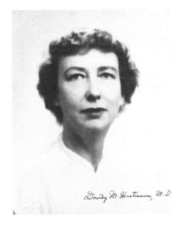

Figure 12.7 Dorothy Horstmann (1911–2001).
Source: National Library of Medicine, http://resource.nlm.nih.gov/101419057.

As a clinician scientist with expertise in virology and epidemiology in the mid-1900s, she worked when polio was at its height with limited capacity for medicine to respond. At that time, it was believed that polio affected the nervous system directly—excluding the possibility of an oral vaccine. Dr. Horstmann and the Yale Study Unit monitored the outbreaks happening in the Eastern United States to understand how the virus was being transmitted. Trained in clinical epidemiology, they systematically set about to determine from which portals of exit the virus was recoverable.[35] They collected samples from water and insects and human blood and fecal samples, pharyngeal swabs, and oropharyngeal washings. It was through this meticulous work and willingness to question the prevailing paradigm that Dr. Horstmann and her colleagues proved that the GI system (fecal-oral transmission) was most likely. Further, they identified poliovirus in the blood. The discovery that poliovirus reached the brain by the bloodstream through infection of the gastrointestinal tract led directly to the development of the oral polio vaccine.

Her reach went beyond polio to include other childhood infections, including rubella, Coxsackie, and Echo viruses.[35] Read more about Professor Dorothy Horstmann here: https://medicine.yale.edu/profile/115700/

CONCLUSION

In this chapter, we discussed how vaccines work, including how they stimulate the immune system. We also discussed the epidemiology of vaccination including the effective reproductive number and herd immunity. While we use VE and effectiveness along with coverage rates and reduced incidence and mortality as measures of vaccine success, the broader effects such as educational attainment and fewer days lost from employment are harder to quantify.

While vaccination is among the greatest public health achievements, vaccine program successes create challenges to disease eradication and elimination programs. Considering the community context in which vaccine programs are implemented and actively engaging with affected communities are integral to achieving vaccine coverage goals.

TEACHING CORNER

DID YOU KNOW?

In infectious diseases, we developed ID-specific terminology associated with core epidemiologic concepts. One of them is the idea of an *attack rate (AR)* where other epidemiologists might use cumulative incidence. Like incidence, the AR has the number of new cases in the numerator, and the denominator is the group or population at risk.

In the example shown in Figure 12.8, tan individuals are uninfected individuals. Those with a shot are vaccinated and those without are not. Purple indicates those individuals who become infected after the study (denoted by the arrow). Using this information, calculate the ARs for the vaccinated group and the unvaccinated group.

TRY THIS

Did you notice that when you calculated the AR, it was the same as the cumulative incidence: new cases over the group denominator you are investigating. Since we have incidence, we can calculate a relative risk (RR) to quantify the protective effect of the vaccine. Recall that RR is the *Incidence in the exposed* over the *Incidence in the unexposed*, and have the *Exposure* be those "exposed" to the vaccine.

$$RR = \left(\frac{I_E}{I_U} \right)$$

Calculate the RR and be sure to put your answer into a sentence.

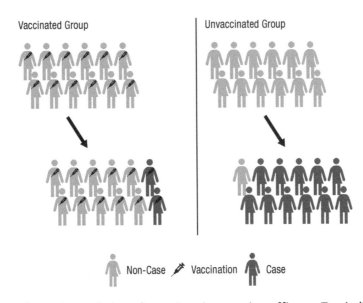

Figure 12.8 Hypothetical populations for estimating vaccine efficacy. Tan individuals are uninfected. Those with a shot are vaccinated and those without are not. Purple indicates those individuals who become infected after the study (denoted by the arrow).

TAKE IT A STEP FURTHER

Tying it back to this chapter, VE is also known as the preventive fraction (PF) or the relative risk reduction (RRR). VE is measured by comparing the ARs of disease among vaccinated and unvaccinated persons and determining the percentage reduction in the incidence rate of disease among vaccinated persons relative to unvaccinated persons. The greater the percentage reduction of illness in the vaccinated group, the greater the VE:

$$VE = \left(\frac{AR_u - AR_v}{AR_u} \right) \times 100; \ PF = \left(\frac{I_u - I_E}{I_u} \right) \times 100 \text{; and, using algebra, } RRR = 1 - RR$$

Notice that VE and PF are the same formula just using different nomenclature: attack rate versus incidence. VE, PF, and RRR are all the proportion of cases that could be prevented if they had been exposed (i.e., vaccinated). (a) Calculate the VE using either the VE or PF formulas and, using the RR you previously calculated, calculate RRR. (b) Make a prediction: If the vaccine showed higher VE, what happens to the RR.

QUESTIONS FOR FURTHER DISCUSSION

1. A beautiful timeline for vaccinations was developed for the history of vaccines by the College of Physicians of Philadelphia. Go to https://historyofvaccines.org/vaccines-101 and identify one misconception you had about vaccinations that is explained there. For instance, epidemiology likes to talk about Edward Jenner's cowpox vaccine, but was he the first to effectively combat smallpox? Be sure to explain not only the correction, but what your misconception was and why.

2. What are the 5 As of vaccine uptake? Take each and list one way you could help support vaccine uptake.

3. Are vaccine hesitancy and vaccine uptake antonyms?

A robust set of instructor resources designed to supplement this text is located at http://connect.springerpub.com/content/book/978-0-8261-5674-7. Qualifying instructors may request access by emailing textbook@springerpub.com.

REFERENCES

1. Centers for Disease Control and Prevention. Global immunization: our progress against polio. https://www.cdc.gov/polio/progress/index.htm
2. Nathanson N, Kew OM. From emergence to eradication: the epidemiology of poliomyelitis deconstructed. *Am J Epidemiol.* 2010;172(11):1213–1229. doi:10.1093/aje/kwq320
3. Martinez-Bakker M, King AA, Rohani P. Unraveling the transmission ecology of polio. *PLoS Biol.* 2015;13(6):e1002172. doi:10.1371/journal. pbio.1002172
4. World Health Organization. Immunization. December 5, 2019. https://www.who.int/news-room/facts-in-pictures/detail/immunization
5. Ellner PD. Smallpox: gone but not forgotten. *Infection.* 1998;26(5):263–269. doi:10.1007/BF02962244
6. Pearce JMS. Salk and Sabin: poliomyelitis immunization. *J Neurol Neurosurg Psychiatry.* 2004;75:1552. https://jnnp.bmj.com/content/75/11/1552

7. Shimabukuro T, Nguyen M, Martin D, DeStefano F. Safety monitoring in the Vaccine Adverse Event Reporting System (VAERS). *Vaccine*. 2015;33(36):4398–4405. doi:10.1016/j.vaccine.2015.07.035

8. World Health Assembly. *Global eradication of poliomyelitis by the year 2000: resolution 41.28.* World Health Organization. 1988. https://apps.who.int/iris/bitstream/handle/10665/226729/WER6322_161-162.PDF

9. Ozawa S, Clark S, Portnoy A, Grewal S, Brenzel L, Walker DG. Return on investment from childhood immunization in low and middle income countries, 2011–20. *Health Aff.* 2016;32(2):199–207. doi:10.1377/hlthaff.2015.1086

10. Centers for Disease Control and Prevention. *CDC Global Immunization Strategic Framework 2021–2030.* Centers for Disease Control and Prevention; 2021. https://www.cdc.gov/global-health/immunization/framework/index.html

11. Doherty M, Buchy P, Standaert B, Giaquinto C, Prado-Cohrs D. Vaccine impact: benefits for human health. *Vaccine*. 2016;34:6707–6714. doi:10.1016/j.vaccine.2016.10.025

12. Rodrigues CMC, Plotkin SA. Impact of vaccines: health, economic and social perspectives. *Front Microbiol.* 2020;11:1526. doi:10.3389/fmicb.2020.01526

13. Historic Ipswich. The Great Dying 1616–1619, "By God's visitation, a wonderful plague." https://historicipswich.org/2021/04/21/the-great-dying

14. de Vries RD, McQuaid S, van Amerongen G, et al. Measles immune suppression: lessons from the Macaque model. *PLOS Pathogens.* 2012;8(8):e1002885. doi:10.1371/journal.ppat.1002885

15. Holmes A, Tildesley MJ, Solomon AW, et al. Modeling treatment strategies to inform yaws eradication. *Emerg Infect Dis.* 2020;26(11):2685–2693. doi:10.3201/eid2611.19149

16. Roberts L. Battle to wipe out debilitating Guinea work parasite hits 10 year delay. *Nature.* 2019;574:157–158. doi:10.1038/d41586-019-02921-w

17. Shretta R, Liu J, Cotter C, et al. Malaria elimination and eradication. In: Holmes KK, Bertozzi S, Bloom BR, Jha P, eds. Diseases Control Priorities. 3rd ed., vol 6. The International Bank for Reconstruction and Development/The World Bank; 2017. doi:10.1596/978-1-4648-0524-0_ch12

18. World Health Organization. WHO recommends groundbreaking malaria vaccine for children at risk [News Release]. October 6, 2021. https://www.who.int/news/item/06-10-2021-who-recommends-groundbreaking-malaria-vaccine-for-children-at-risk

19. World Health Organization. Meeting of the Strategic Advisory Group of Experts on Immunization, October 2016: conclusions and recommendations. *Wkly Epidemiol Rec.* 2016;91(48):561–582. https://www.who.int/publications/i/item/WER9148

20. Han S. Clinical vaccine development. *Clin Exp Vaccine Res.* 2015;4(1):46–53. doi:10.7774/cevr.2015.4.1.46

21. Gouglas D, Le TT, Henderson K, et al. Estimating the cost of vaccine development against epidemic infectious diseases: a cost minimisation study. *Lancet Glob Health.* 2018;6(12):e1386–e1396. doi:10.1016/S2214-109X(18)30346-2

22. Madewell ZJ, Dean NE, Berlin JA, et al. Challenges of evaluating and modelling vaccination in emerging infectious diseases. *Epidemics.* 2021;37:100506. doi:10.1016/j.epidem.2021.100506

23. Burgos RM, Badowski ME, Drwiega E, et al. The race to a COVID-19 vaccine: opportunities and challenges in development and distribution. *Drugs Context.* 2021;10:2020-12-2. doi:10.7573/dic.2020-12-2

24. Jean-Jacques M, Bauchner H. Vaccine distribution—equity left behind? *JAMA.* 2021;325(9):829–830. doi:10.1001/jama.2021.1205

25. Mills M, Salisbury D. The challenges of distributing COVID-19 vaccinations. *EClinical Medicine.* 2020;31:100674. https://www.thelancet.com/journals/eclinm/article/PIIS2589-5370(20)30418-1/fulltext

26. Acharya KP, Ghimire TR, Subramanya SH. Access to and equitable distribution of COVID-19 vaccine in low-income countries. *npj Vaccines.* 2021;6:54. doi:10.1038/s41541-021-00323-6

27. Hershied H, Brody I. How Elvis got Americans to accept the polio vaccine. *Scientific Americana.* January 18, 2021. https://www.scientificamerican.com/article/how-elvis-got-americans-to-accept-the-polio-vaccine

28. Hotez P. America and Europe's new normal: the return of vaccine-preventable diseases. *Pediatr Res*. 2019;85:912–914. doi:10.1038/s41390-019-0354-3

29. Phadke VK, Bednarczyk RA, Salmon DA, Omer SB. Association between vaccine refusal and vaccine-preventable diseases in the United States: a review of measles and pertussis. *JAMA*. 2016;315(11):1149–1158. doi:10.1001/jama.2016.1353

30. Scobie HM, Johnson AG, Suthar AB, et al. Monitoring incidence of COVID-19 cases, hospitalizations, and deaths, by vaccination status — 13 U.S. jurisdictions, April 4–July 17, 2021. *MMWR Morb Mortal Wkly Rep*. 2021;70:1284–1290. doi:10.15585/mmwr.mm7037e1

31. Thomson A, Robinson K, Vallée-Tourangeau G. The 5As: a practical taxonomy for the determinants of vaccine uptake. *Vaccine*. 2016;34(8):1018–1024. doi:10.1016/j.vaccine.2015.11.065

32. Larson H. *Stuck: How Vaccine Rumors Start—and Why They Don't Go Away*. Oxford University Press; 2020.

33. Abad N, Ballester Bon H, Betsch C, et al. *Data for action: achieving high uptake of COVID-19 vaccines*. World Health Organization; 2021. https://www.who.int/publications/i/item/WHO-2019-nCoV-vaccination-demand-planning-2021.1

34. Nyhan B, Reifler J. Does correcting myths about the flu vaccine work? An experimental evaluation of the effects of corrective information. *Vaccine*. 2015;33(3):459–464. doi:10.1016/j.vaccine.2014.11.017

35. Carleton HA. Putting together the pieces of polio: how Dorothy Horstmann helped solve the puzzle. *Yale J Biol Med*. 2011;84(2):83–89. https://www.ncbi.nlm.nih.gov/pmc/articles/PMC3117421

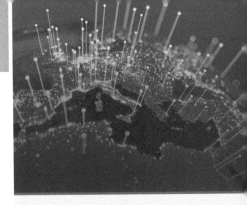

CHAPTER 13

ADVANCES IN DISEASE CONTROL

INTRODUCTION

From 1918 to 1920, the world experienced the most severe influenza pandemic in history, caused by an H1N1 virus, and going on to kill about 50 million worldwide and infect about one-third of the world's population. At the time, there was no vaccine to protect against influenza and no antivirals or antibiotics for secondary infections. In addition, control efforts were limited to nonpharmaceutical measures such as hygiene, isolation, and quarantine. Unfortunately, even technology could not save the day. Wireless telegraphy was supposed to allow for frequent messaging of health information around the world so that information about new cases could be transmitted before they arrived in a new location. However, numerous obstacles came up: some countries did not sign up. Others, like Japan, used the technology to gather military intelligence during World War I. Additionally, while disease statistics became more readily available, there was little support for recommending public health measures to stem the pandemic. The League of Nations Health Organization, which ran the technology, couldn't even declare an outbreak because that was under the authority of various countries and not centralized. Some technologies, however, did help, with radio communication and telephones allowing for more rapid communication to help keep the world informed as influenza spread, and allowing for rapid responses such as quarantines.

LEARNING OBJECTIVES

By the end of this chapter, readers will be able to:

- List advances in disease control in the 21st century.
- Justify how social media, big data, and search tools are used to improve disease control.
- Hypothesize how personalized medicine and technologies can be used to control disease.
- State the role of the P-value and confidence intervals in data analysis.

DIGITAL TRACE DATA IN THE 21ST CENTURY

In 2009, Google and the U.S. Centers for Disease Control and Prevention (CDC) published a methodology to estimate flu activity by region using Google search queries. The basic idea is that there will be more searches for flu when more people are sick with flu-like symptoms. However, search queries frequently overestimated the incidence of illness. For example, Google flu trends forecasted twice as many influenza cases as actually occurred in the United States during the 2012 to 2013 flu season. Additionally, since the case data were not publicly available, there was no way to validate the estimates being produced.[1]

The 21st century and its digital revolution has ushered in a new era of electronic data use for disease tracking and monitoring. By 2019, 67% of the global population had subscribed to mobile devices. The data sources available for epidemiologic surveillance have subsequently increased exponentially, ranging from survey apps and news websites, to search data, to wearable sensors and social media platforms (Figure 13.1).

Digital epidemiology is simply epidemiology that uses digital data. What is unique about this subfield, however, is that it uses data that was generated outside the public health system. Data is often processed to either forecast or nowcast infectious disease outbreaks. Whereas **nowcasting** is a short-term prediction that attempts to track incidence in near real-time, *forecasting* aims to predict the future. One of the potential advantages of digital data sources is early disease detection: the strategy of rapid identification of undetected cases to quickly understand both the magnitude of an outbreak and to reduce transmission. Regular surveillance data of all cases through traditional public health sources is cumbersome, can be delayed (especially if relying on passive surveillance),

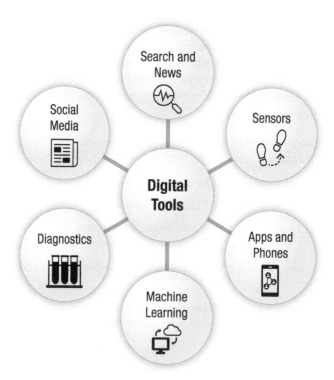

Figure 13.1 **Examples of digital tools used in disease control and surveillance.**

or requires a lot of follow-up (if active surveillance or contact tracing) and may miss cases in which healthcare is not sought. A large proportion of sick people search for relevant health information using the internet. This information is often then available to others, sometimes even with the time and location of the search; that is, with a *time-stamp* and *geo-tag*. Epidemiologists and researchers can then study real-time population health using these **digital traces**. Another potential advantage to these methodologies is the ability to study individual or population behavior and reactions.[2] Using digital data for **mining**, analysis, and information aggregation to inform public health is known as **infodemiology**, or more specifically, when used for surveillance purposes, it is termed **infoveillance**.[3]

Novel Data Sources

In the age of technology, numerous data sources beyond traditional medical/health data have been harnessed for disease control. Search data provides useful information that can potentially uncover a disease outbreak, reveal what the public thinks, or predict future health events. Search terms can be scanned and analyzed, and are often geolocatable, which allows for local or regional analyses of public health issues. For example, a strong positive correlation has been shown between Google search queries and official data on chikungunya and Zika virus cases in South America.[4] Even before increases in cases are noticed by the health authorities, the searches may provide an indicator of possible disease outbreaks. Similarly, Google Trends has allowed for examination of search volume bursts around certain key words. One of these bursts occurred in the second half of 2016 for a rare arbovirus responsible for Mayaro virus disease, resulting in fevers and possible severe complications.[5] Since the disease is typically rare and hard to distinguish from other diseases (e.g., from dengue virus), search data helped to shine a light on a diagnosis and identify next steps. Searches can also be used in predictive modeling. Using the frequency of Yahoo searches for flu-like symptoms, models predicted an increase in positive influenza cultures 1 to 3 weeks in advance and an increase in mortality from pneumonia and influenza up to 5 weeks in advance.[6] While Google and Yahoo are well-known search engines, data from numerous other international search engines such as Baidu, Yandex, Daum, and Parsijoo have also been successfully linked to disease outbreaks.

Online news provides another data source mentioning specific diseases or conditions where clustering of information may represent a new disease outbreak. One of the ways in which these work is that they scan news articles from all over for key disease terms and then aggregate and locate the citations. A number of news aggregators have been developed to monitor or track these types of events. For example, HealthMap uses online news aggregators, eyewitness reports, discussions, and validated official reports using automated processes to facilitate early disease detection by location, time, and agent, and the Global Public Health Intelligence Network (GPHIN) was established to connect experts around the globe and track disease outbreaks, bioterrorism, exposures to chemicals, natural disasters, and more.[7,8] Program for Monitoring Emerging Diseases (ProMED) was launched in 1994 as an internet service to identify unusual health events and, through its mailing list, provides real-time information about outbreaks.[9] Members scan and respond to news and information from across the world. ProMED was the first to report outbreaks of SARS, anthrax, Zika, and more.

Digital data sources leave digital footprints or traces so the data can be aggregated in time and space. Internet of things (IoT)-enabled devices allow for obtaining real-time data streams from readings and measurements. IoT usually refers to connected computing devices, sensors, objects, or even animals or humans who are given unique identifiers and can transfer network data without requiring actual human–human or human–computer interaction. Examples include an individual with an implant, or a sensor that detects a pathogen in the water.

Mobile phones can be used to analyze travel patterns, as was done for nearly 15 million people in Kenya over the course of a year to map routes of dispersal of *Plasmodium falciparum*, the parasite responsible for malaria. Researchers found patterns of local transmission in urban settings, which could provide key signals for local malaria surveillance efforts.[10]

These technologies can be linked to novel analytic approaches to find geographic hotspots of infectious disease transmission that can be utilized to reduce overall levels of community infection and transmission. For example, sensor or mobile phone data can be used to map activity spaces, which are used in epidemiologic studies to represent geographic spaces where people spend most of their daily activities. These analyses have been particularly useful in obesity and greenspace/park use research or when mapping social interactions and certain communicable diseases. Mobile Global Positioning Systems, enabled through mobile phone location data, can be used to examine where people or animals go, and where their activity spaces overlap. This type of work has shown that activity space overlap can be greatest among those individuals who have the greatest genetic similarity in tuberculosis strains, indicating that transmission may be occurring in small overlapping community settings.[11]

infodemiology: Analyzing and disseminating real-time health information from news and social media.

THOUGHT QUESTION

What would you consider an additional novel digital trace not mentioned in this section that could be used for disease control?

PUBLIC PARTICIPATION IN DISEASE CONTROL

Participatory surveillance occurs when disease and symptoms are reported directly by people rather than by health departments (Figure 13.2).[12] These sometimes allow for more rapid, high-volume data collection. Broader designs allow country residents to become volunteers to support ongoing disease surveillance. Influenzanet is a participatory monitoring system for influenza-like illness based on data reported by internet users from the general population. This has allowed for over 36,000 volunteers to provide information in a given season across 10 countries in Europe. The data closely correlate with those obtained through medical provider networks.[13] An app and dashboard known as the "Guardians of Health" were created in Brazil during the 2016 Olympic Games, allowing spectators to provide information about symptoms and to look for possible symptom and syndrome clusters in space and time. The app was downloaded 59,312 times, with 1,745 reports noting a symptom. Fortunately, no major outbreaks were detected throughout the Olympic Games.[14] One of the limitations of crowdsourcing is the reliability of information coming from users. In this example, to mitigate fake postings, spam was tracked and excluded from analyses.

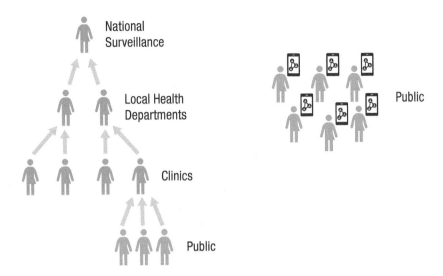

Figure 13.2 Contrasting traditional surveillance systems (left) and participatory surveillance (right).

Particularly during COVID-19, apps with tracing functionalities using Bluetooth and other technologies were used, with countries including Singapore, South Korea, Israel, Italy, Germany, and China fully implementing digital contact tracing. In Singapore, the government developed the TraceTogether app—every time the contact-tracing app came within the proximity of another app, it would save the information locally and issue an alert if a person came close to an infected individual. Individuals who are alerted to a possible exposure can then voluntarily get tested and report their outcome.[15] Companies such as Google and Apple created platforms to collect location-based data from millions of users, which was aggregated and used to track mobility, allowing for hotspot identification and assessment of mitigation strategy effectiveness. Other novel uses of digital trace data include balloons or drones equipped with infrared cameras and sensors to warn those who might be infected with a pathogen.[16]

Sensors can collect detailed information about humans as well as their environment. Low-cost sensors, for example, can measure personal exposures to identify asthma triggers in children. These can be triggered by environmental exposures, specific behaviors (e.g., exercise), or even stress. They are often wearable devices, such as smartwatches, that allow for processing and storing data in real-time and integrating a variety of different information feeds. Similarly, wearable devices have been used to characterize physical activity and sedentary behavior in over 16,500 older women who participated in the Women's Health Study. These data both show the feasibility of using devices and can inform the evidence base on which physical activity guidelines are based.[17] More recently, there are examples of studies that combine a variety of data sources, search queries, social media data, digital data from internet-based sources, and so on.[18]

digital traces: Digital "footprints," or records of activity left behind through online information systems.

participatory surveillance: Participants provide voluntary health-related information through surveys or others sources to monitor disease trends.

Social Media Approaches

Social media data can be used in numerous ways, whether in outbreaks, disease monitoring, prediction, understanding public reactions to an event or policy, or in understanding behaviors.

In 2019, Twitter reported almost one-third of the total notifications related to an avian influenza outbreak earlier than public health surveillance reports.[19] Tweets examining influenza have been compared to CDC national weekly Influenza-Like Illness (ILI) rates. As shown in Figure 13.3, comparing the weekly national ILI rates to the aggregated weekly flu Tweet rate reveals that the two were highly correlated ($r = 0.845$).[20] In evaluating Twitter data and COVID-19 in the United Kingdom, temporal Twitter trends showed a precision of over 80% as they related to case numbers.[21] Twitter has been relatively available to researchers, allowing public access to a 1% random sample of raw Tweets, providing location information if the account has the location turned on.[22]

Tweets can be used for not just the content but also the sentiment. **Content analysis** of Tweets allows for qualitative coding and comparison of themes used in online posts through examination of popular hashtags and key words. It has been used to identify key trends during the 2009 H1N1 swine flu outbreak that may have correlated with outbreak incidence.[23] Tweets were primarily used to disseminate information from credible sources about the outbreak. **Sentiment analysis** is another analytic technique that identifies and classifies particular sentiments (subjective opinions or feelings) in social media texts. One can then classify statements as positive, negative, or neutral, thus allowing to cap-

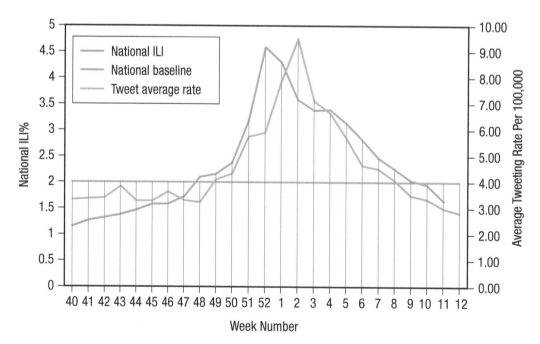

Figure 13.3 Weekly national ILI rates and weekly combined flu Tweet rates across 31 cities over the 2013 to 2014 flu season.

Source: Allen C, Tsou M-H, Aslam A, Nagel A, Gawron J-M. Applying GIS and machine learning methods to Twitter data for multiscale surveillance of Influenza. *PLoS One*. 2016;11(7):e0157734. doi:10.1371/journal.pone.0157734

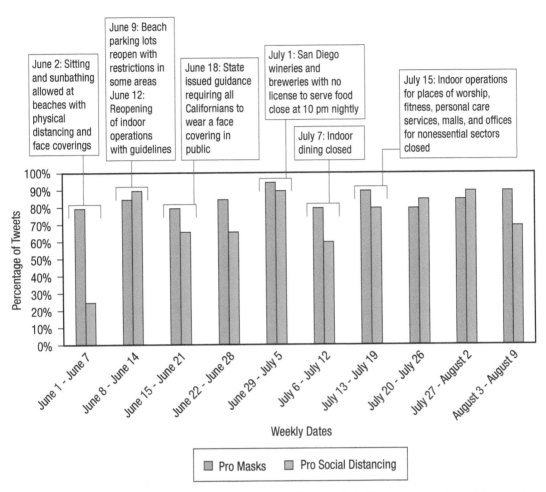

June 2: Sitting and sunbathing allowed at beaches with physical distancing and face coverings

June 9: Beach parking lots reopen with restrictions in some areas June 12: Reopening of indoor operations with guidelines

June 18: State issued guidance requiring all Californians to wear a face covering in public

July 1: San Diego wineries and breweries with no license to serve food close at 10 pm nightly

July 7: Indoor dining closed

July 15: Indoor operations for places of worship, fitness, personal care services, malls, and offices for nonessential sectors closed

Figure 13.4 Sentiment analysis on Twitter regarding social distancing and masking during COVID-19. The text boxes illustrate local policy changes over time.

ture not just what people were Tweeting, but also how they felt about it. When exploring public opinion and sentiment toward certain COVID-19 mitigation policies, one can look at sentiments expressed in relation to broader policy or regulatory decisions (Figure 13.4).

Sentiment in social media has been a particularly useful data source in exploring the role of misinformation during an infectious disease outbreak. Being able to ascertain the sentiment of messages can alert public health to areas where messaging may be counterproductive to public health. Social media data may not routinely misalign with public health messaging on various themes.[24] However, in the aggregate, even a small amount of misinformation can lead to the public not following public health orders, as was experienced during COVID-19, where information was distorted, often intentionally (known as disinformation), due to political agendas, prevailing health myths, or constitutional beliefs.[25] Those regions where there is a misalignment can then be examined for future interventions.

Despite all these examples of successful mining of social media and wearable technologies, there are also examples where social media data has incorrectly predicted upcoming flu seasons.[26] Twitter data indicated a typical flu season from 2011 to 2012, but the season peaked 3 months late. There were also many flu misdiagnoses based on Twitter data prior to flu seasons in 2012 to 2013 and 2013 to 2014. The extent to which the characteristics of reported events can accurately represent the incidence of actual health events is thus debatable. Given the limited length of data (e.g., a Tweet), different language styles between internet users, and no restriction on their writing style, user-generated content often contains a high amount of noise. Data is often cross-sectional and limited by sample size and subjectivity of interpretation. Importantly, the content generated by users is also inherently biased as it reflects only the information that people are comfortable revealing and tracks the people who are using social media. Demographics for most digital platforms are not nationally representative and are skewed toward younger, more educated individuals.

content analysis: Analysis of text content and comparison of major themes.

sentiment analysis: Analysis of how people feel and respond.

THOUGHT QUESTION

What might be content and sentiment analysis one could undertake to examine whether students feel anxious during a pandemic?

IMPROVING PREDICTIONS THROUGH MACHINE LEARNING AND BIG DATA

Every year the CDC runs an annual competition known as FluSight in which teams of researchers compete to develop the most accurate weekly ILI predictions possible. This has created a lot of interest in influenza modeling using digital data.[27] One year, nearly a dozen researchers collected almost 160,000 Tweets containing the key word "flu" from 11 U.S. cities. The study concluded that compared to Tweet analyses in the previous influenza season, there was increased accuracy in using Twitter as a supplementary surveillance tool for influenza as better filtering and classification methods yielded higher correlations for the 2013 to 2014 influenza season than those found for Tweets in the previous influenza season.[28]

Given the large volumes of data that can now be collected and the potential it holds for disease detection, there is a need to harness, verify, and interpret its use. This includes complex data that is rapidly collected in massive amounts, known as **big data**. Digital sources of big data can include many of the data sources already mentioned as well as electronic medical records, genomics, imaging data, or data from social networks.

Machine learning is broadly defined as the ability for computers to learn patterns from data without being explicitly programmed. Typically, subsets of data are used to train complex algorithms to classify or predict various outcomes and then the algorithm can be fed larger data sets to process. **Training data** refers to a data set that is used to teach the machine learning model, and then the trained model is unleashed on the primary data set. Using machine learning techniques, Toronto's surveillance system was first to detect the COVID-19 epidemic outbreak in the epicenter of Wuhan.[29] The BlueDOT web-based startup that uses various models and algorithms, along with a variety of unique data sources, including airline data, population density, news, climate, and disease reservoir reports, was initially able to correctly predict H1N1 influenza spread in

2009 through air travel data. During COVID-19, BlueDOT announced 9 days before any official information was released that the world was experiencing a new outbreak.[30] Other companies such as Metabiota have also used advanced computational methods to predict COVID-19 outbreaks, predicting outbreaks a week early in several Asian countries.[31]

Artificial intelligence methods can be particularly useful in predicting how an outbreak might be affected by seasonality, for example, in noting whether warmer or cooler weather facilitates disease spread. Models can use data to predict the most likely scenarios when a novel agent arrives next. Machine learning was also used to create an evidence-based application to inform the general population and healthcare providers of updated, evidence-based Ebola guidelines based on evolving data.[32] These machine learning techniques are sometimes called "black boxes" because while their predictions may be quite accurate, the predictors that go into the models can be complex and challenging to interpret (Figure 13.5).

It is clear that large and open data sets will be increasingly useful in the field of digital epidemiology. Some of the current issues include having access to large, high-quality data sets that are publicly available. In addition, fake or nonrepresentative data may be harder to spot. However, big data provides a complement to traditional epidemiologic data sources that suffer from challenges related to sample size, limited geographic distribution, and lack of data or certainty in multiple timepoints. The need for large, global data sets during

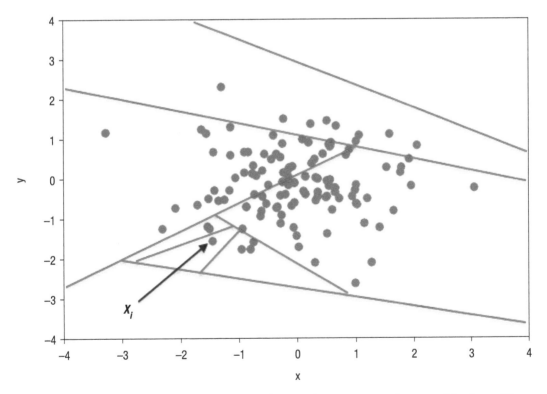

Figure 13.5 A complex machine learning technique known as random partitioning with extended isolation forests uses decision trees to pick random intercept and slope features of data sets. Imagine that the x-axis is a normalized age, and the y-axis is a normalized obesity score. How would you define the point marked with X to a clinician to use the information to make a diagnosis?

Source: Courtesy of Sal Borrelli.

the COVID-19 pandemic propelled some landmark initiatives that created better data sharing models. These include the World Health Organization's (WHO's) Global Research on Coronavirus Disease Database and the GISAID Initiative (Global Initiative on Sharing All Influenza Data). Microsoft, Facebook, Semantic Scholar, the Allen Institute for AI, and five other collaborators made the COVID-19 Open Research Dataset (CORD-19) openly available, which contains about 44,000 scholarly articles free for use (allenai.org/data/cord-19).

 machine learning: Algorithmic approaches that adapt to patterns in data without programming a prediction task.

THOUGHT QUESTION

What are some ways in which machine learning can be used to improve the public's health?

PERSONALIZED MEDICINE

Influenza can evolve into a severe infection resulting in exaggerated inflammation, respiratory failure, and mortality among some young adults. However, steroids to reduce inflammation do not improve survival among all patient populations. Given what we now know about the role of immunity and the response of the host to influenza, individualized biomarkers of severe infection can be increasingly monitored. This in turn can result in targeted therapeutics that help to restore a normal immune response, which can reduce severity and also shorten recovery periods.

Precision medicine, sometimes known as "personalized medicine," is an approach to tailoring disease prevention and treatment that takes into account differences in people's genes, environments, and lifestyles. In contrast, population health requires directing efficient use of resources toward those most at risk. A newer term, **precision public health**, has been loosely defined as "an emerging discipline that uses extensive population-specific data to provide the right intervention to the right population at the right time."[33] For example, genome sequencing and molecular tests can provide more timely and precise identification of pathogens, as well as insights into their sources, spread, and susceptibility to antibiotics. The CDC's Advanced Molecular Detection (AMD) initiative uses molecular techniques to quickly detect a pathogen. Nucleic-based tests amplify and detect target organisms' nucleic acids, and multiplex tests can detect multiple pathogens at once, allowing for quick differentiation among different pathogens. Studying changing influenza virus genomic sequences can be used to select and design seasonal influenza vaccines.[34] Data on transmission patterns during COVID-19 have helped to inform decisions regarding specific home and school closures.[35] Similarly, precise geographic information allows for identification of disease hotspots and subsequent public health interventions. In many ways, this work is not new; rather, the large quantities of data and new technologies have allowed for better predictive analytics and use of data to address upstream social factors that lead to poor health. However, this arena is not without controversy. Since the core of public health is to improve population health, if precision is about the individual, through improved clinical medicine, then these two approaches are

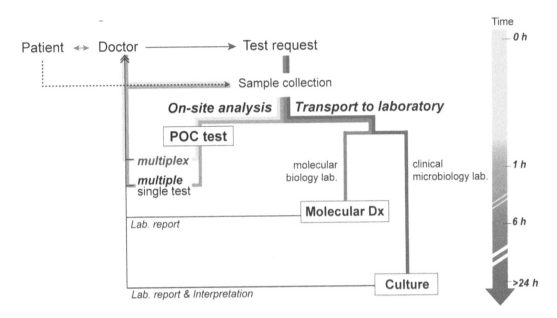

Figure 13.6 Point-of-care (POC) testing that can lead to a more rapid clinical diagnosis and response. Note that the left side of the graphic shows the time to response with POC, in contrast to a molecular diagnosis (Dx) in the middle and traditional culture-based methods on the right. *Source*: Kim H, Huh HJ, Park E, et al. Multiplex molecular point-of-care test for syndromic infectious diseases. *BioChip J*. 2021;15:14–22. doi:10.1007/s13206-021-00004-5

at odds. Large social questions, such as universal healthcare, may not be easily addressed through data-heavy techniques.

Personalized medicine does mean that specific tools can provide personalized clinical care because of their specificity and speed. This paradigm has led to development and deployment of point-of-care (POC) diagnostics for screening, which have shown to help slow the spread of the disease (Figure 13.6). In the time of COVID-19, POC testing has allowed for effective remote monitoring or telemedicine approaches. New technologies such as the mobile nucleic acid amplification testing (mobiNAAT) screen for gonorrhea, can determine antibiotic susceptibility in just 15 minutes; that is, before the patient leaves the clinic.[36] Tests can also detect microorganisms that may not be cultured through more traditional techniques and require only a small amount of a specimen. The goal is that these tests can lead to pathogen-specific treatment and the use of more specific antibiotics.

precision public health: Using population-specific data to provide the right intervention to the right population at the right time.

THOUGHT QUESTION

What might be some of the pitfalls of personalized medicine when applied to population health?

APPLICATIONS OF NEW TECHNOLOGIES

Pandemic influenza is often nonseasonal, with less distinct clinical features, and may disproportionately harm a variety of population groups. However, when a pandemic occurs, the virus is typically novel, making it impossible to create and stockpile vaccines in advance. Thus, once vaccines are manufactured and made available, there are typically insufficient quantities for everyone. Vaccine rationing creates an ethical dilemma in terms of who to vaccinate first. Those subgroups at greatest risk may not be obvious at first. Despite this, different justifications have been proposed.[37] Some proposed that healthcare workers be prioritized given the nature of their work with affected patients. Others have proposed frontline workers who are likely to be exposed. Some note that children should receive highest priority given their life trajectory as well as to minimize community transmission. Similarly, others would say that the sickest or the most medically or socially vulnerable should receive priority vaccination. Another approach is to consider social clusters based on family or social connections. Finally, some argue for a standard procedure such as a lottery. Underlying the rationale for these decisions is the motivation: whether to improve individual health outcomes, increase fairness and equity, or maximize the overall health of the population.

Ethics

Numerous new ethical dilemmas have come up with the advent of new technologies. When collecting data on an individual in the context of an outbreak, consent is most commonly limited to data that will be used only for monitoring purposes, that they will not be transferred to any public or private company, and that they remain anonymized. There may be an inherent conflict of interest between open access to large data sets and privacy protection, given that access can result in more unregulated use. Frameworks to collect, share, and access data without compromising individual security and privacy are still in their infancy. This is clearly essential when considering personal identifiers and unique genomic data.

Some ethical issues are quite specific to infectious disease outbreaks. On a broader basis, governments have an ethical obligation to ensure that they can carry out effective epidemic prevention and response efforts, including relevant public health laws and economic and scientific resources. During an outbreak, some population groups might be particularly vulnerable—for example, certain marginalized groups may lack access to clean water—and identifying their heightened risk may further marginalize them. Ethical decisions also arise due to resource constraints, such that not all patients can get needed care. During the Ebola outbreak, access to general healthcare services decreased, resulting in documented increases in deaths from TB, HIV, and malaria.[38] Ethical dilemmas can occur when public health measures are instituted that restrict personal freedoms, as happened in the COVID-19 pandemic. For example, stay-at-home measures were instituted to keep community transmission levels down but required individuals to at times forsake their own individual needs. These measures may play an important role in controlling infectious disease outbreaks, and in protecting the community, but also lead to increased resistance to other disease control measures.[39]

Data Visualization

With new advances has come a need to better communicate data and information. Data visualization has a long history, dating back to John Snow, when he hand-plotted cholera cases on a map and found them to cluster around the Broad Street pump. More advanced tools now allow public health professionals and researchers to integrate, synthesize, and visualize complex reams of data. With the advent of spatially explicit data, either from geocoded social media or remotely sensed satellite data, comes the increased use of mapping as a way to visualize and analyze disease. Humans are visual organisms and maps are intuitive. Modern-day uses of data include geo-coding electronic health records and then mapping them to better visualize the spread of methicillin-resistant *Staphylococcus aureus* (Figure 13.7).[40] While we typically think of mapping as just consisting of data visualization, spatial epidemiologists also use mapping as a precursor to spatial analyses like cluster detection and spatio-temporal modeling.

Social network analyses provide another way of visualizing networks of people and disease spread. In the field of molecular epidemiology, relationships between different strains of a virus or bacteria can be calculated and shown through phylogenetic trees called **dendrograms** (Figure 13.8). The field of phylo-geography is specifically concerned with understanding the relationship between the population biology and geography of a pathogen species. These tools link spatial aggregation with the genetic similarity of different isolates. Molecular epidemiologists can identify not just which pathogens are circulating but also link back to likely sources based on the genetic similarity of the pathogen and the social network of the individuals.

With all this information available, data dashboards have also evolved to provide real-time public health data. These often include confirmed cases, hospitalizations, and deaths, to help keep the public and key decision-makers informed. Most often they will display not only rates, but visualizations including line graphs indicating temporal trends,

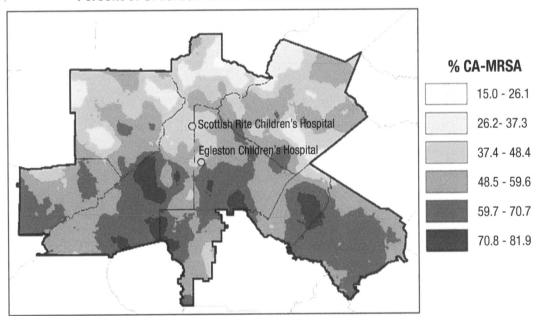

Percent of *S. aureus* cases that are CA-MRSA

% CA-MRSA

15.0 - 26.1
26.2 - 37.3
37.4 - 48.4
48.5 - 59.6
59.7 - 70.7
70.8 - 81.9

Scottish Rite Children's Hospital

Egleston Children's Hospital

Figure 13.7 *Staphylococcus aureus* cases that have community-associated methicillin-resistant infections across Atlanta, Georgia.

Source: Immergluck LC, Leong T, Malhotra K, et al. Geographic surveillance of community associated MRSA infections in children using electronic health record data. *BMC Infect Dis*. 2019;19:170. doi:10.1186/s12879-019-3682-3

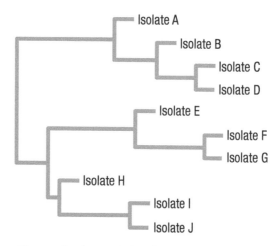

Figure 13.8 Dendrogram illustrating how viral or bacterial isolates may be related to each other through genetic drift or mutation.

Source: Carroll LN, Au AP, Detwiler LT, Fu TC, Painter IS, Abernethy NF. Visualization and analytics tools for infectious disease epidemiology: a systematic review. *J Biomed Inform*. 2014;51:287–298. doi:10.1016/j .jbi.2014.04.006

and maps indicating the spatial location. Importantly for researchers, very often the underlying data are shared so that additional analysis can be conducted. In the time of COVID-19, these included maps as well as epidemic curves showing data over time. The NextStrain open repository uses viral sequences to show global maps of spread of the infection.[41]

dendrogram: A diagram showing hierarchies between similar data, particularly as they relate to phylogenies and taxonomies.

While we cannot underestimate the importance of data sharing across platforms, data sharing creates additional problems. In order to combine data collected by differing entities, they have to be measuring the same thing and at the same resolution. Explicitly stated case definitions help by ensuring that, even if the same definitions are not used, researchers can make an informed decision about whether the data can be combined or if there are possible ways to modify the data so that they can be combined. Spatial resolution refers to the level of aggregation that data may take, for example, point data if address or latitude/longitude are available. Temporal resolution refers to both the frequency and duration over which the data were collected. All of these can influence the validity of combining data sets. Increasingly, there are attempts to standardize how data are collected and reported such that combinations across data sets can be valid.

THOUGHT QUESTION

During the COVID-19 pandemic, numerous data dashboards were created for public use. Find two of these and identify what specific data elements they included, and what was most effective in their presentation.

HYPOTHESIS TESTING AND CHANCE IN INFECTIOUS DISEASES

Exposure to influenza has been associated with an increased risk of both hospitalizations and deaths among older adult residents living in long-term care facilities.[42] Specifically, in one set of findings, 9.2% of residents were exposed to influenza compared to 7.4% of the residents who were not exposed. This resulted in the following findings: relative risk (RR [95% confidence interval, CI] = 1.24 [1.05; 1.47]) and the risk of death (5.8% vs. 4.3%; RR [95% CI] = 1.36 [1.10; 1.70]).

When we study infectious diseases, we are often interested in population-level outcomes such as infection prevalence or intensity. These relate to exposure patterns, immunity, genetics, age, and a wide variety of other factors such as diet and coinfections. To examine whether these associations are true or due to chance, **statistical inference** uses observed data to draw conclusions about populations. That is, how much uncertainty there might be in a given sample, and how generalizable sample findings might then be to a broader population. **Point estimates** are the statistics calculated from the sample data, which in turn are used to estimate the underlying **population parameter**; for example, reporting the mean age in a sample as a measure of the population mean age.

The **P-value** is a measure of how likely it is that observed data in an experiment would have occurred by chance. Thus, what is the likelihood of getting an observed data value given the null hypothesis? Consider a graph with data on the distribution of hours of work in a week in the United States (Figure 13.9). The mean value (point estimate) is 40. Given this is a normal distribution, the likelihood of someone working 40 hours is higher closer to the mean and lower toward the extreme ends of the curve. The chances of someone doing 40 hours at this point or more are seen in the area to the right of the point.

The P-value is the probability of getting a value at least as extreme as the observed value when picking values randomly from the population distribution. Thus, the smaller the P-value, the stronger the evidence against the null hypothesis. As an example, imagine a randomized trial examining the use of a new vaccine for flu compared to the existing one, which finds a relative risk of 0.78. The authors report a P-value that tests the hypothesis of no association between the intervention (flu vaccination) and the outcome (flu infection). The authors report a P-value of 0.9. A large P-value indicates that chance is a likely reason for this finding. Based on the study findings, it is very likely that

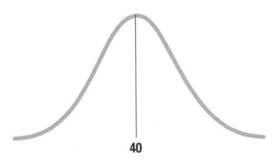

40

Figure 13.9 Normally distributed graph showing a distribution of working hours per week, with a mean of 40.

a finding with this relative risk, or one more extreme, would have happened based on chance alone, so we would not reject the null hypothesis. The study authors could thus note that "the chance (or probability) of getting a result more extreme than the one we observed is 90% if the null hypothesis is true." It would not be correct to say that "there is a 90% chance that the null hypothesis is true." A study result is considered **statistically significant** if the P-value is less than a prespecified significance level. Studies often use a P-value cutoff of 0.05 as statistically significant, which tells us that the null hypothesis is rejected when the chance of the outcome is less than 5%. This means that there is a 5% risk of an error (and the findings being incorrect), such that the null is rejected when it should not have been. Choosing what significance level is somewhat arbitrary and based on a preset cutoff point on which we call our findings true or false. This threshold P-value is also known as α (alpha), or the probability of a type I error. A type I error refers to the mistake of rejecting the null hypothesis when it is true. As previously noted, a P-value of 0.05 is indicative of a 95% significance level, and an α of 5%.

Two factors that may determine the role of chance are the study sample size and the variability of what is being examined. If all else is equal, a P-value will be smaller when there is a larger observed difference between two groups, less variation within groups, or a larger sample size. With a large enough sample size and a decrease in sample variability, the null hypothesis is likely to be rejected. Larger groups are likely to be more representative of the underlying population. This is particularly important in an era of big data. Additionally, for the P-value to be meaningful in significance testing, the null hypothesis must be true, while this is not the case for the critical value in hypothesis testing. Although the critical value comes from α based on the null hypothesis, rejecting the null hypothesis is not a mistake when it is not true. P-values do not measure the actual size of an effect and replication of an experiment is difficult because of the variability we might see in reporting across samples.

To better account for chance, **confidence intervals (CI)** can be used. This means that if we test an intervention an infinite number of times, drawing participants randomly from the same population each time, the 95% CI will include the true effect estimate in 95% of the trials. The CI of the estimate can range across a wide range of possible points, that, with a certain degree of probability, contain the true population parameter. For example, for the previously noted relative risk of 0.78, the interval might range from a beneficial 0.35 to an adverse 1.81, in which case we are 95% certain that the data don't support strong benefit for the intervention, but rather the range of possible effects that are compatible with the observed data. The 95% confidence interval range can also be used to decide whether a point estimate is statistically different than the null value of 1.0. A wider CI means that the sample size is either too small or the sample variability too great to know the true parameter, whereas a tighter CI allows for a more precise sample estimate (Figure 13.10).

P-value: A measure of how likely it is that observed data in an experiment would have occurred by chance.

confidence interval (CI): The range of probabilities within which a true effect lies. The interval provides the measure of uncertainty in a sampling method.

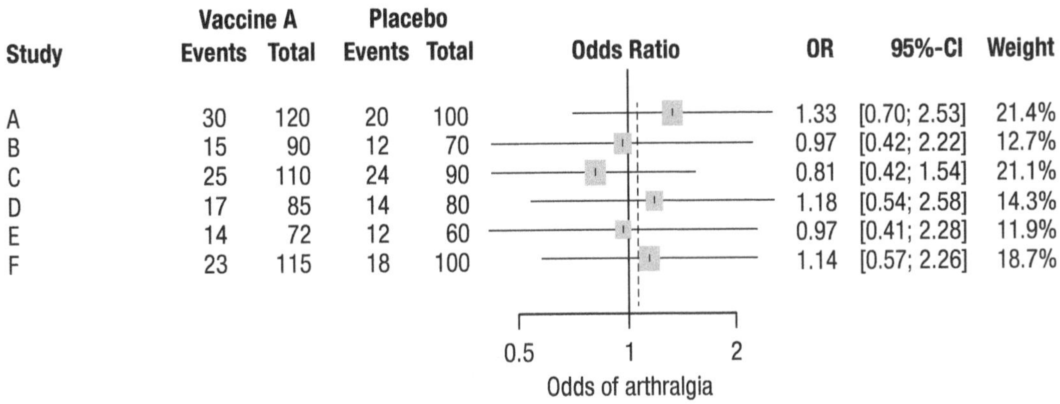

Study	Vaccine A		Placebo		Odds Ratio	OR	95%-CI	Weight
	Events	Total	Events	Total				
A	30	120	20	100		1.33	[0.70; 2.53]	21.4%
B	15	90	12	70		0.97	[0.42; 2.22]	12.7%
C	25	110	24	90		0.81	[0.42; 1.54]	21.1%
D	17	85	14	80		1.18	[0.54; 2.58]	14.3%
E	14	72	12	60		0.97	[0.41; 2.28]	11.9%
F	23	115	18	100		1.14	[0.57; 2.26]	18.7%

0.5   1   2

Odds of arthralgia

Figure 13.10 A range of sample 95% confidence intervals comparing a vaccine to placebo across studies (A-F).

Source: Tawfik GM, Dila KAS, Mohamed MYF, et al. A step by step guide for conducting a systematic review and meta-analysis with simulation data. *Trop Med Health*. 2019;47:46. doi:10.1186/s41182-019-0165-6

THOUGHT QUESTION

How is statistical significance related to hypothesis testing?

HEADS UP!

But it's significant to me! It is important not to confuse statistical significance with clinical significance. A highly significant statistical finding may actually have limited clinical significance. For example, COVID-19 has led to multisystemic disease. A study reported statistically significantly elevated lipase among 17% of COVID-19 patients and the elevation was reported as associated with worse clinical outcomes. Lipase is an enzyme manufactured in the pancreas (and other locations) the body uses to break down fats. However, in subsequent review, patients who were part of the testing panel were likely to be sicker to begin with. Since pancreatic involvement in COVID-19 has been rare, the evidence does not support a clinical role of lipase as a marker of more severe disease and may in fact lead to unnecessary testing and diagnosis.[43]

CASE STUDY

Professor Michael Selgelid has been studying ethical issues raised by infectious diseases for the past two decades. After obtaining a BS in Biomedical Engineering at Duke University, Selgelid completed his PhD in Philosophy at the University of California, San Diego. His work in bioethics has taken him to numerous institutions and has covered a range of infectious diseases. The 2002 to 2003 SARS pandemic raised questions of how to plan for and respond to a worldwide pandemic, and Selgelid then worked on the big three killers of HIV/AIDS, TB, and malaria. All of these point to the conflict between protecting individuals and improving public health, which sometimes infringes on individual rights. Selgelid contributed to key WHO guidelines on public health surveillance ethics, including the importance of privacy and informed consent, and has also advised the Australian and U.S. governments on how to ethically conduct biological research that might be used to create more pathogenic organisms. One of his key papers examined ethical and self-interested reasons why wealthy developed nations should be motivated to do more to improve healthcare in developing countries. After working on key emergency committees on Ebola, he was then well-primed to lead a WHO Working Group developing *Key criteria for the ethical acceptability of COVID-19 human challenge studies*. This document synthesizes ethical guidance regarding the role of controlled human infection studies in testing the many vaccine candidates for SARS-CoV-2. In 2004, Selgelid was a finalist for the prestigious Mark S. Ehrenreich Prize in Healthcare Ethics Research.

CONCLUSION

Digital tools have proliferated in the past decades, with questions about whether to adopt tools based on benefits, such as more rapid surveillance and subsequent public health response, and drawbacks, which may be ethical in nature. New data sources include mobile phones, wearables, search data, social media, crowdsourcing, and more. In response the analysis tools that an epidemiologist might use are growing and adapting as well. There is growing potential to use machine learning and big data to forecast disease spread, and personalized medical and public health approaches to customize care and disease response. Applications of these technologies also include improved data visualization and communication but must be weighed with the protection of individual rights and the challenges of combining data sets created for different purposes. Importantly, for studies using new technologies and big data, appropriate data management and analytic techniques are more important than ever.

END-OF-CHAPTER RESOURCES

TEACHING CORNER

DID YOU KNOW?

Flu vaccines vary from year to year depending on how well-matched circulating flu viruses are to those used to make the vaccines as well as the characteristics of the person being vaccinated. Recent studies show that flu vaccination reduces the risk of illness by 40% to 60% among the overall population. There has been shown to be better protection against some subtypes, such as influenza B and influenza A (H1N1) viruses. During the 2019 to 2020 season, flu vaccination prevented an estimated 7.5 million influenza illnesses, 3.7 million influenza-associated medical visits, 105,000 influenza-associated hospitalizations, and 6,300 influenza-associated deaths.[44]

TRY THIS

Imagine a survey conducted to find out what people thought about the effectiveness of the flu vaccine. People are asked to report their thoughts through social media, email links, and online ads. How would you characterize the survey sample? Is it representative of the population?

TAKE IT A STEP FURTHER

What kinds of questions might the survey ask to best get at flu vaccine effectiveness perceptions? The survey also wanted to know whether the vaccine was seen as helpful. The null hypothesis was that 50% of the public would view the vaccine as helpful. The survey found that 61% actually saw it as helpful with a 95% CI ranging from 53% to 69%. Would you reject the null hypothesis? How would you interpret these findings?

QUESTIONS FOR FURTHER DISCUSSION

1. What are some limitations of digital disease surveillance?

2. Consider at least one novel or innovative technological advance not covered in this chapter used for disease control in the past 5 years. What might make a technology more promising? How could it be made more generalizable to the broader public? Some suggested technologies include use of nanotechnology, telemedicine, self-testing, and targeted public health messaging.

3. What are some additional ethical issues that have arisen in recent years with the advent of digital tool use during outbreaks and pandemics?

4. List two strengths and limitations in using social media during a disease outbreak.

A robust set of instructor resources designed to supplement this text is located at http://connect.springerpub.com/content/book/978-0-8261-5674-7. Qualifying instructors may request access by emailing textbook@springerpub.com.

REFERENCES

1. Lazer D, Kennedy R, King G, Vespignani A. The parable of Google Flu: traps in big data analysis. *Science*. 2014;343:1203–1205. doi:10.1126/science.1248506
2. Samerski S. Individuals on alert: digital epidemiology and the individualization of surveillance. *Life Sci Soc Pol*. 2018;14:13. doi:10.1186/s40504-018-0076-z
3. Eysenbach G. Infodemiology and infoveillance: tracking online health information and cyberbehavior for public health. *Am J Prevent Med*. 2011;40:S154–S158. doi:10.1016/j.amepre.2011.02.006
4. Strauss R, Lorenz E, Kristensen K, et al. Investigating the utility of Google trends for Zika and chikungunya surveillance in Venezuela. *BMC Public Health*. 2020;20(1):947. doi:10.1186/s12889-020-09059-9
5. Adawi M, Bragazzi NL, Watad A, Sharif K, Amital H, Mahroum N. Discrepancies between classic and digital epidemiology in searching for the Mayaro virus: preliminary qualitative and quantitative analysis of Google trends. *JMIR Public Health Surveill*. 2017;3(4):e93. doi:10.2196/publichealth.9136
6. Polgreen PM, Chen Y, Pennock DM, Nelson FD, Weinstein RA. Using internet searches for influenza surveillance. *Clin Infect Dis*. 2008;47(11):1443–1448. doi:10.1086/593098
7. HealthMap. https://healthmap.org/en
8. Government of Canada. About GPHIN. https://gphin.canada.ca/cepr/aboutgphin-rmispenbref.jsp?language=en_CA
9. International Society for Infectious Diseases.. About ProMED. https://promedmail.org/about-promed
10. Wesolowski A, Eagle N, Tatem AJ, et al. Quantifying the impact of human mobility on malaria. *Science*. 2012;338:267–270. doi:10.1126/science.1223467
11. Bui DP, Chandran SS, Oren E, et al. Community transmission of multidrug-resistant tuberculosis is associated with activity space overlap in Lima, Peru. *BMC Infect Dis*. 2021;21:275. doi:10.1186/s12879-021-05953-8
12. Guerrisi C, Turbelin C, Blanchon T, et al. Participatory syndromic surveillance of influenza in Europe. *J Infect Dis*. 2016;214:S386–S392. doi:10.1093/infdis/jiw280
13. Koppeschaar CE, Colizza V, Guerrisi C, et al. Influenzanet: citizens among 10 countries collaborating to monitor influenza in Europe. *JMIR Public Health Surveill*. 2017;3:e66. doi:10.2196/publichealth.7429
14. Leal Neto O, Cruz O, Albuquerque J, et al. Participatory surveillance based on crowdsourcing during the Rio 2016 Olympic games using the guardians of health platform: descriptive study. *JMIR Public Health Surveill*. 2020;6:e16119. doi:10.2196/16119
15. Government of Singapor. Trace together. https://www.tracetogether.gov.sg
16. Edoh T. Risk prevention of spreading emerging infectious diseases using a hybrid crowdsensing paradigm, optical sensors, and smartphone. *J Med Syst*. 2018;42(5):91. doi:10.1007/s10916-018-0937-2
17. Lee IM, Shiroma EJ, Evenson K, Kamada M, LaCroix A, Buring J. Using devices to assess physical activity and sedentary behavior in a large cohort study: The Women's Health Study. *J Meas Phys Behav*. 2018;1(2):60–69. doi:10.1123/jmpb.2018-0005
18. Aslam AA, Tsou M, Spitzberg BH, et al. The reliability of Tweets as a supplementary method of seasonal influenza surveillance. *J Med Internet Res*. 2014;16(11):e250. doi:10.2196/jmir.3532
19. Yousefinaghani S, Dara R, Poljak Z, Bernardo TM, Sharif S. The assessment of Twitter's potential for outbreak detection: avian influenza case study. *Sci Rep*. 2019;9:18147. doi:10.1038/s41598-019-54388-4
20. Allen C, Tsou M-H, Aslam A, Nagel A, Gawron J-M. Applying GIS and machine learning methods to Twitter data for multiscale surveillance of influenza. *PLoS One*. 2016;11(7):e0157734. doi:10.1371/journal.pone.0157734
21. Cheng IK, Heyl J, Lad N, et al. Evaluation of Twitter data for an emerging crisis: an application to the first wave of COVID-19 in the UK. *Sci Rep*. 2021;11:19009. doi:10.1038/s41598-021-98396-9
22. Twitter Developer Platform. Overview: sample realtime Tweets. https://developer.twitter.com/en/docs/tweets/sample-realtime/overview.html

23. Chew C, Eysenbach G. Pandemics in the age of Twitter: content analysis of Tweets during the 2009 h1N1 outbreak. *PLoS One*. 2010;5:e14118. doi:10.1371/journal.pone.0014118

24. Oren E, Martinez L, Hensley RE, et al. Twitter communication during an outbreak of hepatitis A in San Diego, 2016–2018. *Am J Public Health*. 2020;110(S3):S348–S355. doi:10.2105/AJPH.2020.305900

25. Gabarron E, Oyeyemi SO, Wynn R. COVID-19-related misinformation on social media: a systematic review. *Bull World Health Organ*. 2021;99(6):455–463A. doi:10.2471/BLT.20.276782

26. Seo DW, Shin SY. Methods using social media and search queries to predict infectious disease outbreaks. *Healthc Inform Res*. 2017;23:343–348. doi:10.4258/hir.2017.23.4.343

27. Centers for Disease Control and Prevention. CDC competition encourages use of social media to predict flu. November 25, 2013. https://www.cdc.gov/flu/news/predict-flu-challenge.htm

28. Mowery J. Twitter influenza surveillance: quantifying seasonal misdiagnosis patterns. *Online J Public Health Inform*. 2016;8:7011. doi:10.5210/ojphi.v8i3.7011

29. McCall B. COVID-19 artificial intelligence: protecting health-care workers and curbing the spread. *Lancet Digital Health*. 2020;2:e166–e167. doi:10.1016/S2589-7500(20)30054-6

30. Bowles J. How Canadian AI start-up BlueDot spotted coronavirus before anyone else had a clue. March 10, 2020. https://diginomica.com/how-canadian-ai-start-bluedot-spotted-coronavirus-anyone-else-had-clue

31. Rossi B. The Metaboita story. April 9, 2019. https://medium.com/@billrossi/the-metabiota-story-d553f41d03bd

32. Colubri A, Hartley MA, Siakor M, et al. Machine-learning prognostic models from the 2014–16 Ebola outbreak: data-harmonization challenges, validation strategies, mHealth applications. *EClinicalMed*. 2019;11:54–64. doi:10.1016/j.eclinm.2019.06.003

33. Rasmussen SA, Khoury MJ, del Rio C. Precision public health as a key tool in the COVID-19 response. *JAMA*. 2020;324(10):933–934. doi:10.1001/jama.2020.14992

34. Neher RA, Bedford T, Daniels RS, Russell CA, Shraiman BI. Prediction, dynamics, and visualization of antigenic phenotypes of seasonal influenza viruses. *Proc Natl Acad Sci USA*. 2016;113:E1701–E1709. doi:10.1073/pnas.1525578113

35. Oude Munnink BB, Nieuwenhuijse DF, Stein M, et al; Dutch-COVID-19 response team. Rapid SARS-CoV-2 whole-genome sequencing and analysis for informed public health decision-making in the Netherlands. *Nat Med*. 2020;26(9):1405–1410. doi:10.1038/s41591-020-0997-y

36. Gaydos CA, Manabe YC, Melendez JH. A narrative review of where we are with point-of-care sexually transmitted infection testing in the United States. *Sex Transm Dis*. 2021;48(8S):S71–S77. doi:10.1097/OLQ.0000000000001457

37. Williams JH, Dawson A. Prioritising access to pandemic influenza vaccine: a review of the ethics literature. *BMC Med Ethics*. 2020;21:40. doi:10.1186/s12910-020-00477-3

38. Parpia AS, Ndeffo-Mbah ML, Wenzel NS, Galvani AP. Effects of response to the 2014–2015 Ebola outbreak on deaths from malaria, HIV/AIDS, and tuberculosis, West Africa. *Emerg Infect Dis*. 2016;22(3): 433–441. doi:10.3201/eid2203.150977

39. World Health Organization. *Guidance for Managing Ethical Issues in Infectious Disease Outbreaks*. World Health Organization; 2016.

40. Immergluck LC, Leong T, Matthews K, et al. Geographic surveillance of community associated MRSA infections in children using electronic health record data. *BMC Infect Dis*. 2019;19:170. doi:10.1186/s12879-019-3682-3

41. Nextstrain team. Genomic epidemiology of novel coronavirus—global subsampling. https://nextstrain.org/ncov/global

42. Gaillat J, Chidiac C, Fagnani F, et al. Morbidity and mortality associated with influenza exposure in long-term care facilities for dependent elderly people. *Eur J Clin Microbiol Infect Dis*. 2009;28(9):1077–1086. doi:10.1007/s10096-009-0751-3

43. Rathi S, Sharma A, Patnaik I, Gupta R. Hyperlipasemia in COVID-19: statistical significance vs clinical relevance. *Clin Transl Gastroenterol*. 2020;11(12):e00261. doi:10.14309/ctg.0000000000000261

44. Centers for Disease Control and Prevention. Estimated influenza illnesses, medical visits, and hospitalizations averted by vaccination in the United States—2019–2020 influenza season. https://www.cdc.gov/flu/about/burden-averted/2019-2020.htm

GLOSSARY

acquired immunity: Immune response acquired over the lifetime by natural infection or immunity and is specific to specific antigens.

active surveillance: Systematic identification and location of cases of disease, including screening, diagnosis, and treatment.

acute: Short-lived infection, usually with a rapid onset, often severe, and usually resolves.

adaptation: The actions we must engage in in response to expected climate effects on health.

administrative controls: Altering the way the work is done, including timing of work, policies and other rules, and work practices such as standards and operating procedures.

airborne precautions: Preventing transmission of infectious agents that remain infectious in air over long distances.

analytic epidemiology: Studies that measure the association between a particular exposure and a disease and aim to further examine known associations or hypothesized relationships.

animalcules: Microscopic animals (often protozoans), as observed by Leeuwenhoek for the first time under a microscope.

asymptomatic: *a-* (without) symptoms. Individuals who are infected but do not show clinical symptoms of the disease. This is in contrast to symptomatic individuals.

attack rate: A synonym for incidence usually reserved for acute disease and often reported as a percent of those at risk.

bacteria: Small, single-celled organisms. They can be beneficial or detrimental. Examples include *Helicobacter pylori* (strongly associated with stomach cancer), *and Mycobacterium tuberculosis* (causative agent of tuberculosis).

basic reproduction number (R_0): The number of secondary infections that will arise from a single case in a fully susceptible population.

behavioral immune system: Psychological processes that facilitate immune responses that enter the body through responses to specific disease-avoidance behaviors.

bias: Systematic error resulting in incorrect associations.

big data: Complex data collected in large amounts.

built environment: Areas created by humans and used by people for living, working, and recreation.

carrier: An individual who is infected and able to spread an infection to others.

case-control studies: A prevalence study which starts with cases and compares risk factors to matched controls.

case definition: A set of criteria used to classify individuals as having the health condition being assessed; they may include only symptomology or may include laboratory confirmation.

case fatality rate (CFR): A measure of disease severity considering the deaths due to a disease as a proportion of the total number of cases of that disease.

causal inference: Technique to assess whether a relationship exists or does not exist between a particular exposure and an outcome.

causative agent: The agent, or pathogen, responsible for an illness.

chain of infection: Path, or route, taken by a pathogen through the host.

chronic: Longer-lasting infections.

climate refugee: A person who is displaced because of climate change effects.

clinical trials: An experimental study design in which individuals are assigned to exposure or unexposed and monitored for disease outcome.

cluster: An unusual aggregation of cases or health events grouped together by place and time.

cohort study: An incidence study where two groups, exposed and not exposed, are followed over time to compare the risk of developing a disease. The relative risk is the commonly calculated measure of effect.

colonization: The presence of organisms on a body surface (like on the skin, mouth, intestines, or airway) without causing disease in the person.

community immunity: See herd immunity.

comorbidities: Other diseases or conditions simultaneously present in an individual.

component cause: Each participating factor in a sufficient cause that in itself does not cause disease.

confidence interval (CI): The range of probabilities within which a true effect lies. The interval provides the measure of uncertainty in a sampling method.

confounding: A third factor, not the exposure or outcome variable, that is a common cause of both the exposure and the outcome, that may result in a spurious association between the exposure and outcome. It is biologically important to understand given its role.

contact investigations: Also known as contact tracing, they provide a systematic process to identify people, known as contacts, who have been exposed to cases of an infectious disease.

contact patterns: Patterns of contacts, such as those between different groups of people (such as age groups) and in different social settings.

contact precautions: Precautions intended to prevent the spread of infectious agents that are transmitted by direct or indirect contact.

contact tracing: Also known as contact investigations, they provide a systematic process to identify people, known as contacts, who have been exposed to cases of an infectious disease.

contacts: Persons exposed to an organism by sharing air space with a person with (potentially) infectious disease.

content analysis: Analysis of text content and comparison of major themes.

control: A comparison group or individual who is similar to the cases with respect to known demographic information, comorbidities, and could, under knowable situations, have contracted the disease, but did not.

coverage: The percentage of people in a population who are receiving the vaccine of interest.

cross-sectional study: A class of observational study where, after defining the population to be studied, information is collected from individuals about both their exposures and outcomes, usually at the same time.

dendrogram: A diagram showing hierarchies between similar data, particularly as they relate to phylogenies and taxonomies.

descriptive epidemiology: Epidemiology that describes person, place, and time and often will summarize data in tables and graphs.

digital traces: Digital "footprints," or records of activity left behind through online information systems.

direct contact transmission: Transmission through physical contact between an infected person and a susceptible one.

disability-adjusted life years (DALY): An alternative measure of the burden of disease which combines years of life lost to premature mortality with the years of life lost due to living in less than full health (i.e., healthy life lost due to disability).

droplet nuclei: Droplets less than 5 microns (μm) in diameter and often implicated in airborne transmission due to their tiny size.

droplet precautions: Precautions intended to prevent the spread of infectious agents that are transmitted by respiratory secretions or mucous membrane contact.

ecological fallacy: An error made in thinking that relationships observed for groups also hold for the individuals within those groups.

ecological studies: Studies conducted at the population or group level, rather than at the individual level.

economic injury level: The lowest level of insects (the injury) where the loss productivity equals the cost for insect management.

effective reproduction number $(R_e, sometimes\ called\ R_t)$**:** The number of secondary infections, this estimate changes over the course of an epidemic as the number of susceptible individuals, and therefore the contact between infectious and susceptible individuals, changes.

endemic: Usual or constant prevalence of a disease in a population within a geographic area.

engineering controls: Strategies designed to protect workers from hazardous conditions by removing hazardous conditions or by placing a barrier between the worker and the hazard.

entomologic risk: Probability of encountering a disease vector.

epidemic: An increase, or higher than expected numbers, in the prevalence of a disease in a population within a geographic area. Distinguished from an outbreak in its greater geographic or temporal reach.

epidemiologic curve: A graph where time is on the x-axis and number of cases on the y-axis to show the progression of an epidemic. The shape of the curve informs the probable type of exposure.

epidemiologic data: Data describing the person, place, and time of an exposure or outcome of interest.

epidemiologic links: Characteristic that links two cases, such as close contact between two people or a common exposure, such as spending time in the same place together.

ethnographic data: Direct observation of users in a natural environment that allows one to gain insights into understanding how people interact. Methods are qualitative and allow for observing what is of direct significance to a community.

etiology: The cause(s) of a disease and how it is acquired.

experiment: A series of observations performed prospectively under control of the researcher.

experimental study: A study where the researcher introduces an intervention and studies the subsequent effects.

exposure: Any factor that may be associated with an outcome of interest. This may be the primary independent variable or risk factor of interest in an epidemiologic study.

extrinsic incubation period: The time for a vector to become infectious (able to transmit) after becoming infected.

food and environmental testing data: Laboratory data used to confirm the pathogen from food and environmental samples.

food safety: Access to contaminant-free foods.

food security: A steady and reliable access to food.

fomites: Inanimate objects contaminated with some microorganism.

fungus: Fungi represent their own kingdom. A few of the millions of fungi may infect hosts. Examples include *Candida spp.* (yeast infections) and *Coccidioides spp.* (causative agent of Valley fever).

generalizability: A measure of how study results can be applied to a broader group or alternative locations.

generation time: The interval from the moment one person becomes infected until that person infects another person.

germ theory: The science-backed explanation that infectious diseases arise from exposure to microorganisms and germs.

health disparities: Health differences closely linked with social, economic, and/or environmental disadvantage.

health equity: Individuals achieve their full health potential through reduction of barriers that drive different health outcomes.

herd immunity: Indirect protection to groups when enough of the group is immunized such that those unable to be vaccinated or those who did not develop sufficient immunity to thwart the infection are still protected.

horizontal transmission: The passage of an agent from one individual to another of the same "generation."

incidence proportion: A measure of the risk of developing the outcome of interest. It is calculated as the number of new cases in a given population at a given time period over the total population at risk for developing a disease during the same time period.

incubation period: The time between exposure to an infected individual and the onset of symptoms.

indirect contact transmission: Transmission without direct contact. Contact occurs through contaminated surfaces or objects, or through a vector.

infectivity: The likelihood a disease infects others, commonly examined using the proportion of exposed individuals who become infected.

infodemiology: Analyzing and disseminating real-time health information from news and social media.

information bias: A systematic error in the way that information is collected.

infoveillance: A type of surveillance using information found online to better understand human behaviors and health.

innate immunity: Nonspecific immune response that we are born with and includes physical, chemical, and certain immune cells.

intention to treat: Analyzing results in a manner where all participants who are randomized are included in the statistical analysis and analyzed according to the group they were originally assigned, regardless of what treatment they received.

international health regulations: An overarching legal framework that defines countries' rights and obligations in handling public health events and emergencies that cross borders across the globe.

latent period: Time from acquiring infection to the onset of infectiousness.

line listing: A table containing key information about each case in an outbreak, with each row representing a case and each column representing a variable such as demographic, clinical, and epidemiologic information.

machine learning: Algorithmic approaches that adapt to patterns in data without programming a prediction task.

mining: Sorting through large data sets to identify patterns and relationships.

mitigation: The actions that can be taken to limit the effects of climate change by reducing or preventing greenhouse gas emissions into the atmosphere.

mode of transmission: Method that a pathogen uses to get from a starting point to a destination.

mortality rate: A measure of deaths in a population at a given time period.

multilevel modeling: Statistical modeling techniques that recognize a clustered interdependent data structure. For example, individuals may be nested within a geographical area or students within a school.

natural history of a disease: Natural course of a disease from the time immediately prior to its inception, progressing through its presymptomatic phase and different clinical stages to the point where it has ended and the patient is either cured, chronically disabled, or deceased without external intervention.

necessary cause: A component cause that must be present in every sufficient cause of a given outcome.

negative predictive value (NPV): The proportion of healthy individuals truly diagnosed as negative out of all those individuals who have a negative test result.

nowcasting: Short-term prediction that attempts to track disease incidence in near real-time.

observational study: Study design where the researchers do not intervene in the exposure (e.g., case-control or cohort study).

odds ratio: The ratio of the odds of exposure among cases over the odds among non-exposed. It is the commonly calculated measure of effect for case-control studies.

One Health: A transdisciplinary approach that considers the linkages between animal and human health in their shared environment.

outbreak: A sudden increase in the occurrence of disease in a population, usually with limited geographic spread and time limited.

P-value: A measure of how likely it is that observed data in an experiment would have occurred by chance.

pandemic: An epidemic that is widespread or has global spread and impact and may infect a great number of people.

parasites: An organism that lives in or on other organisms. Like a virus, parasites need hosts to survive, but unlike a virus, they do not require the host machinery to reproduce. Examples include *Taenia spp.* (tapeworms) and *Plasmodium spp.* (malaria).

participation bias: A systematic error that occurs when the characteristics of those who agree to participate are different from those who do not.

participatory surveillance: Participants provide voluntary health-related information through surveys or other sources to monitor disease trends.

passive surveillance: Detection of cases among those seeking medical care and who are both aware of their own symptoms and have access to healthcare facilities.

pathogenicity: The likelihood of developing clinical disease, commonly examined through the proportion of infected individuals who develop disease.

pathotype: A further classification of microorganism which distinguishes within species based on differences in virulence and the pathology (i.e., disease it causes).

per protocol: Analyzing results based on who actually received treatment, removing data from patients who didn't comply with the protocol.

point estimates: The statistics calculated from sample data.

population parameter: The statistics that describe the entire group or underlying population.

portal of entry: Sites through which infectious pathogens get into the body, often mucous membranes, injuries, or the respiratory, gastrointestinal, or genitourinary tracts.

portal of exit: The means, or body site, through which a pathogen exits from a (human) reservoir.

positive predictive value (PPV): The proportion of cases who have a truly positive test result/event out of all those who have positive test results/are detected.

power: The smallest sample size needed to detect the effect of a given test or intervention at a desired level of statistical significance.

precision public health: Using population-specific data to provide the right intervention to the right population at the right time.

prevalence: A measure of the burden of disease in a population. It is calculated as the number of existing cases over the population able to get the disease during a given time period. It may be represented as a rate or a percentage.

prions: Transmissible proteins that induce abnormal folding of normal cellular proteins. Examples include Creutzfeld-Jakob disease and scrapie.

proportionate mortality ratio (PMR): A measure of the proportion of deaths due to a given cause from all deaths in a population.

quality-adjusted life years (QALY): An alternative measure of the burden of disease which is a measure of the quality and quantity of life lived.

reservoir: Where the agent normally resides, be it humans, other animals, or the environment.

risk difference: The difference in incidence among exposed and the incidence among unexposed.

risk ratio: Also known as the incidence proportion ratio or relative risk, the ratio between two risks observed in exposed and unexposed groups.

seasonality: Regular and predictable annual changes not just in weather but also in host behavior and disease trends.

selection bias: A systematic error that occurs when the individuals selected for the sample do not accurately represent the source population.

sensitivity: Proportion of cases correctly detected/tested positive. A higher sensitivity implies fewer false-negative results.

sentiment analysis: Analysis of how people feel and respond.

sentinel surveillance: A system of ongoing data collection and monitoring from selected sites or populations that allows for rapid identification of possible outbreaks and public health events.

sexually transmitted infection (STI): A viral or bacterial infection usually transmitted from person to person during vaginal, anal, or oral intercourse or genital touching.

snowball sampling: A methodology by which individuals recruited into a study are asked to recruit additional participants, thereby *snowballing* the effect of the sampling.

social desirability bias: A systematic error that occurs when individuals answer questions in a way that may reflect more favorably on them.

social determinants of health: The conditions in which people are born, grow, live, work, and age, including the healthcare system, which influence their achieving health and well-being.

social epidemiology: The discipline within epidemiology that emphasizes the study of mechanisms and processes that produce social inequalities as they are related to health.

social network analysis (SNA): A methodology to map and analyze the connections between individuals within groups.

social network-based intervention (SNI): A methodology to use social networks in order to influence healthy behavior.

social protection policies: Initiatives designed to reduce vulnerability to poverty through education, investments, job placement, and protecting the aging population.

social stigma: The judging or condemning of individuals based on their social characteristics, in this case having an infection.

spatiotemporal: In the context of epidemiology, data collected across time (temporal) as well as space (spatio), allowing for an assessment or, when mapped, visualization of changes in disease patterns across a landscape or other surface.

specificity: Proportion of healthy individuals who are correctly detected/tested negative. A higher specificity implies fewer false-positive results.

spillover event: A single event during which a pathogen from one species moves into another species, potentially resulting in a new disease outbreak.

stakeholders: Those individuals with a personal stake in the project or outcome.

Standard Precautions: The minimum infection prevention practices that apply to all patient care, regardless of suspected or confirmed infection status of the patient, in any setting where healthcare is delivered.

statistical inference: Using observed data to draw conclusions about populations.

statistical significance: Attributable to a specific factor, as opposed to due to chance; that is, unlikely to have occurred given the null hypothesis.

sufficient cause: A complete causal mechanism that will inevitably produce disease.

superspreader: A phenomenon where few people account for the majority of disease transmission, through behavior, biology, or the environment.

sylvatic cycle: The portion of a transmission cycle that naturally occurs in animals, also referred to as enzootic cycle.

symptomatic: Individuals infected who exhibit clinical symptoms of the disease.

syndromic surveillance: Categorizing symptoms and diagnoses into syndromes to identify illness clusters early, often before diagnoses are confirmed and reported to public health agencies, and to mobilize a rapid response.

traceback data: Data generated by tracing back from the marketplace to the source which describes the distribution chain in an effort to identify the contamination course.

training data: A data set that is used to teach a machine learning model.

vaccine effectiveness: A measure of the ability of a vaccine to prevent disease under "real-world" conditions.

vaccine efficacy: A measure of the reduction in incidence in a vaccinated group compared to an unvaccinated group under ideal conditions.

vaccine hesitancy: Reluctance or refusal to vaccinate despite the availability of services.

validity: The degree to which the information collected answers the research question.

vectorial capacity: The daily average number of infectious bites resulting from a vector biting an initial index case

vector competence: A measure of whether a mosquito is able to acquire and transmit a pathogen.

vector-borne diseases: Diseases where the pathogen is transmitted between hosts by an intermediary or vector. Vectors are blood-feeding arthropods, including mosquitoes, fleas, ticks, lice, midges, and certain blood-feeding bugs and flies.

vector-borne zoonotic diseases: Diseases of non-human animals which require an intermediary to transmit to humans.

vehicles: Objects that serve as carriers of infection from an infected individual to a healthy one.

vertical transmission: The passage of an agent from mother to offspring.

virulence: The likelihood of developing severe disease, commonly examined through the proportion of diseased individuals who develop more severe or fatal outcomes.

virus: Viruses are generally the smallest pathogens and are encapsulated DNA or RNA. They require a host (cellular machinery) to replicate. Examples include HIV (causative agent of AIDS) and SARS-CoV-2 (causative agent of COVID-19).

whole genome sequencing: A laboratory process used to determine a complete DNA or RNA sequence, which can be useful in tracking disease outbreaks.

zoonotic diseases: Diseases of non-human animals, which can be transmitted to humans.

INDEX